AF556771

Stentless Bioprostheses

Second Edition

Stentless Bioprostheses

Second Edition

Edited by

Hans A. Huysmans MD PhD
Professor of Cardiothoracic Surgery, Department of Cardiothoracic Surgery, University Hospital Leiden, The Netherlands

Tirone E. David MD FRCS(c) FACS
Professor of Surgery, Division of Cardiovascular Surgery, The Toronto Hospital, Toronto, Canada

Stephen Westaby BSc FRCS MD
Consultant Cardiac Surgeon, Oxford Heart Centre, John Radcliffe Hospital, Oxford, UK

ISIS
MEDICAL
MEDIA

59 St. Aldates
Oxford OX1 1ST, UK

1st Edition 1995
2nd Edition 1999

British Library Cataloguing in Publication Data.
A catalogue record for this title is available from the British Library

ISBN 1 899066 18 7

Huysmans, H. A. (Hans)
Stentless Bioprostheses (2nd Edition)
Hans A. Huysmans, Tirone E. David and Stephen Westaby (eds)

Always refer to the manufacturer's Prescribing Information before prescribing drugs cited in this book.

Design
Design Online, UK

Typesetting
Chandos Electronic Publishing, Oxon, UK

Image reproduction
Track Direct, UK

Cover photograph (lower): courtesy of
St Jude Medical, Inc. All rights reserved

Isis Medical Media staff
Commissioning Editor: John Harrison
Senior Editorial Controller: Catherine Rickards
Production Controller: Geoff Holdsworth

Printed and bound by
Book Print, S.L. Spain

Distributed in the USA by
Books International Inc., PO Box 605
Herndon, VA 20172, USA

Distributed in the rest of the world by
Plymbridge Distributors Ltd., Estover Road,
Plymouth, PL6 7PY, UK

Contents

List of contributors

Sandy M. Adair
Department of Cardiothoracic Surgery, Bowman Gray School of Medicine of Wake Forest University, Winston-Salem, NC, USA

R. Autschbach
Heart Centre, Department of Cardiac Surgery, University of Leipzig, Leipzig, Germany

Juscelino T. Barbosa
Department of Cardiac Surgery, Biocor Institute, Belo Horizonte-MG, Brazil

J. Barlow
Department of Cardiology, University of Witwatersrand, Witwatersrand, South Africa

Leo Baur
Department of Cardiothoracic Surgery, University Hospital Leiden, Leiden, The Netherlands

K. Black
CryoLife Inc., Kennesaw, GA, USA

Y. De Bruyne
Department of Cardiac Surgery, CHU de Charleroi, Site de Jumet, 6040 Jumet, Belgium

Michael Buche
Cliniques Universitaires UCL, Mont Godinne, Yvoir, Belgium

Paul C. Cartier
Department of Cardiovascular Surgery, Laval Hospital, 2725 Chemin Sainte-Foy, Quebec G1V 4G5, Canada

Marcelo Frederique de Castro
Department of Cardiac Surgery, Biocor Institute, Belo Horizonte-MG, Brazil

K. Chandrasekaran
Section of Cardiology, University of Oklahoma Health Sciences Center, P. O. Box 26901, Oklahoma City, OK 73190, USA

George T. Christakis
Division of Cardiac Surgery, Sunnybrook Health Science Centre, University of Toronto, Toronto, Ontario, Canada

Richard P. Cochran
Division of Cardiothoracic Surgery, University of Wisconsin, 600 Highland Avenue, Madison, WI 53792-3226, USA

Maria Alzira Ribeiro Alves Coelho
Department of Cardiac Surgery, Hospital Luxemburgo and Hospital Socor, Belo Horizonte-MG, Brazil

A. Robert Cordell
Department of Cardiothoracic Surgery, Bowman Gray School of Medicine of Wake Forest University, Winston-Salem, NC, USA

Tirone E. David
Department of Surgery, University of Toronto, 200 Elizabeth Street, Toronto, Ontario M5G 2C4, Canada

Denis Desaulniers
Department of Cardiovascular Surgery, Laval Hospital, 2725 Chemin Sainte-Foy, Quebec G1V 4G5, Canada

Anno Diegeler
Heart Centre, Department of Cardiac Surgery, University of Leipzig, Leipzig, Germany

Luis Diodato
Cardiovascular Surgery Service, Hospital Italiano, Buenos Aires, Argentina

John E. Dobbins
Department of Cardiothoracic Surgery, Bowman Gray School of Medicine of Wake Forest University, Winston-Salem, NC, USA

V. Doisy
Department of Cardiac Surgery, Cardiologic Hospital, Lille, France

Donald B. Doty
Division of Thoracic and Cardiovascular Surgery, Department of Surgery, LDS Hospital, Salt Lake City, UT, USA

Daniel Doyle
Department of Cardiovascular Surgery, Laval Hospital, 2725 Chemin Sainte-Foy, Quebec G1V 4G5, Canada

Jean G. Dumesnil
Department of Cardiology, Laval Hospital, 2725 Chemin Sainte-Foy, Quebec G1V 4G5, Canada

T. Edwards
Wessex Cardiothoracic Centre, Southampton General Hospital, Southampton, UK

Gebrine El Khoury
Cliniques Universitaires St.-Luc – UCL, Avenue Hippocrate 10, 1200 Brussels, Belgium

R. C. Elkins
Section of Thoracic and Cardiovascular Surgery, University of Oklahoma Health Sciences Center, P. O. Box 26901, Oklahoma City, OK 73190, USA

Volkmar Falk
Heart Centre, Department of Cardiac Surgery, University of Leipzig, Leipzig, Germany

Fernando A. Fantini
Department of Cardiac Surgery, Biocor Institute, Belo Horizonte-MG, Brazil

Jean H. Flores
Division of Thoracic and Cardiovascular Surgery, Department of Surgery, LDS Hospital, Salt Lake City, UT, USA

R. W. M. Frater
Department of Cardiothoracic Surgery, Montefiore Medical Center, Montefiore, NY, USA

Stephen E. Fremes
Division of Cardiac Surgery, Sunnybrook Health Science Centre, University of Toronto, 2075 Bayview Avenue H410, Toronto, Ontario M4N 3M5, Canada

Bernard S. Goldman
Division of Cardiac Surgery, Sunnybrook Health Science Centre, University of Toronto, 2075 Bayview Avenue H410, Toronto, Ontario M4N 3M5, Canada

S. Goldstein
CryoLife Inc., Kennesaw, GA, USA

Bayard Gontijo
Department of Cardiac Surgery, Biocor Institute, Belo Horizonte-MG, Brazil

Beatrice Günther
Heart Centre, Department of Cardiac Surgery, University of Leipzig, Leipzig, Germany

J. Hamby
CryoLife Inc., Kennesaw, GA, USA

Mark G. Hazekamp
Department of Cardiothoracic Surgery, University Hospital Leiden, P. O. Box 9600, 2300 RC Leiden, The Netherlands

Marcelo Hermeto
Department of Cardiology, Biocor Institute, Belo Horizonte-MG, Brazil

Paul A. Hutter
Department of Cardiology, Wilhelmina's Children's Hospital, Utrecht, The Netherlands

Hans A. Huysmans
Department of Cardiothoracic Surgery, University Hospital Leiden, P. O. Box 9600, 2300 RC Leiden, The Netherlands

Ulrik Hvass
Hôpital Bichat, 46 Rue H. Huchard, Paris 75019, France

Xu Y. Jin
Oxford Heart Centre, John Radcliffe Hospital, Headington, Oxford OX3 9DU, UK

Marc Joris
Department of Cardiac Surgery, CHU de Charleroi, Site de Jumet, 6040 Jumet, Belgium

Cameron Joyner
Division of Cardiac Surgery, Sunnybrook Health Science Centre, University of Toronto, Toronto, Ontario, Canada

Arie Pieter Kappetein
Department of Cardiothoracic Surgery, University Hospital Leiden, Leiden, The Netherlands

Dalane W. Kitzman
Section of Cardiology, Bowman Gray School of Medicine of Wake Forest Universisty, Winston-Salem, NC, USA

C. J. Knott-Craig
Section of Thoracic and Cardiovascular Surgery, University of Oklahoma Health Sciences Center, P. O. Box 26901, Oklahoma City, OK 73190, USA

Neal D. Kon
Department of Cardiothoracic Surgery and Cardiology, Bowman Gray School of Medicine of Wake Forest University, Winston-Salem, NC 27157, USA

Karyn S. Kunzelman
Division of Cardiothoracic Surgery and Bioengineering, 600 Highland Avenue, Madison, WI 53792-3236, USA

M. M. Lane
Section of Thoracic and Cardiovascular Surgery, University of Oklahoma Health Sciences Center, P. O. Box 26901, Oklahoma City, OK 73190, USA

Michel Lemieux
Department of Cardiovascular Surgery, Laval Hospital, 2725 Chemin Sainte-Foy, Quebec G1V 4G5, Canada

S. A. Livesey
Wessex Cardiothoracic Centre, Southampton General Hospital, Southampton, UK

Cristiane Nunes Martins
Department of Paediatric Cardiology, Biocor Institute, Belo Horizonte-MG, Brazil

Idail Costa Martins Jr
Department of Echocardiography, Biocor Institute, Belo Horizonte-MG, Brazil

Roberto Max
Department of Paediatric Cardiology, Biocor Institute, Belo Horizonte-MG, Brazil

Erik-Jan Meijboom
Department of Cardiology, Wilhemina's Children's Hospital, Utrecht, The Netherlands

Jacques Métras
Department of Cardiovascular Surgery, Laval Hospital, 2725 Chemin Sainte-Foy, Quebec G1V 4G5, Canada

S. Middlemost
Department of Cardiology, University of Witwatersrand, Witwatersrand, South Africa

Roger C. Millar
Division of Thoracic and Cardiovascular Surgery, Department of Surgery, LDS Hospital, Salt Lake City, UT, USA

William Mirsch
Tissue Development Programs, St. Jude Medical Valve Division, St. Paul, MN 55117, USA

Friedrich W. Mohr
Heart Centre, Department of Cardiac Surgery, University of Leipzig, Leipzig, Germany

D. Moreau
Department of Cardiac Surgery, Cardiologic Hospital, Lille, France

Giancarlo Grossi Mota
Department of Cardiac Surgery, Hospital Luxemburgo and Hospital Socor, Belo Horizonte-MG, Brazil

José Antonio Navia
Cardiovascular Surgery Service, Hospital Italiano, Gascon 450, Buenos Aires, Argentina

José Luis Navia
Cardiovascular Surgery Service, Hospital Italiano, Gascon 450, Buenos Aires, Argentina

C. Nojek
Hospital Español, Buenos Aires, Argentina

Abdel-Mohsen Nomeir
Section of Cardiology, Bowman Gray School of Medicine of Wake Forest University, Winston-Salem, NC, USA

Mark O'Brien
Prince Charles Hospital, Brisbane, Queensland, Australia

Ozanam Cesar de Oliveira
Department of Echocardiography, Biocor Institute, Belo Horizonte-MG, Brazil

Jaap Ottenkamp
Department of Paediatric Cardiology, University Hospital Leiden, Leiden, The Netherlands

Pietro Pascotto
Division of Cardiology, Mirano Hospital (VE), Italy

Carlos Hector Passerino
Department of Cardiac Surgery, Hospital Luxemburgo and Hospital Socor, Belo Horizonte-MG, Brazil

João Alfredo de Paula e Silva
Department of Cardiac Surgery, Biocor Institute, Belo Horizonte-MG, Brazil

Rodolfo Pizarro
Cardiovascular Surgery Service, Hospital Italiano, Buenos Aires, Argentina

Elvio Polesel
Department of Cardiac Surgery, Umberto 1° Hospital, Mestre-Venice, Italy

A. Prat
Department of Cardiac Surgery, Cardiologic Hospital, 59037 Lille, France

Raul Corrêa Rabelo
Department of Cardiac Surgery, Hospital Luxemburgo and Hospital Socor, Belo Horizonte-MG, Brazil

Thomas Rauch
Heart Centre, Department of Cardiac Surgery, University of Leipzig, Leipzig, Germany

Gilles Raymond
Department of Cardiovascular Surgery, Laval Hospital, 2725 Chemin Sainte-Foy, Quebec G1V 4G5, Canada

Dario F. Del Rizzo
Department of Surgery, University of Manitoba, Health Sciences Centre, Winnipeg, Manitoba R3A 1R9, Canada

Donald N. Ross
Guy's and National Heart Hospitals, 25 Upper Wimpole Street, London W1M 7TA, UK

Jean E. Rubay
Cliniques Universitaires, St-Luc – UCL, Avenue Hippocrate 10, Brussels 1200, Belgium

J. Saez de Iribarra
Department of Cardiac Surgery, Cardiologic Hospital, Lille, France

Erik Schampaert
Division of Cardiology, Sunnybrook Health Science Centre, University of Toronto, Toronto, Ontario, Canada

L. Schilling
Heart Centre, Department of Cardiac Surgery, University of Leipzig, Leipzig, Germany

Paul H. Schoof
Department of Cardiothoracic Surgery, University Hospital Leiden, Leiden, The Netherlands

Jeri Sever
Division of Cardiac Surgery, Sunnybrook Health Science Centre, University of Toronto, Toronto, Ontario, Canada

G. Shaaban
Department of Cardiac Surgery, Cardiologic Hospital, Lille, France

I. A. Simpson
Wessex Cardiothoracic Centre, Southampton General Hospital, Southampton, UK

C. Stankowiak
Department of Cardiac Surgery, Cardiologic Hospital, Lille, France

P. C. Strike
Wessex Cardiothoracic Centre, Southampton General Hospital, Southampton, UK

M. Sussman
Department of Cardiothoracic Surgery, University of Witwatersrand, Witwatersrand, South Africa

Bert E. Suys
Department of Paediatric Cardiology, University Hospital Leiden, Leiden, The Netherlands

V. T. Tsang
Wessex Cardiothoracic Centre, University of Southampton, Southampton, UK

Carlo Valfrè
Department of Cardiac Surgery, Regional Hospital, Treviso, Italy

Han H. van Krieken
Department of Cardiothoracic Surgery, University Hospital Leiden, Leiden, The Netherlands

Jaques A. M. van Son
Heart Centre, Department of Cardiac Surgery, University of Leipzig, Leipzig, Germany

A. Vincentelli
Department of Cardiac Surgery, Cardiologic Hospital, Lille, France

Ektor Vrandecic
Research and Development, Biocor Institute, Belo Horizonte-MG, Brazil

Erika Vrandecic
Department of Paediatric Cardiology, Biocor Institute, Belo Horizonte-MG, Brazil

Mario P. Vrandecic
Department of Cardiac Surgery, Biocor Institute, Belo Horizonte-MG, Brazil

T. Walther
Heart Centre, Department of Cardiac Surgery, University of Leipzig, Leipzig, Germany

James G. Warner
Section of Cardiology, Bowman Gray School of Medicine of Wake Forest University, Winston-Salem, NC, USA

C. Weigl
Heart Centre, Department of Cardiac Surgery, University of Leipzig, Leipzig, Germany

E. Weinschelbaum
Funcdación Favaloro, Buenos Aires, Argentina

Stephen Westaby
Oxford Heart Centre, Department of Cardiac Surgery, John Radcliffe Hospital, Oxford OX3 9DU, UK

Claudio Zerio
Division of Cardiology, Mirano Hospital (VE), Italy

Claudio Zussa
Department of Cardiac Surgery, Umberto 1° Hospital, Mestre-Venice, Italy

Preface to the First Edition

Valve prostheses continue to improve towards the goal of optimum haemodynamic function, indefinite durability and a minimal risk of thromboembolism. Most modern mechanical valves have indefinite structural integrity with excellent flow characteristics. Their propensity for thromboembolism remains however, and necessitates continuous anticoagulation. The current objective for bioprostheses is improved haemodynamics with prolonged durability and mitigation from early calcification in the young patients. They do not need anticoagulants but the stent of a bioprosthesis is both obstructive and a focus for stress on the tissue component. Stents were adopted when the effects of prolonged cardiopulmonary bypass were prevalent and myocardial protection poorly developed. The stent and sewing ring facilitate implantation with a short ischaemic time but at a price. Stentless valves (epitomised by the autogenous pulmonary valve and aortic homograft) require a more complex surgical approach but leave the valve cusps within their natural environment and provide non-obstructive central flow. In addition to reduced stress on the tissue component, the use of zero pressure fixation, together with antimineralization agents should translate into improved durability. The potential benefit of this technology is to allow bioprosthetic valve replacement in patients over 65 years of age without the risk of early tissue failure and reoperation.

Recently there has been a resurgence of interest in the use of aortic homograft and pulmonary autograft aortic valve replacement. The use of stentless porcine valves was further stimulated by the work of Tirone David and his group. Others followed this lead with both aortic and mitral stentless bioprostheses, the majority of which appear to provide haemodynamic superiority over their stented counterparts. Only time will tell if improved flow characteristics will translate into less calcification and greater durability.

In January 1994 the proponents and manufacturers of stentless bioprostheses came together in Paris to discuss the role and relative merits of these devices. A great deal of information and lively discussion are contained in the book from the Symposium and we are grateful to the contributors for providing their manuscripts. This information forms the baseline against which further developments in stentless valve technology may be compared.

Stephen Westaby and Armand Piwnica

Preface to the Second Edition

Bioprosthetic heart valve replacement began in the 1960's with the use of aortic homografts and then stentless porcine valves. At this time, the added difficulty of freehand sewn implant techniques was an important source of morbidity through the damaging effects of cardiopulmonary bypass and poorly developed myocardial protection. Stent mounting of both human and xenograft valves greatly facilitated the implant technique and allowed widespread adoption of bioprostheses. However, with the continued use of freehand aortic homografts and the evolution of the Ross procedure the benefits of stentless over stented valves were increasingly obvious. Stent mounting produces unnecessary left ventricular outflow tract obstruction and applies excessive stresses on the biological tissue. Renewed interest in stentless xenografts was stimulated by the editors and authors of this book and there is mounting clinical evidence to support the theoretical advantages of this approach.

This edition of Stentless Bioprostheses follows the Second International Symposium on Stentless Bioprostheses, in Noordveg, Holland. The text provides a comprehensive and state-of-the-art evaluation of those valves currently available in Europe and the USA. The content is completely different from the First Edition and provides valuable information for all surgeons and cardiologists with an interest in valve replacement.

Stephen Westaby

I Paediatric Applications of Stentless Bioprostheses

CHAPTER 1

Long-term results of the porcine aortic valve monocusp graft in right ventricular outflow tract reconstruction

M. P. Vrandecic, F. A. Fantini, B. Gontijo, C. N. Martins, R. Max, O. C. de Oliveira, I. C. Martins Jr, J. T. Barbosa, J. A. de Paula e Silva, M. F. de Castro, E. Vrandecic and E. Vrandecic

The use of a transannular patch for right ventricular outflow tract reconstruction in patients with inadequate pulmonary annulus has shown immediate changes in haemodynamics, changing from a pressure-loaded to a volume-loaded right ventricle, due to the pulmonary regurgitation that generally occurs. Several methods have been used to abolish or decrease pulmonary insufficiency.[1–4] The use of monocusp grafts for right ventricular outflow tract reconstruction remains controversial. The purpose of this chapter is to present results using a porcine monocusp graft, which has been employed at the authors' institution during the last seven years.

Materials and methods

Retrospective data analysis was carried out in 45 patients who underwent porcine aortic valve monocusp grafts, mounted onto a bovine pericardial patch (PAMG), for a variety of congenital heart malformations, between June 1989 and April 1996.

There were 13 female and 32 male patients, whose ages ranged between 2 weeks and 18 years (mean 4.8 ± 4.7 years). There were eight infants in the first year of life and six patients over 12 years. The patients' weights ranged from 2.78 to 48 kg (mean 16.9 ± 10.8 kg). The preoperative diagnosis is shown in Table 1.1.

Table 1.1 Preoperative diagnosis

	No.	(%)
Tetralogy of Fallot	28	(62.2)
Pulmonary valve dysplasia	6	(13.3)
Pulmonary atresia and VSD	4	(8.9)
Absent pulmonary valve syndrome	3	(6.7)
Hypoplastic right ventricle syndrome	2	(4.4)
Double outlet right ventricle	1	(2.2)
Truncus arteriosus	1	(2.2)
	45	(100)

VSD, ventricular septal defect.

Fifteen patients (33.3%) had imperfect pulmonary arterial anatomy, eight patients presented with some degree of distortion of the pulmonary branch caused by a previous shunt. Seven patients had true stenosis of the left pulmonary branch, five had absence of the left branch and three had huge dilatation of the pulmonary trunk and branches.

A previous palliative operation was performed in 15 patients (33.3%), including two classical Blalock–Taussig shunts, 12 modified Blalock shunts with the interposition of a polytetrafluoroethylene prosthesis (Gore-Tex Shunt, W. L. Gore & Associates, Inc., Newark, DE, USA) and one surgical pulmonary valvulotomy.

The monocusp used consisted of a glutaraldehyde-treated select aortic porcine cusp tailored and attached to the bovine pericardial smooth surface without stent (Biocor Industria e Pesquisas Ltda, Belo Horizonte, Brazil). Monocusp sizes used are shown in Table 1.2. Monocusp graft size was manufactured in accordance with Biocor stented valve size.

Table 1.2 Monocusp size used in 45 patients

Size (mm)	No. of patients	(%)
19	7	(15.6)
21	17	(37.8)
23	14	(31.1)
25	5	(11.1)
27	1	(2.2)
29	1	(2.2)

Standard cardiopulmonary bypass, moderate hypothermia and crystalloid cardioplegia were used in all cases. Ventricular septal defect, whenever present, was corrected with a bovine pericardial patch. The right ventricular outflow tract incision used began at the right ventricular infundibulum up to the left pulmonary artery onset. Inverted 'T' right ventriculotomy with extension close to the septal infundibular inferior edge was used.

Monocusp graft size was selected taking into account the patch width and total area to be covered by the new cusp. The patch was then tailored to the desired shape and attached by two stay sutures placed at its lateral aspect, matching the monocusp graft to the native patient's cusps in order to obtain satisfactory valve coaptation.

The anastomosis between the monocusp patch and the patient's pulmonary artery wall was approximated by a continuous Prolene 5/0 suture, starting at the upper corner. After the procedure was completed, gradients were measured across the right ventricular outflow tract by a pull-back recording.

During each patient's late follow-up, monocusp function was assessed by physical examination, serial electrocardiography, chest radiograph and echo-Doppler cardiography on a biannual basis. Cardiac catheterization was also performed if new findings were encountered during the patient's follow-up.

Results

There were five early deaths (11.1%); however, death was not related to the monocusp graft implant in any of these cases. All deaths were due to a low cardiac output related to poor preoperative clinical condition.

Follow-up was complete in 37 (92.5%) of the hospital survivors and ranged from 6 to 88 months (mean 38.5 ± 19.0 months). There were no late deaths. Two children were reoperated.

Of the 37 patients who survived, one, for whom correction of an absent pulmonary valve was performed, developed dyspnoea at exertion. This was confirmed 2 years after the operation by symptom-limited work capacity-assessed ergometry. The patient's echo-Doppler cardiography and cardiac catheterization studies disclosed no gradient across the right ventricular outflow tract but a severe pulmonary regurgitation, with a moderate right ventricular dilatation.

At reoperation a monocusp free of the degenerative process was found, well adapted to the site of implantation, but insufficient to cover the whole valvular area, since there were no valve remnants on the natural annulus. That monocusp was replaced by a Biocor stentless aortic valve with a good result.

Another patient with a corrected tetralogy of Fallot was found to be asymptomatic but with increasing systolic murmur discovered during follow-up. This patient's echo and cardiac catheterization studies showed a severe infundibular stenosis with a normal function of the monocusp graft. Again, at reoperation an intact, flexible monocusp without degeneration was found and a new monocusp graft was implanted. The patient did well and has been followed since then. The histopathological studies of the explanted monocusp have shown well-preserved collagen fibres without any evidence of calcification on the leaflet and with minimal calcium along the suture line.

The remaining 35 patients were all asymptomatic. Five patients are taking medication at the time of writing.

Thirty-six patients have undergone echo-Doppler cardiographic analysis in the last 6 months (Table 1.3). The monocusp remained mobile in every case, without any signs of calcification, dilatation or retraction, and therefore without significant stenosis. The peak systolic pressure gradient measured across the right ventricular outflow tract ranged from 0 to 32 mmHg, with a mean of 19.0 ± 5.8 mmHg. Pulmonary valve insufficiency was absent in 12 (33%), mild in 15 (42%) and moderate in 9 (25%) patients.

Table 1.3 Late postoperative echo-Doppler cardiographic data in 36 patients

RV outflow tract gradient		
Range : 0–32 mmHg		
Mean : 19.0 ± 5.8 mmHg		
Pulmonary regurgitation	**No. patients**	**(%)**
Absent	12	(33)
Mild	15	(42)
Moderate	9	(25)

Discussion

Lillehei and associates[5] introduced transannular patch enlargement of the right ventricular outflow tract in 1955 as a method of relieving stenosis and re-establishing right ventricle–pulmonary artery continuity. This procedure has been one of the most used techniques in congenital heart surgery. The immediate haemodynamic consequence is predictable, but controversy exists regarding the short- and long-term influence of the pulmonary insufficiency on the right ventricular function.

The short-term postoperative period is characterized by an acute change from a pressure-loaded to a volume-loaded right ventricle, increasing end-diastolic volume, depressing the function of the right side of the heart and finally decreasing the overall cardiac output.[6] Mortality and morbidity have been related to this situation.[7]

The hospital mortality observed in our series was slightly higher than that usually reported, even though improvement in pulmonary valve function was achieved.

Nevertheless, it is important to emphasize that our study population consisted of a group of selected patients with complex congenital pathologies who were generally in a poor preoperative clinical condition. The deaths observed were not related to the use of a monocusp.

The acute change observed soon after correction generally requires a period of time for adaptation, as shown experimentally by Ellison,[8] Bender,[9] Austen[10] and their associates and clinically by Kirklin[11] and Poirier.[12] Although some authors have stated that the chronic pulmonary insufficiency is well tolerated,[12–14] others have demonstrated that long-standing pulmonary regurgitation is associated with ventricular dysfunction.

Bove and collaborators,[15] using radionuclide ventriculography, have shown that the pulmonary regurgitation may adversely affect right ventricular function following repair of tetralogy of Fallot, leading to enlargement of the heart, right and left ventricular dysfunction and development of arrhythmias.

Meijboom,[16] Jonsson[17] and their associates stated that the exercise capacity of patients with dilatation of the right ventricle due to pulmonary regurgitation was significantly decreased, when compared with patients with small degrees of pulmonary valve insufficiency. In another study, Jonsson[18] found that moderate and severe pulmonary valve incompetence had a negative influence on lung function.

Thus, the use of a mechanism to decrease pulmonary valve incompetence is important in general and essential in some circumstances.[19] Our current policy is to indicate electively implantation of a monocusp in patients requiring transannular patch reconstruction with pulmonary artery abnormalities, as with absence of left branch, primary branch stenosis, distortion caused by previous shunts and dilatation, seen in absent pulmonary valve syndrome. We also include patients with a previous right ventricular dysfunction, elevated pulmonary vascular resistance or exuberant collateral circulation to the lungs.

Our current clinical experience with the use of porcine monocusp grafts has shown satisfactory functional performance of the cusp up to 7 years after implantation. The cusp motion appeared flexible and synchronous with the cardiac cycle in every case, without signs of any significant obstruction of the right ventricular outflow tract. The residual regurgitation noted was low and there was no evidence of tissue degeneration.

Conclusion

The porcine aortic valve monocusp graft provided excellent late results in selected patients, effectively reducing or abolishing pulmonary valve regurgitation without evidence of late stenosis. Although the test of time is required, the satisfactory haemodynamics and excellent clinical performance, with no monocusp-related complications within 7 years, have made this the graft of choice in the authors' institution whenever it is indicated.

References

1. Abdulali S A, Silverton P, Yakirevich V S, Ionescu M I 1985 Right ventricular outflow tract reconstruction with a bovine pericardial monocusp patch. J Thorac Cardiovasc Surg 89: 764–771
2. Ionescu M I, Macartney F J, Wooler G H 1972 Reconstruction of the right ventricular outlet with fascia lata composite graft. J Thorac Cardiovasc Surg 63: 60–74
3. Maluf M A, VerdeJ L, Leal J C *et al* 1993 Reconstituição da valva pulmonar e via de saída do ventrículo direito, com prótese bivalvular e prótese tubular valvada de tronco pulmonar de porco: estudo experimental e aplicação clínica. Rev Bras Cir Cardiovasc 8(1): 20–38
4. Clarke D R, Campbell D N, Pappas G 1989 Pulmonary allograft conduit repair of tetralogy of Fallot. J Thorac Cardiovasc Surg 98: 730–737

5. Lillehei C W, Cohen M, Warden H E 1995 Direct vision intracardiac surgical correction of tetralogy of Fallot, pentalogy of Fallot and pulmonary atresia defects: report of first ten cases. Ann Surg 42: 418–452
6. Hugel W, Hannekum A, Schreiber S, Dalichau H 1984 The hemodynamics and contractility of the right ventricle in the early postoperative phase following correction of tetralogy of Fallot. Thorac Cardiovasc Surg 32: 253–255
7. Equchi S, Irisawa T, Asano K 1972 Use of valve-retaining homograft and heterograft patch for reconstruction of right ventricular outflow tract. Clinical experience in tetralogy of Fallot. Ann Thorac Surg 14: 615
8. Ellison R G, Brown W, Yeh T J, Hamilton W F 1970 Surgical significance of acute and chronic pulmonary valvular insufficiency. J Thorac Cardiovasc Surg 60: 549
9. Bender H W, Austen W G, Ebert P A *et al* 1963 Experimental pulmonic regurgitation. J Thorac Cardiovasc Surg 45: 451–459
10. Austen W G, Greenfield L J, Ebert P A, Morrow A G 1962 Experimental study of right ventricular function after surgical procedures involving the right ventricle and pulmonic valve. Ann Surg 155: 606–613
11. Kirklin J W, Blackstone E H, Jonas R A *et al* 1992 Morphologic and surgical determinants of outcome events after repair of tetralogy of Fallot and pulmonary stenosis. J Thorac Cardiovasc Surg 103: 706–723
12. Poirier R A, McGoon D C, Danielson G K 1977 Late results after repair of tetralogy of Fallot. J Thorac Cardiovasc Surg 73: 900–909
13. Kirklin J K, Kirklin J W, Blackstone E H *et al* 1989 Effect of transannular patching on outcome after repair of tetralogy of Fallot. Ann Thorac Surg 48: 783–791
14. Jones E L, Conti C R, Neill C A *et al* 1973 Long-term evaluation of tetralogy patients with pulmonary valvular insufficiency resulting from outflow-patch correction across the pulmonic annulus. Circulation 48: Suppl 3: 11–8
15. Bove E L, Byrum C J, Thomas F D *et al* 1983 The influence of pulmonary insufficiency on ventricular function following repair of tetralogy of Fallot. J Thorac Cardiovasc Surg 85: 691–696
16. Meijboom F, Szatmari A, Deckers J W *et al* 1995 Cardiac status and health-related quality of life in the long term after surgical repair of tetralogy of Fallot in infancy and childhood. J Thorac Cardiovasc Surg 110: 883–891
17. Jonsson H, Ivert T, Jonasson R *et al* 1995 Work capacity and central hemodynamics thirteen to twenty-six years after repair of tetralogy of Fallot. J Thorac Cardiovasc Surg 110: 416–426
18. Jonsson H, Ivert T, Jonasson R *et al* 1994 Pulmonary function thirteen to twenty-six years after repair of tetralogy of Fallot. J Thorac Cardiovasc Surg 108: 1002–1009
19. Ilbawi M N, Idriss F S, Muster A S *et al* 1981 Tetralogy of Fallot with absent pulmonary valve. Should valve insertion be part of the intracardiac repair? J Thorac Cardiovasc Surg 81: 906–915

CHAPTER 2

Switchback: using the pulmonary autograft to replace the aortic valve after the arterial switch operation

M. G. Hazekamp, P. H. Schoof, B. E. Suys, P. A. Hutter, E.-J. Meijboom, J. Ottenkamp and H. A. Huysmans

Aortic valve insufficiency has been described to occur following the arterial switch operation. Valve insufficiency is mild in most cases. In some patients valve repair or root reconstruction may solve the problem, but in others the valve will have to be replaced. As the number of patients surviving long term after the arterial switch operation is growing, valve insufficiency may be seen more often. In infants the ideal way to replace the aortic valve is using the pulmonary autograft. Our experience with aortic valve replacement using the pulmonary autograft (former aortic valve) in one infant with a previous arterial switch is described.

Case report

A girl aged 3 years and 4 months was referred to us from another institution. At the age of 2 days an arterial switch operation had been performed for simple transposition of the great arteries. The coronary anatomy was normal (1LCx-2R, Leiden classification).[1] The aorta was anterior to the pulmonary artery. Both semilunar valves were tricuspid and normal. The coronary arteries were excised together with U-shaped aortic wall buttons and implanted in the pulmonary artery base using the trap-door technique. The neopulmonary root was reconstructed with a pantaloon-shaped patch of autologous pericardium. A Lecompte manoeuvre was part of the procedure. The postoperative course was complicated by ischaemia, frequent ventricular extrasystoles and periods of ventricular fibrillation. Left hemidiaphragm paresis necessitated later diaphragm plication.

Following an extended intensive care period the patient gradually recovered and eventually could be discharged from the hospital. Progressive dilatation of the aortic root with valvular insufficiency was observed during follow-up. Insufficiency was considered to be significant (2/4) at the age of 1 year; the left ventricle was dilated. The girl's condition deteriorated gradually, leading to fatigue at slight exertion.

Physical examination at the age of 3 years and 4 months showed a girl weighing 12.5 kg with an aortic insufficiency murmur at auscultation and a blood pressure of 105/45 mmHg. The electrocardiogram demonstrated a sinus rhythm with left ventricular hypertrophy and left precordial ST-segment inversions. The left ventricle had deteriorated at echocardiography with an end-diastolic dimension of 52 mm. The shortening fraction was calculated to be 25%. Aortic valve regurgitation was severe (4/4). The pulmonary valve was normal. Cardiac catheterization confirmed these findings. Pulmonary artery pressure was 25/10 mmHg. Both coronary arteries were visualized angiographically without evident stenoses. Angiography showed an aneurysm on the anterior aspect of the aortic root (Figure 2.1). Left ventricular contractions were diminished with diffuse hypokinesia.

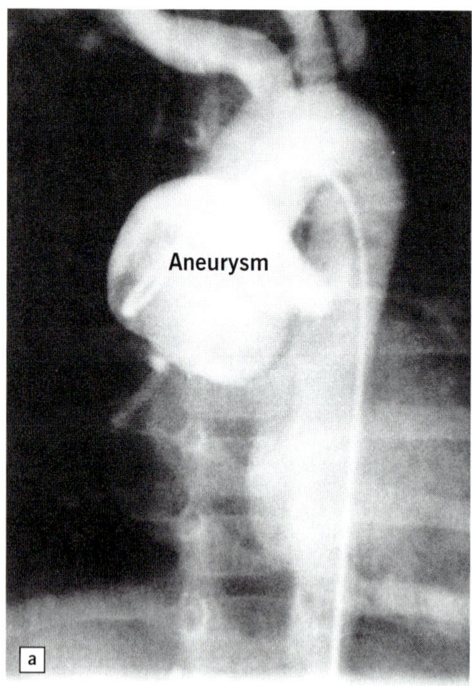

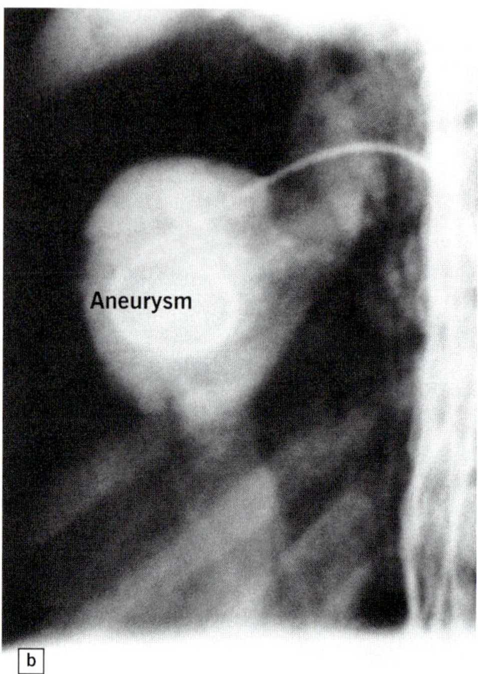

Figure 2.1 Large aneurysm of the aortic root following arterial switch operation. (a) Anteroposterior view; (b) lateral view.

Surgical procedure

The anatomy was as expected after an arterial switch procedure with the pulmonary artery in front of the aorta. The proximal part of the ascending aorta was aneurysmatic. Cannulation was high in the ascending aorta and in the right auricle with a right-angled cannula. Cardiopulmonary bypass with moderate hypothermia was started. A left vent was inserted and the aorta was cross-clamped. Retrograde St Thomas cardioplegia was repeated every 30 min combined with external myocardial cooling. The pulmonary artery was transected just proximal to the bifurcation, which facilitated exposure of the aortic root. The pulmonary valve was tricuspid without signs of degeneration. The pericardium used to reconstruct the neopulmonary trunk had fused with the rest of the pulmonary artery. The aorta was transected distal to the aneurysmatic root. The aortic valve was tricuspid with fibrosis and retraction of all three leaflets. The coronary buttons had grown after the switch procedure without evidence of coronary stenosis. The aortic valve and root were resected leaving generous coronary buttons. Next the pulmonary trunk was dissected from the right ventricle. The external diameter was 18 mm whereas the aortic annular diameter was 1 mm larger. The autograft was used to reconstruct the resected aortic root. In an effort to prevent distension the autograft was inserted slightly deeper into the left ventricle than the original aortic valve. The coronary buttons were inserted as ‘U’s after having excised equal U-shaped parts from the pulmonary autograft in order to avoid widening of the intercommissural distances. All suture lines were with running 5 or 6/0 Prolene (Ethicon GbmH, Nordtstedt, Germany). After 100 min of myocardial arrest, the pulmonary trunk was reconstructed with a 21 mm cryopreserved pulmonary homograft (Heart Valve Bank, Berlin, Germany) on a beating heart. Cardiopulmonary bypass was discontinued after rewarming. After modified ultrafiltration, the cannulas were removed and protamine was given. Epicardial echocardiography showed a well-functioning new aortic valve with no or minimal insufficiency. Haemodynamics were good with dopamine 5 mg/kg per min.

The patient was extubated the next day and discharged from the intensive care unit on the second post-operative day. She was discharged from the hospital 9 days after surgery. Echocardiography showed a still dilated left ventricle and a well-functioning pulmonary autograft with a minimal central jet of insufficiency, which was not considered to be of any haemodynamic importance.

Discussion

Aortic valve insufficiency is seen more frequently in patients after pulmonary artery banding previous to the arterial switch operation. Dilatation of the pulmonary trunk is the cause of insufficiency of the neoaortic valve following an arterial switch procedure. Even without previous pulmonary artery banding, aortic insufficiency sometimes occurs following the arterial switch procedure. The neoaortic valve diameter has been reported to be higher than in the normal population, which may explain the mild valvular regurgitation that is observed in some patients after the arterial switch procedure.[2] The exact pathogenesis of the increase in aortic annulus diameter in switch patients is not fully understood.

Surgical technical aspects may play a role. An increased intercommissural distance should theoretically lead to a loss of central coaptation of the valve cusps. Yamaguchi *et al.* indicated that the use of coronary buttons may reduce the incidence of insufficiency as compared to the use of trap-door incisions and U-shaped coronary transfers.[3]

The aortic insufficiency was mainly caused by the aortic root aneurysm in the patient described, although the thickening and retraction of the leaflets remain unexplained. A too-wide pericardial patch may have been used at the time of the arterial switch operation to adapt the wider neoaortic root to the smaller distal ascending aorta.

Aortic valve replacement by mechanical valve prosthesis following arterial switch for transposition has been performed (personal communication, J. M. Quaegebeur, 1996) and reported earlier.[4] Aortic valve repair following the arterial switch procedure has also been described.[5] In this infant we chose to replace the aortic valve with a pulmonary autograft for several reasons. Besides the known advantages of the pulmonary autograft in children as compared to other valve prostheses, some specific reasons were present in this special situation. Resection of the aneurysmatic aortic root was necessary and the relatively difficult access to the aortic root made the choice of a homograft less preferable in view of the inevitable reoperation.

The operation turned out to be straightforward. The anterior placement of the pulmonary trunk made its harvesting easy. Coronary artery problems were not encountered. Transposition may, however, be combined with coronary artery patterns that make harvesting of the pulmonary trunk more difficult, especially if the right coronary artery crosses the right ventricular outflow tract. No important mismatch between the diameters of pulmonary trunk and aortic annulus existed, which further encouraged us to choose the pulmonary autograft for aortic root replacement.

Conclusion

The Ross procedure (arterial switch operation) is technically feasible following an arterial switch operation and may be a particularly attractive alternative for this special population. This may be even more true as it is the original aortic valve that is used to replace the insufficient neoaortic valve.

Acknowledgement

Reproduced from J Thorac Cardiovasc Surg 1997 114: 844–6, with permission from Mosby–Year Book Inc.

References

1. Gittenberger-de Groot A C, Sauer U, Oppenheimer-Dekker A, Quaegebeur J M 1983 Coronary arterial anatomy in transposition of the great arteries: a morphological study. Pediatr Cardiol 4(Suppl 1): 15–24
2. Klautz R J M, Ottenkamp J, Quaegebeur J M, Buis-Liem T N, Rohmer J 1989 Anatomic correction for transposition of the great arteries: first follow-up (38 patients). Pediatr Cardiol 10: 1–9
3. Yamaguchi M, Hosokawa Y, Imai Y *et al* 1990 Early and midterm results of the arterial switch operation for transposition of the great arteries in Japan. J Thorac Cardiovasc Surg 100: 261–269
4. Ungerleider R M, Gaynor J W, Israel P, Kanter R J, Armstrong B E 1992 Report of neoaortic valve replacement in a ten year old girl after an arterial switch procedure for transposition. J Thorac Cardiovasc Surg 104: 213–215
5. Serraf A, Roux D, Lacour-Gayet F *et al* 1995 Reoperation after arterial switch operation for transposition of the great arteries. J Thorac Cardiovasc Surg 110: 892–899

CHAPTER 3

Pulmonary root replacement with the Freestyle stentless aortic xenograft in growing pigs

P. H. Schoof, M. G. Hazekamp, H. H. van Krieken and H. A. Huysmans

Reconstruction of the right ventricular outflow tract for congenital cardiac defects, including the Ross operation, is generally performed with the use of a homograft. Its limited availability, however, keeps us searching for a readily available alternative with comparable haemodynamic characteristics and longevity. The stentless aortic xenograft with its superior haemodynamics and expected favourable durability appears a promising substitute.[1–3] Before embarking on its clinical use for right ventricular outflow reconstruction, we decided to assess the valve in the growing pig, in which the results of left-sided implantation have been shown to produce excellent, reproducible results.[4]

Materials and methods

During a period of 15 months, 18 Dutch Landrace piglets weighing 26.6 ± 3.2 kg (mean ± SD; range 22.0–31.2 kg) were operated on. Pulmonary root replacement with the Medtronic Freestyle aortic root bioprosthesis (Medtronic, Minneapolis, MN, USA) was performed in all 18 animals, four of whom also underwent a complete Ross procedure.

Operation

After overnight fasting, premedication, shaving and weighing, anaesthesia was induced and endotracheal intubation performed. Through a median sternotomy, the aorta and right atrium were cannulated and normothermic cardiopulmonary bypass was initiated. Cardioplegic arrest was induced using antegrade St Thomas crystalloid cardioplegia. The pulmonary root was excised from the bifurcation down to and including a 5 mm muscular ridge below the valve. Subsequently, an oversized 21 (n = 13) or 23 (n = 5) mm stentless porcine aortic xenograft was tailored obliquely at its distal end to accommodate the natural pulmonary artery curvature and was positioned with the coronary stumps pointing sidewards. Both distal and proximal anastomoses were made with 5/0 Prolene (Ethicon, Somerville, NJ, USA) in a continuous fashion. In 4 piglets, the pulmonary autograft was used to replace the aortic root. At normothermia, cardiopulmonary bypass was discontinued, the heart decannulated, heparin antagonized and the chest closed, leaving drains in the pericardium and substernally.

Postoperative course

All animals were extubated primarily or within a few hours after the operation and brought to a temperature- and oxygen-regulated intensive care unit. Core temperature and ECG were monitored, chest drains were intermittently aspirated and arterial blood gases sampled. Anaesthetics were administered and blood transfusions or diuretics were given if necessary. After 1 or 2 days, the animals returned to their stalls. Jugular and carotid lines as well as skin sutures were removed after 1 week using light general anaesthesia. All animals stayed for 2–3 weeks before they were returned to the farm, where they were left to grow as much as possible and fed unrestrictedly. Throughout the whole study period, all animals received humane care in compliance with the Dutch Animal Welfare Act. The experimental protocol was reviewed and approved by the University of Leiden Committee on the Care and Use of Laboratory Animals.

Euthanasia

Animals not dying of a natural cause were put to death when symptoms of heart failure developed, or when they reached more than 160 kg. Euthanasia was carried out with the use of metomidate hydrochloride, azaperone, pancuronium and potassium chloride.

Autopsy

In all animals, a thoracolaparotomy was performed and a cause of death was established. The heart and proximal great vessels were excised and after inspection of the transected ventricles, the xenograft was excised, rinsed in Ringer's solution and photographed. All specimens were fixed in 3.6% formaldehyde and representative specimens were sectioned and stained (hematoxylin and eosin, elastin van Gieson, Gram). Stained sections were assessed by our histopathologist (Dr Han H. van Krieken).

Results

There were no operative deaths. Early mortality occurred in one pig that accidentally pulled out its carotid line during the night and died from exsanguination.

Three pigs were well at more than 160 kg and were sacrificed. Fourteen pigs died or were euthanized prematurely because of heart failure after 2 weeks to 11 months (Figure 3.1).

At gross examination of the autopsy specimens, xenograft endocarditis was diagnosed in two pigs. Both grafts showed destruction of the valve cusps characterized by tears and perforations with loosely adherent fibrinous material causing severe insufficiency. These valves looked markedly different from the other explants. One of the pigs with endocarditis had a Ross operation and showed destruction of the autograft as well.

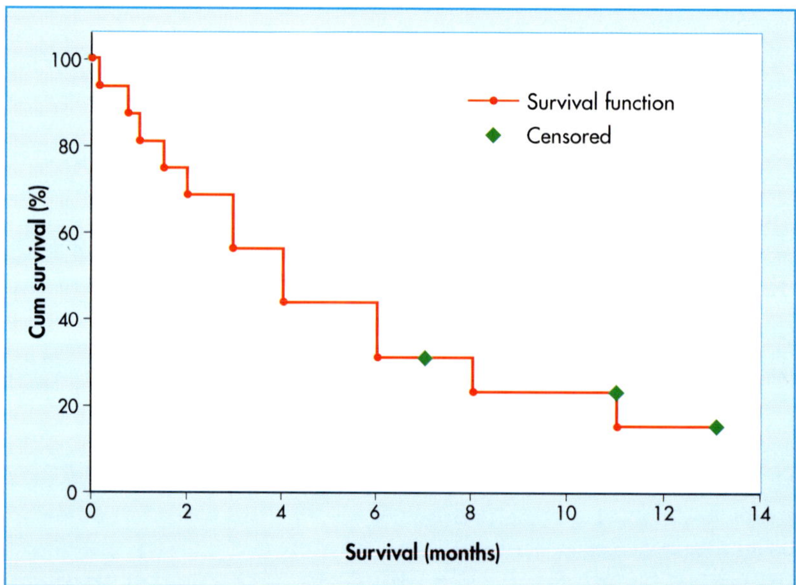

Figure 3.1 Cumulative (Cum) survival of the studied animals after operation. Three animals that were healthy at euthanasia were censored.

In the other 12 animals, again more of less pronounced signs of right ventricular failure were found at autopsy, with hepatomegaly, ascites and oedematous tissues. All xenograft explants showed severe gross cuspal pathology with large, smooth, and thick immobilizing nodular structures representing the remnants of former cusps. The functional orifice was significantly reduced in all pigs (Figure 3.2). The tubular portion of the xenograft felt calcified in most explants and showed a smooth and shiny inner surface in all. Death and severe heart failure were apparently valve related in all 14 animals.

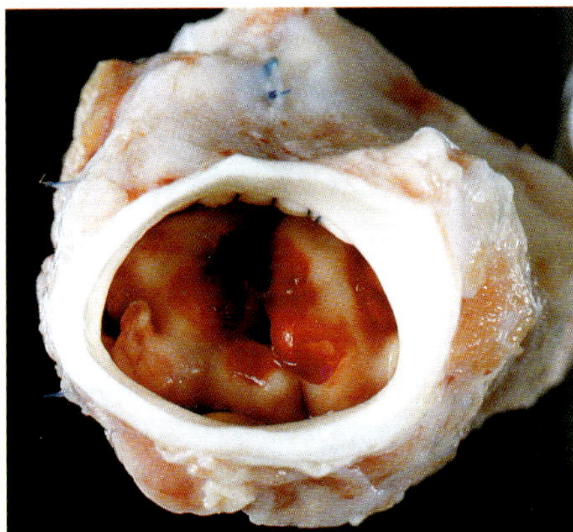

Figure 3.2 Macroscopic photograph of explanted xenograft showing the typical deformations of the valve as found in most animals.

The explants of the three electively sacrificed pigs showed similar changes but less pronounced in two animals and a relatively unaffected valve in one.

At microscopy, large cuspal masses of degenerating collagen and fibrin were found with focal calcifications and nodules of various inflammatory cells but without microorganisms (Figure 3.3). In two explants, solitary colonies of bacteria were found within the collagen-fibrin nodules, without inflammatory cells.

Discussion

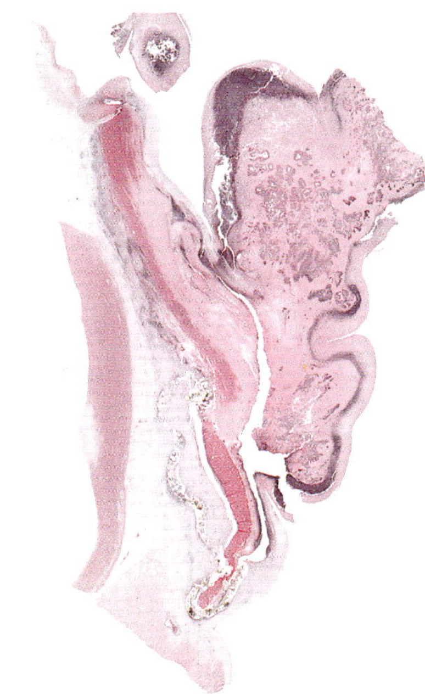

Figure 3.3 Hematoxylin- and eosin-stained section showing the prosthetic wall (left) and the severely malformed valve (right) with large areas of collagen and fibrin. (× 10 before 55% reduction.)

In earlier days, the favourable experience with the stented porcine bioprosthesis for adult valve replacement prompted its use for right ventricular outflow tract repair in children with subsequent disappointing results.[5–8] Nowadays, the favourable early results in adults of the unstented porcine bioprosthesis or stentless xenograft again seem to prompt us to use this valve for right ventricular outflow tract reconstruction, including the Ross operation.[9] With the experience of this study, we doubt whether the Freestyle stentless xenograft can be considered an alternative to the pulmonary homograft or even the old porcine valved conduit. The Freestyle stentless xenograft is a relatively straight stiff tube, not well shaped to be inserted in the pulmonary position, and needs to be tailored to prevent it from deformation at implantation. Furthermore, the coronary buttons may hinder proper positioning of the graft in the right ventricular outflow tract. Although early clinical results of the Freestyle stentless xenograft in the pulmonary position in adults were good,[9] we were concerned about long-term results and reluctant to use this valve electively for this indication. When homografts are not available and a Ross operation is performed on an emergency basis in a young adult, the stentless xenograft is probably the second best alternative for right ventricular outflow tract recontruction. On the basis of our experimental findings, use of this valve in children would not be recommended.

Because the Freestyle stentless xenograft has been shown to perform well in the aortic position in growing Dutch Landrace pigs,[4] the mechanism of early degeneration in the pulmonary position is probably determined by the different haemodynamics in the right ventricular outflow tract and the intrinsic characteristics of the aortic xenograft valve. The reduced extensibility of the valve cusps due to glutaraldehyde fixation, without influence in the high pressures of the left ventricular outflow tract, may play a critical role in the lower pressures of the right ventricular outflow tract. It may cause an unfavourable opening–closing behaviour of the valve, accelerating valve dysfunction due to platelet–fibrin depositions and subsequent cuspal immobilization and degeneration. The gross architecture of the xenograft explants differed markedly from homograft explants used as fresh implants for Ross operations in piglets of comparable weight and same species. The explants (n = 12) showed mild cuspal thickening and retraction with fine, probably calcific, nodular structures causing valve insufficiency and little or no wall calcification after 3 to 11 months (6.6 ± 2.3 months, mean ± standard deviation) (Schoof P *et al.*, unpublished results).

The mode of degeneration of the xenograft explants was unfamiliar to us with various inflammatory cells found at microscopy, as a possible expression of a non-bacterial thrombotic endocarditis. An infectious cause could not be excluded in two of four samples because small colonies of bacteria were found, although without inflammatory cells.

Possibly the stentless pulmonary xenograft will be a better valve for pulmonary reconstruction. It might approach the haemodynamic performance and longevity of the pulmonary homograft. The theoretical advantages of the pulmonary over the aortic xenograft have already been alluded to by Donald Ross[10] and the superior function of fixed pulmonary valves was also suggested by Christie and Barratt-Boyes.[11] They showed that the glutaraldehyde-fixed pulmonary valve has the advantage of decreased stiffness, increased radial extensibility, and better preserved anisotropy probably due to a significantly lower collagen content.[11] These characteristics may be of particular benefit in the low pressure pulmonary position because the fixed pulmonary leaflets can be expected to offer significantly less haemodynamic resistance to blood flow, which possibly prevents the valve from early failure.

Conclusion

The Freestyle stentless aortic xenograft implanted in the pulmonary position in piglets showed early failure in the majority of animals. Presuming the juvenile pig to be a representative experimental model, clinical use of this valve in children would not be recommended.

Acknowledgement

The Department of Research and Development of Medtronic Incorporated, Minneapolis, MN, is gratefully acknowledged for financial support of this study.

Reprinted with permission from the Society of Thoracic Surgeons (Ann Thorac Surg 1998; 65: 1726–9).

References

1. Westaby S, Amarasena N, Omerod O *et al* 1995 Time related haemodynamic changes after aortic valve replacement with the Freestyle stentless valve. Ann Thorac Surg 60: 1633–1639
2. Sintek C F, Fletcher A D, Khonsari S 1995 Stentless porcine aortic root: valve of choice for the elderly patient with the small aortic root? J Thorac Cardiovasc Surg 109: 871–876
3. Stelzer P, McCabe J C, Subramanian V A 1994 Aortic valve replacement with the stentless porcine aortic root. Abstr. 6th International Symposium on Cardiac Bioprostheses, Vancouver

4. Hazekamp M G, Goffin Y A, Huysmans H A 1993 The value of the stentless biovalve prosthesis. An experimental study. Eur J Cardiothorac Surg 7: 514–519
5. Bisset G S, Schwartz D C, Benzing G, Helmsworth J A, Schreiber J T, Kaplan S 1981 Late results of reconstruction of right ventricular outflow tract with porcine xenografts in children. Ann Thorac Surg 31: 437–443
6. Ebert P A 1984 Current techniques and results in infancy. In: Moulton A L (ed) Congenital heart surgery. Current techniques and controversies. Appleton Davies, Pasadena, CA, USA, pp 81–90
7. Boyce S W, Turley K, Yee E S, Vernier E D, Ebert P A 1988 The fate of the 12 mm porcine valved conduit from the right ventricle to the pulmonary artery. A ten year experience. J Thorac Cardiovasc Surg 95: 201–207
8. Schaff H V, DiDonato R M, Danielson R M *et al* 1984 Reoperation for obstructed pulmonary ventricle–pulmonary artery conduits: early and late results. J Thorac Cardiovasc Surg 88: 334–343
9. Konertz W, Sidiropoulos A, Hotz H, Borges A, Baumann G 1996 Ross operation and right ventricular outflow tract reconstruction with stentless xenografts. J Heart Valve Dis 5: 418–420
10. Ross D N 1995 From homograft to stentless bioprosthesis. In: Piwnica A, Westaby S (eds) Stentless bioprosthesis. Isis Medical Media Ltd, Oxford, UK, pp 17–23
11. Christie G W, Barratt-Boyes B G 1995 Mechanical properties of porcine pulmonary valve leaflets; how do they differ from aortic leaflets? Ann Thorac Surg 60: S195–199

II Stentless Prostheses in the Mitral Position

CHAPTER 4

The porcine mitral stentless valve: critical analysis at 5 years

M. P. Vrandecic, B. Gontijo, F. A. Fantini, O. C. de Oliveira, I.C. Martins Jr, M. Hermeto, J. T. Barbosa, J. A. de Paula e Silva, M. F. de Castro, E. Vrandecic and E. Vrandecic

The concept of preserving at least one subvalvar apparatus in order to retain left ventricular geometry after mitral valve replacement is not new.[1] Lillehei *et al.*[2] reported decreased operative mortality after mitral valve replacement when preserving the posteromedial subvalvar apparatus.

Several investigators carried out the task to substantiate Lillehei's claim[3–9] and the procedure is now considered standard. Introduced in 1968, mitral valvuloplasty has recently become the gold standard surgical treatment for the diseased mitral valve.

Carpentier,[10] in spite of the high incidence of early reoperations, eventually mastered the technique and refocused attention on preoperative echo analysis and intraoperative observation of the mitral valve apparatus.

Accurate mitral valve study and adherence to functional classification and segmental valve analysis before and during surgery have led to good results. The use of the mitral annuloplasty ring in this procedure has become necessary to decrease postoperative mitral insufficiency. Several reports have indicated mitral insufficiency in up to 17% of patients during the first postoperative year.[11–16]

Since mitral annuloplasty has limiting factors, such as poor mitral tissue component, mitral valve replacement with mechanical or tissue valve is indicated. Current heart valve substitutes with aortic design, implanted in the mitral position, when analysed over time have provided low patient survival at 10 years.[17–19] Recently, Acar *et al.*[20] have reported satisfactory results in mitral valve replacement using homograft and annuloplasty ring.

Since 1992, we have been using the porcine mitral stentless valve (PMSV) in an attempt eventually to improve current long-term clinical results. The porcine mitral stentless valve has natural anatomical and physiological characteristics similar to the human mitral valve and good clinical results have been obtained, particularly in patients with poor preoperative left ventricular function.

Patients, data and method

Patient selection

One hundred and twenty-five patients underwent mitral valve replacement using PMSV at this institute between March 1992 and December 1996. The decision to use this particular valve was based upon patients' acceptance and preoperative echo analysis of the nature of the mitral valve disease. Only patients above 40 years of age (26) underwent cardiac catheterization. Twenty-five patients (20%) were in atrial fibrillation.

All patients underwent per-operative echo-Doppler cardiography and were followed by clinical, laboratory and echocardiography analysis every 3 months during the first year and biannually thereafter. Patients' ages ranged from 11 to 72 years, with a mean age of 36.5 ± 14.18. There were 73 female (58.4%) and 52 male (41.6%) patients. The most common aetiology indicating mitral valve replacement was rheumatic heart disease sequelae in 108 patients (86.4%), myxomatous degenerations in eight (6.4%), prosthetic dysfunction in six (4.8%), native endocarditis in two (1.6%) and mitral dysfunction due to coronary ischaemia in one (0.8%). The haemodynamic profile showed double valve lesions in 63 patients (50.4%), mitral stenosis and/or mitral insufficiency in 31 patients in equal numbers for each lesion (24.8%). There were 23 patients (18.4%) with previous heart surgery. Six had mitral valve replacement previously, 13 had mitral commissurotomy and four mitral valvuloplasty.

Associated procedures were performed in 11 patients (8.8%): five underwent aortic valve replacement, one myocardial revascularization, two aortic commissurotomy and three mitral stentless chordal shortening.

Total patient follow-up was 3.75 months, with a mean follow-up of 29.5 months. Preoperative functional class (NYHA) showed five patients (4%) in class II, 79 (63.2%) in class III and 41 (32.8%) in class IV (Table 4.1).

Table 4.1 Preoperative clinical data

Number: 125 patients	Total patient follow-up
Age: 36.5 ± 14.18 (mean)	3.75 months
Gender	(mean 29.5 months)
Female: 73 (58.4%)	Functional class (NYHA)
Male: 52 (41.6%)	Class II 5 patients (4.0%)
Aetiology	Class III 79 patients (63.2%)
RHD 108 pts (86.4%)	Class IV 41 patients (32.8%)
Predominant mitral lesion	Atrial fibrillation: 25 patients (20%)
Double valve lesion (50.4%)	Patient follow-up
Previous surgeries: 23 pts (18.4%)	Clinical, Laboratory, Echo-Doppler: Every 3 months for the first year; biannually thereafter
Associated surgeries: 11 pts (8.8%)	

Surgical procedures

Although the principles of the surgical procedure were previously published,[21–23] it is important to review the objective and means to achieve the best intraoperative surgical results.

Standard cardiopulmonary bypass, bubble oxygenator and crystalloid cardioplegia were used in the majority of the patients; recently, blood retrograde cardioplegia is being used.

The purpose of the mitral valve replacement using PMSV was to restore the left ventricular continuity, providing a satisfactory flow pattern and thus improving and preserving the left ventricular function. The procedure designed has guidelines similar to the objective of the mitral valvuloplasty.

Preoperative echo analysis of the mitral valve complex and intraoperative adherence to the functional classification and segmental valve analysis are of paramount importance. Mitral valve analysis includes observation of patients' mitral annulus abnormalities, subvalvar apparatus length, left ventricular cavity determination and chordal origin positioning and possible abnormalities. The critical viewing of those segments may positively add to the correct choice of valve size.

Since the major surgical complication determined was mitral valve insufficiency, a specific mitral stentless sizer of shape, form and measurements similar to the PMSV has recently become available. This sizer may provide the following:

1. Patient's mitral valve annular analysis to determine if annuloplasty in conjunction with the mitral stentless valve implant may be required.
2. The anterolateral and posteromedial papillary muscle to annulus height.
3. Assistance in positioning, angulation, size and number of sutures needed to anchor at a right angle with chordal correct alignment of the new stentless mitral chordal origin using the free pericardial edge for later anchoring suture (Figure 4.1).

Since the measurements are obtained in diastole, the mitral subvalvular apparatus is at its most relaxed state.

Valve leaflets and mitral chord should be entirely inside the left ventricle so as to obtain near-perfect leaflet coaptation. Care should be taken to properly assess patients' mitral annulus (Figures 4.2–4.5).

As with any new product and surgical technique, training is required.

Echocardiography

Preoperative, perioperative and postoperative studies were performed using ATL, ultramark-9 colour Doppler echocardiographic unit with 3.5 and 5.0 MHz phased array ultrasound probes.

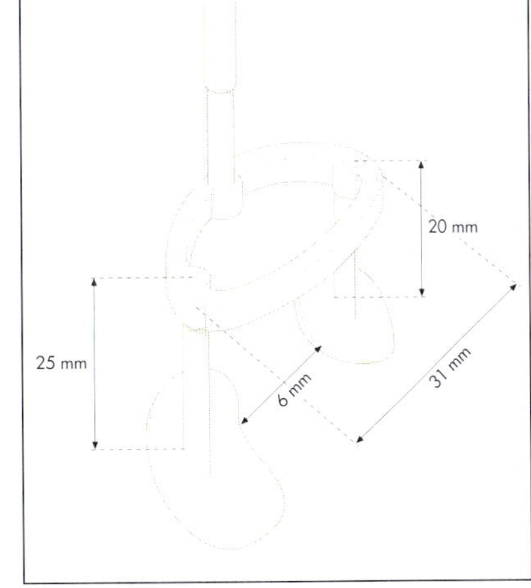

Figure 4.1 Stentless mitral sizer.

Two-dimensional, M-mode, continuous-wave Doppler and colour-flow Doppler echocardiograms were obtained from the parasternal short and long axes, as well as from the apical two and four chamber views, according to the recommendations of the American Society of Echocardiography.

The onset of the Q wave in the ECG defined the end of diastole and the peak downwards motion of the ventricular septum the end of systole.

The following echocardiographic data were assessed: end-systolic, end-diastolic left ventricular (LVESD, LVEDD), left atrial (LASD, LADD), right ventricular (RVESD, RVEDD). Fractional shortening (FS) was calculated according to the usual mathematical formulae.

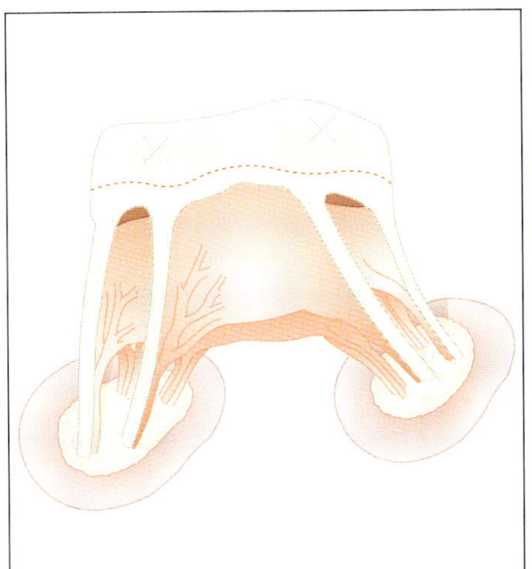
Figure 4.2 Mitral stentless valve – front view at relaxing state (diastole).

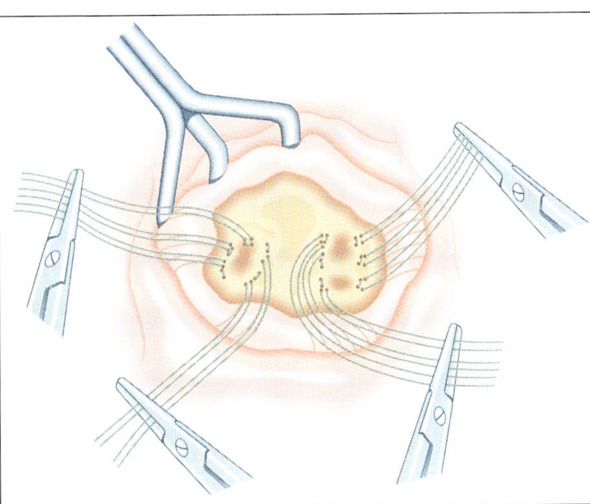
Figure 4.3 Diagrammatic papillary muscle U-type suture placement.

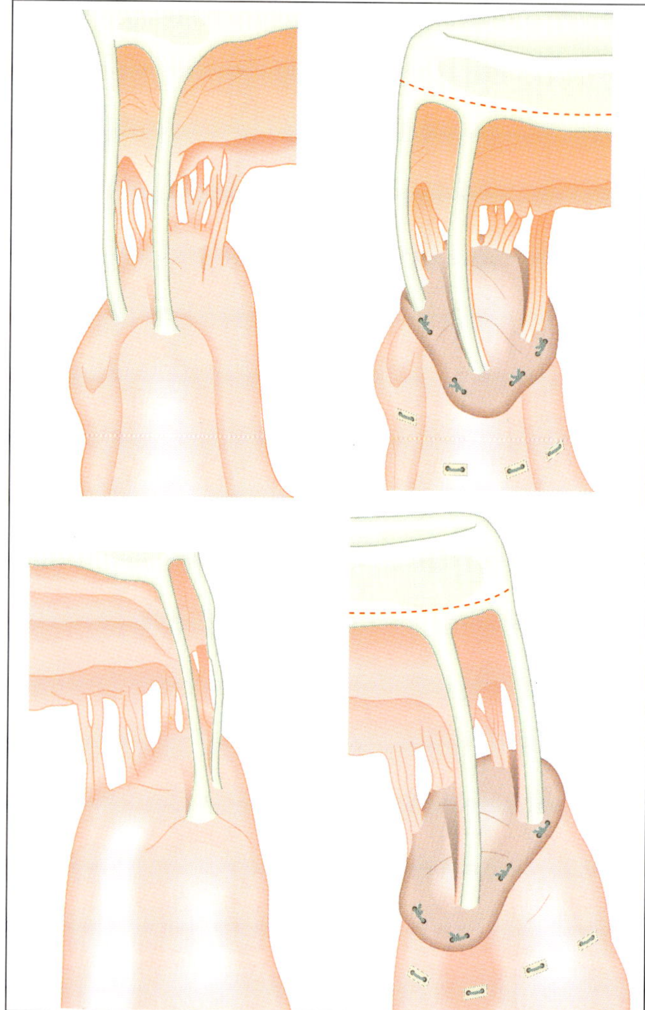

Figure 4.4 New chordal origin placement over patient's own chordal origin.

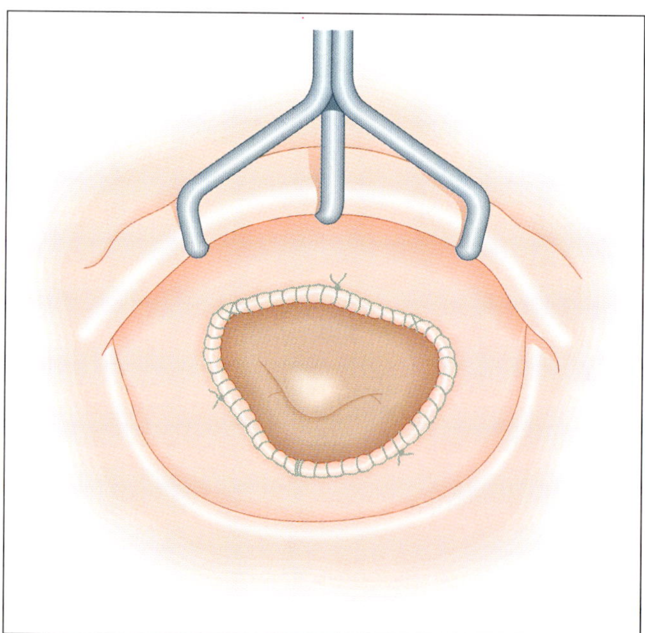

Figure 4.5 Completed annular suture; note 'D' annular shape and subannular leaflet closure.

Statistical analysis

Statistical software used were SAS system and the STS system. Data were presented as mean and standard deviation of numerical and absolute and/or relative numbers for discrete parameters. Univariate analysis of variance was first performed and a t-test for differences within a group was performed; $p < 0.05$ was considered significant.

Results

The overall patient hospital mortality was 5.6% (seven patients) and none was valve related. Patient death was due to low cardiac output in three patients, acute cerebral vascular accident in two, major pulmonary emboli in one and blood dyscrasia in one.

Hospital mortality

Ten patients required reoperations because of surgical bleeding or due to mitral valve dysfunction. In five patients reoperation was performed to establish surgical homeostasis. Five patients required replacement of their PMSV with a porcine stented valve, in two because PMSV mismatched and in three because of early papillary partial dehiscence, noticed before sternal closure in one and within 1 week in the other two patients. There was no hospital mortality in this subgroup.

One hundred and eighteen patients were discharged from hospital, 113 with PMSV. One patient was lost to follow-up (Table 4.2).

Late reoperation

Late reoperations were performed in 23 patients (20.4%). The reoperation was

Table 4.2 Patient follow-up after hospital discharge

Discharged	118
Patients with PMSV	113
Lost to follow-up	–1
Initial follow-up	112
Reoperations	–23
Late death	–4
Late patient follow-up	85

indicated because of PMSV insufficiency in 14 patients (12.4%), PMSV endocarditis in six (5.3%) and PMSV stenosis in three (2.7%). Of these 23 reoperated patients, four died, two because of low cardiac output and two due to cerebral embolic complication and eventual cerebral death.

Late mortality was recorded in four patients, due to progressive ventricular dysfunction in one, acute pancreatitis in one, pneumonia in one and sepsis due to PMSV endocarditis in one.

Total late death was recorded in eight patients (7.1%), including four patients requiring reoperations (reoperative death).

Among 112 patients in follow-up, 23 patients were reoperated, thus the follow-up was restricted to 89 patients. The late non-surgical patient mortality in four further reduced the current follow-up to 85 patients (Figures 4.6–4.9).

Clinical, laboratory and echo-Doppler cardiography of those patients showed the following. Echocardiographic data were in agreement with clinical patient data. Seventy one patients (83.5%) showed competent PMSV, 11 patients (12.9%) with stable mild (+1) mitral insufficiency, two patients (2.4%) with mild paravalvular leak and one (1.2%) being followed because of PMSV stenosis (Tables 4.3, 4.4 and Figures 4.10–4.12).

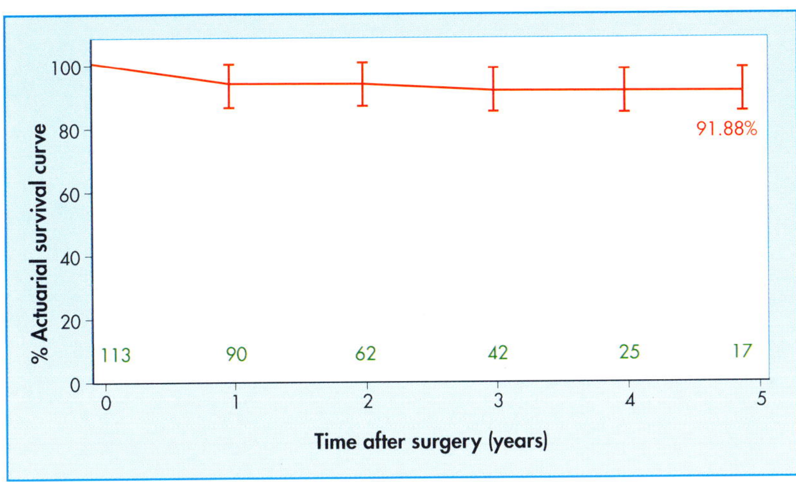

Figure 4.6 Mitral stentless valve – % actuarial survival curve, hospital mortality excluded.

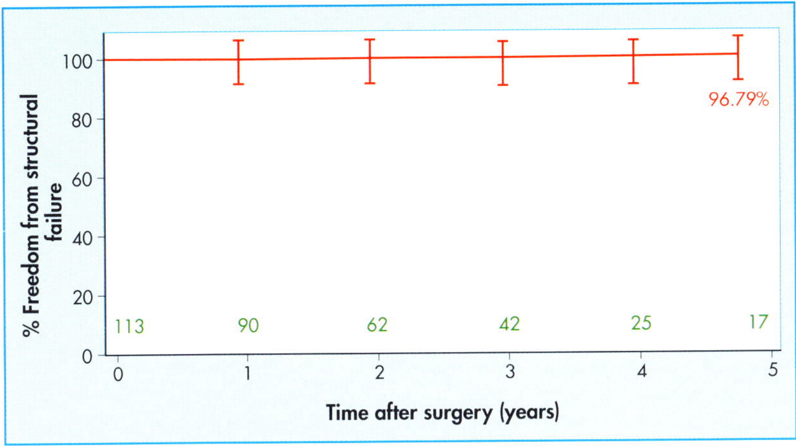

Figure 4.7 Mitral stentless valve – % freedom from structural failure.

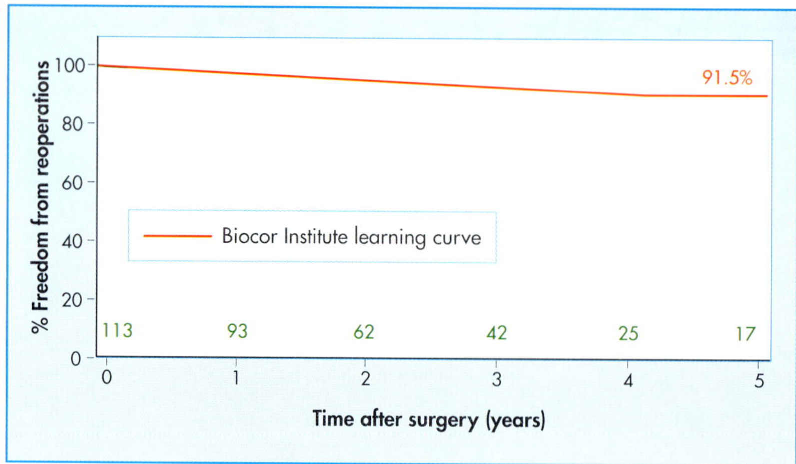

Figure 4.8 Mitral stentless valve – % freedom from re-operation.

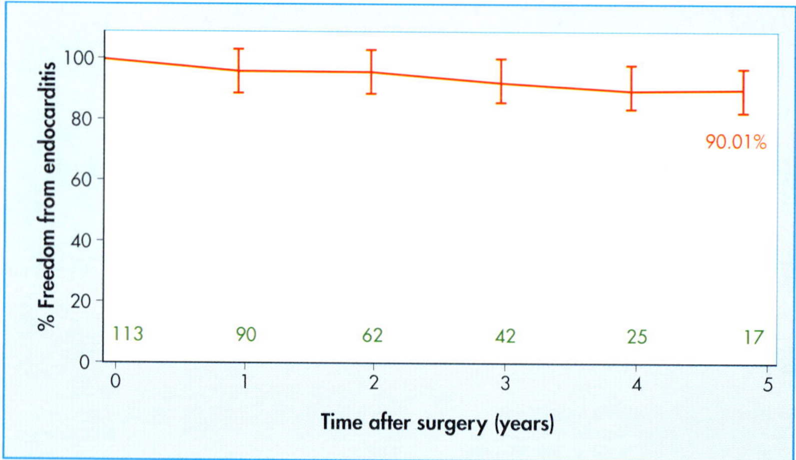

Figure 4.9 Mitral stentless valve – % freedom from endocarditis.

Table 4.3 Results of preoperative and postoperative in-hospital echo-Doppler cardiography

	Preoperative data	Postoperative data
LVESD	50.3±5.1	46.9±7.5
LVEDD	60.8±9.2	54.1±5.3
LASD	62.3±7.1	43.0±9.3
LADD	65.7+8.4	42.4+7.8
RVESD	28.3±7.7	20.2±5.0
RVEDD	37.4±8.2	26.7±4.6
LV-L	103.6±10.0	92.4±7.3

LVESD, left ventricular end-systolic diameter; LVEDD, left ventricular end-diastolic diameter; LASD, left atrial systolic diameter; LADD, left atrial diastolic diameter; RVESD, right ventricular end-systolic diameter; RVEDD, right ventricular end-diastolic diameter; LV-L, left ventricular length.

Current functional class (NYHA) showed 75 patients (88.23%) are currently in functional class I, seven (8.2%) are in class II and three (3.5%) are in functional class III.

Discussion

The mitral heart valve complex is a unique structure that prevents ventricular dysfunction, allowing vortex flow and satisfactory left ventricular haemodynamics. Among heterologous mitral valves, the porcine species is the closest anatomically to

Table 4.4 Long-term echo-Doppler cardiography

	Preoperative data	Postoperative data
LVESD	50.3±5.1	39.0±8.2
LVEDD	60.8±9.2	50.3±7.4
LASD	62.3±7.1	42.7±8.4
LADD	65.7+8.4	40.1±8.5
RVESD	28.3±7.7	21.3±5.3
RVEDD	37.4±8.2	26.9±4.8
LV-L	103.6±10.0	81.4±8.1

LVESD, left ventricular end-systolic diameter; LVEDD,left ventricular end-diastolic diameter; LASD, left atrial systolic diameter; LADD, left atrial diastolic diameter; RVESD, right ventricular end-systolic diameter; RVEDD, right ventricular end-diastolic diameter; LV-L, left ventricular length.

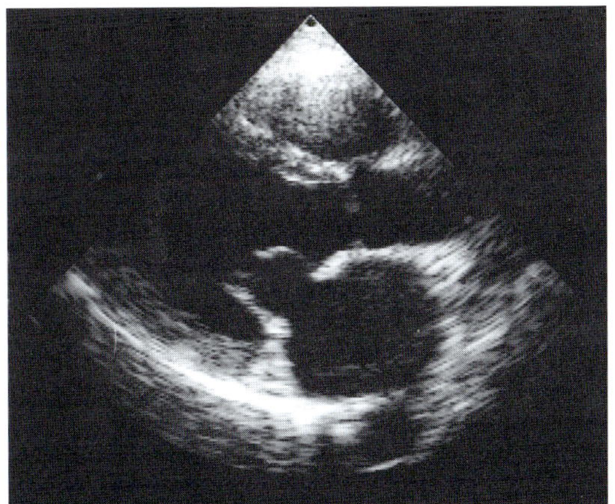

Figure 4.10 Long axis view of wide mitral leaflet opening.

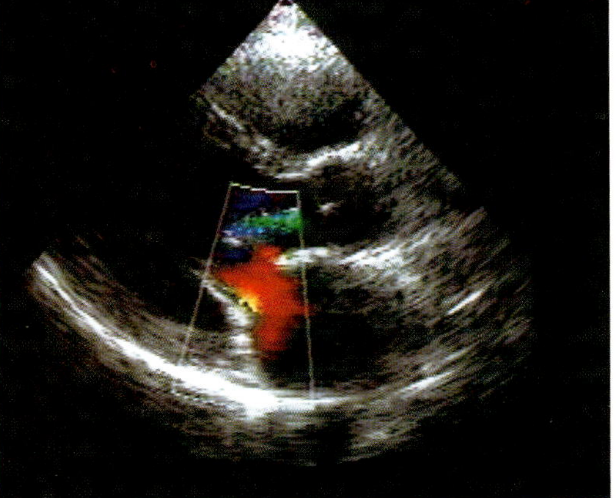

Figure 4.11 Long axis view – colour Doppler flow without turbulence.

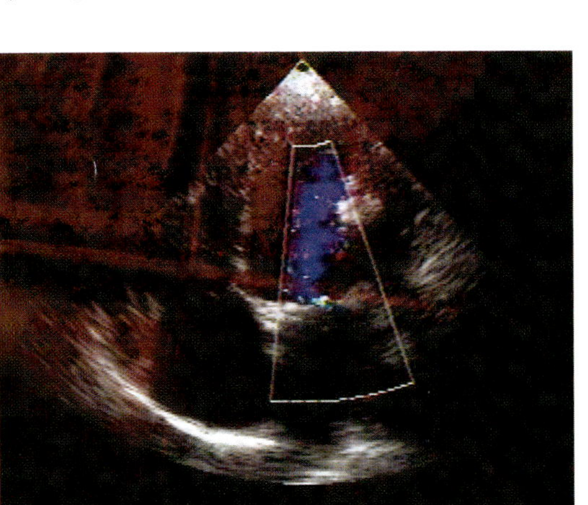

Figure 4.12 Four chamber view of a fully competent valve (systole).

the human mitral valve.[24] Since major ventricular dysfunction has been reported at 5 and 10 years in patients who have undergone mitral valve replacement using aortic designed heart valve substitutes, new options are needed to restore and preserve ventricular function. Mitral valvuloplasty remains the gold standard, followed by papillary preservation. In many instances, because of the severity of mitral disease, previous mitral surgery and papillary excision, the above techniques may not be feasible.

In this sense, the concept of the use of PMSV is a valid one, since it restores left ventricular function, preventing ventricular dilatation. In order to master this new technique and to further teaching to interested surgeons, one has to accept a wider learning curve. Three surgeons have conducted teaching courses that include performing surgery when appropriate. To date, interested surgeons have performed this surgery for the first time under guidance and this may be partially responsible for the higher reoperative rate.

The figure of 23 reoperations in this study is high, yet understandable if the objective is to transmit the surgical steps and to improve technical details. There were

14 reoperations because of mitral insufficiency and at reoperation the following conditions were found. There were eight patients displaying leaflet rupture at the pericardial annular suture line. These findings were related to poor valve length choice. Three patients with paravalvular leak had their annulus severely calcified posteriorly. There were three in whom chordal rupture at mid-length was encountered and rupture was due to excessive stress of the mitral chord. These findings are in accordance with the major surgical difficulty encountered, which was the common difficulty in correctly determining valve length. The other reoperations performed are in accordance with the higher Brazilian incidence of endocarditis found in six patients. Mitral stenoses have shown excessive foreign body reaction and annular pannus formation, which may represent tissue failure. The recent development of the mitral stentless sizer may contribute to the correct assessment of annulus, chordal length and alignment in patients in a positive way, thus providing the correct valve size with adequate annular correction.

This new technique and design has gained acceptance and although there are several drawbacks to overcome, current clinical follow-up has shown excellent results at up to 5 years in 85 patients.

Improvements in design and surgical techniques are possible with the addition of calcificant retardant treatments that may be accomplished with time. Recently a new tool has been added and this new three-dimensional valve sizing device may improve further the choice of the correct mitral stentless valve size, thus decreasing complications and improving the patient's quality of life.

The need for multicentric controlled trials is clear. At this point in time, clear-cut patient indications, new sizer, and reproducible surgical technique allied to 5 years of clinical follow-up, make this heart valve substitute the natural alternative in selected patients requiring mitral valve replacement.

Conclusions

Current experience with the use of PMSV at this institution is valid and although a high reoperation rate was reported, it is necessary to focus on the importance of teaching this new technique. The following conclusions can be drawn:

1. PMSV provides left ventricular remodelling and LV preservation.
2. The LV remodelling is better appreciated in patients with moderate ventricular dilatation.
3. Better patient selection will enhance clinical results.
4. The implanting technique does require training.
5. The use of the new mitral stentless valve sizer may promote closer-to-ideal mitral stentless valve choice.
6. Monitored clinical trials may provide the ultimate answer to mitral stentless valve performance versus time.

References

1. Lillehei C W, Gott V L, Wall R A, Vargo R L 1957 Surgical correction of pure mitral insufficiency by annuloplasty under direct vision. Lancet 77: 446–449
2. Lillehei C W, Levy M J, Bonnabeau R C 1964 Mitral valve replacement with preservation of papillary muscles and chordae tendinae. J Thorac Cardiovasc Surg 47: 532–543
3. Crawford M H, Souchk J, Oprian C A *et al* 1990 Determinants of survival and left ventricular performance after mitral valve replacement. Circulation 81: 1173–1181
4. David T E, Ho T W 1986 The effect of preservation of chordae tendinae on mitral valve replacement for postinfarction mitral regurgitation. Circulation 74(Suppl I): 116–120
5. David T E, Uden D E, Strauss H D 1983 The importance of the mitral apparatus in left ventricular function after correction of mitral regurgitation. Circulation 68(Suppl II): 76–82

6. Gams E, Strauss H D, Meher E, Anderson M J, Macdonald I L, Buda A I 1981 Is it important to preserve the chordae tendinae and papillary muscles during mitral valve replacement ? Can J Surg 24: 326–331
7. Gams E, Hagl S, Schad H, Heimisch W, Mendler N, Sebening F 1991 Significance of the subvalvular apparatus for left-ventricular dimensions and systolic function: experimental replacement of the mitral valve. J Thorac Cardiovasc Surg 39: 5–12
8. Rushmer R F, Finlayson B L, Nash A M 1956 Movements of the mitral valve. Circ Res 4: 337–342
9. David T E, Burns R F, Bacchus C M, Druck M N 1984 Mitral valve replacement for mitral regurgitation with and without preservation of the chordae tendinae. J Thorac Cardiovasc Surg 88: 718–725
10. Carpentier A 1984 Valve reconstruction in predominant mitral valve incompetence. In: Duran C (ed) Recent progress in mitral valve disease. Butterworths & Co (Publishers) Ltd, London, pp 265–274
11. Deloche A, Jebara V A, Relland J Y M *et al* 1990 Valve repair with Carpentier techniques. The second decade. J Thorac Cardiovasc Surg 99: 990–1002
12. Carpentier A 1983 Cardiac valve surgery – the 'French' correction. J Thorac Cardiovasc Surg 86: 323–337.
13. Antunes M J, Magalhães M P, Colsen P R, Kinsley R H 1987 Valvuloplasty of rheumatic mitral valve disease. J Thorac Cardiovasc Surg 94: 44–56
14. Duran C G, Pomar J L, Revuelta J M *et al* 1980 Conservative operation for mitral insufficiency. J Thorac Cardiovasc Surg 79: 326–337
15. Castro J L, Moon M R, Rayhill S C *et al* 1993 Annuloplasty with flexible or rigid ring does not alter left ventricular systolic performance, energetic or ventricular–arterial coupling in conscious, closed-chest dogs. J Thorac Cardiovasc Surg 105: 643–659
16. Carpentier A 1989 The 'reference point'. Le club Mitrale Newsletter 1–6
17. Mykén P 1995 Long term performance of a porcine heart valve prosthesis. A clinical 10-year follow-up with special reference to survival and function. From Department of Thoracic and Cardiovascular Surgery, Sahlgrenska University Hospital, University of Göteborg, Göteborg, Sweden
18. Lytle B W, Cosgrove D M, Gill C C *et al* 1985 Mitral valve replacement combined with myocardial revascularization: Early and late results for 300 patients, 1970 to 1983. Circulation 71: 1179–1190
19. Cohn L H, Allred E N, Cohn L A *et al* 1985 Early and late risk of mitral valve replacement. J Thorac Cardiovasc Surg 90: 872–881
20. Acar C, Farge A, Ramsheyi A *et al* 1994 Mitral valve replacement using a cryopreserved mitral homograft. Ann Thorac Surg 57: 746–748
21. Yankah A C, Sievers H H, Lange P E, Bernhard A 1995 Clinical report on stentless mitral allografts. J Heart Valve Dis 4: 40–44
22. Vrandecic M, Fantini F A, Gontijo B *et al* 1995 Surgical technique of implanting the stentless porcine mitral valve. Ann Thorac Surg 60: S439–S442
23. Vrandecic M, Gontijo B, Fantini F A *et al* 1992 Anatomically complete heterograft mitral valve substitute: surgical technique and immediate results. J Heart Valve Dis 1: 254–259
24. Kunzelman K S, Cochran R P, Verrier E D, Eberhart R C 1994 Anatomic basis for mitral valve modelling. J Heart Valve Dis 3: 491–496

CHAPTER 5

Hemi-homograft replacement of the mitral valve: a finite element model

K. S. Kunzelman and R. P. Cochran

Mitral valve repair, particularly in the last decade, has become the 'gold standard' for the treatment of mitral valve disease. The advantages as compared to standard prosthetic replacement have been well documented. However, even with the continuing improvements and advancements in mitral repair techniques, a certain subset of patients remain whose valvular lesions present tissue which is unsuitable for repair. The number of patients in this category is significant enough that investigators continue to focus on alternatives that would alleviate the necessity for standard prosthetic replacement. Such alternatives have included the use of autologous pericardium to fashion a bicuspid valve,[1,2] the Quadrileaflet pericardial valve[3] the use of porcine mitral heterografts,[4–7] or the use of full[8–14] or partial[15–17] mitral homografts.

Most of the above alternatives are focused on replacement of the entire native mitral valve. However, the use of partial homografts may be considered the ultimate extension of mitral repair techniques, and partial homograft techniques have been recently described in both animal and clinical studies. The current indications for clinical use are a calcified stenotic valve which cannot be suitably debrided or reconstructed in another fashion, or a valve with acute bacterial endocarditis which is localized and severe enough that standard repair techniques would be unsuccessful.[15–17]

Acar, while working with Carpentier at the Broussais Hospital, solved some of the dilemmas associated with both full and partial replacement. Several different uses of partial homografts have been described, including replacement of an entire half of the valve (anterolateral or posteromedial half). We consider these techniques to be an exciting breakthrough in 'extended' or 'radical' mitral repair techniques. However, from a mechanical engineering point of view, some questions are raised. In particular, we were concerned whether any dysynchrony might occur when combining the relatively normal homograft tissue with the remaining diseased native tissue. To begin addressing what is really a series of complex questions, we initially chose to address a 'hemi-homograft' technique, in which the entire anterolateral half of the valve is replaced. We used this model to evaluate leaflet stresses, coaptation, and chordal stresses, to determine the effect of the interaction of the two tissues.

Methods

We have developed a finite element model of the mitral valve and have previously evaluated normal function,[18] the effects of disease,[19,20] and proposed surgical repair.[21–23] In this study, we used the model to evaluate the technique of hemi-homograft replacement.

Finite element analysis is mathematically based and is performed on a computer, due to the large amount of data processing involved. In a typical analysis, the geometry of the system to be studied is first input into the computer. Secondly, the geometry is divided into small pieces (finite elements) interconnected by nodes. Next, the governing equations which relate force, deformation, strain and stress are derived for each of the finite elements. Finally, given the boundary and loading conditions, the governing equations for all the finite elements are solved simultaneously, providing deformation, strain and stress values across the entire system.

A detailed description of the development of our 'first-generation' three-dimensional finite element mitral valve model[18] as well as geometrical and physiological updates to a 'second-generation' model[20] have been reported previously. The model was created using ANSYS structural analysis software (ANSYS Inc., Houston, PA, USA, Version 4.4A) installed on an AST Premium II personal computer. The geometry was based upon porcine anatomy, chosen because of its similarity to human valve anatomy.[24] All of the structural components of the natural valve were included: the annulus, anterior and posterior leaflets, marginal and basal chordae (including strut chordae), and papillary muscles (Figure 5.1). Since chordal classification varies widely in the literature, for this model, chordal definition was based simply on the level of insertion at the leaflet, consistent with our previous studies. Marginal chordae are defined as those inserting directly into the free edge, and basal chordae are defined as inserting further back towards the annulus. The 'strut' chordae are the two particularly strong and thick chordae stretching from each papillary muscle to the undersurface of the anterior leaflet. (These have been alternately called 'intermediate'[25] or 'principal'[26] chordae.)

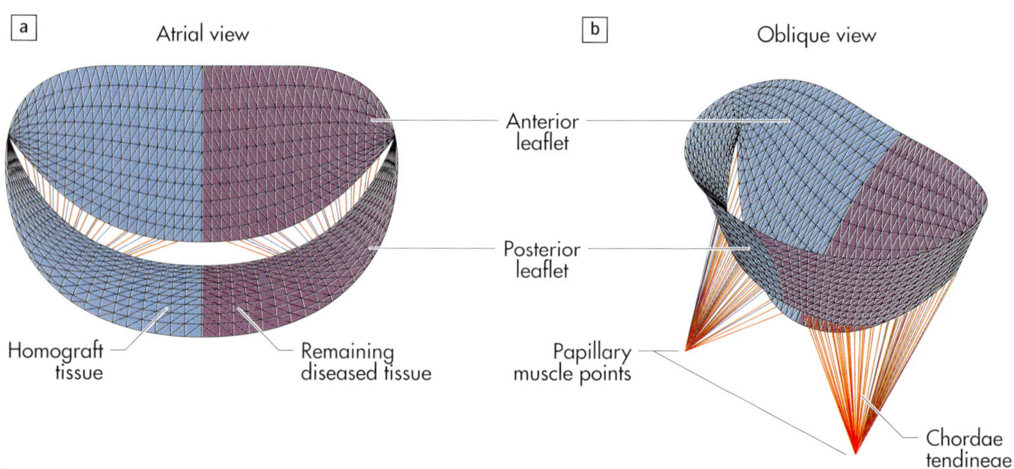

Figure 5.1 Hemi-homograft model geometry. (a) View from atrial side. (b) Oblique view.

Component representation and boundary conditions

The various structural components of the valve were represented by finite elements having the material properties of the physical valve (Table 5.1). Within the leaflet elements, collagen fibres were simulated by defining a direction of greater stiffness corresponding to the known orientation of collagen fibres.[27] Once the elements were defined, several boundary conditions were necessary for the model to properly simulate the physical constraints on the *in situ* valve. First, a hinge condition was defined at the annulus, allowing the leaflet to rotate at the annular nodes. Secondly, the basal and marginal chordae were attached to the leaflet and papillary muscle points, and were free to rotate. Thirdly, the boundary condition between the anterior and posterior leaflets was defined by interface elements, which could translate and rotate with changing leaflet position at the coapting leaflet surfaces.

Table 5.1 Mitral valve physical and material properties of homograft tissue in the finite element model (native tissue values are the same, except thickness of leaflet and chordal tissue was increased by 20%)

	Units	Anterior leaf	Trigone	Posterior leaf	Marginal chordae	Basal chordae	Strut chordae	Gap
t	mm	1.31	1.45	1.26	–	–	–	–
A	mm^2	–	–	–	0.40	0.79	1.15	–
E_x	kPa	6230	6230	2090	40 700	22 100	22 100	–
E_y	kPa	2350	2350	1890	–	–	–	–
ν	–	0.45	0.45	0.45	–	–	–	–
G_{xy}	kPa	1370	1370	690	–	–	–	–
ρ	g/cm	10.4	10.4	10.4	10.4	10.4	10.4	–
K_n	kPa	–	–	–	–	–	–	20 000
μ	g/mm/s	–	–	–	–	–	–	0.0

t, thickness; A, cross-sectional area; E_x, Young's modulus in x direction; E_y, Young's modulus in y direction; ν, Poisson's ratio; G_{xy}, shear modulus; ρ, density; K_n, gap stiffness; μ, friction coefficient.

Modifications in order to simulate hemi-homograft replacement

First, we assumed that in the native tissue, alterations have occurred which necessitate surgical intervention. In this study, we assumed both the leaflet and chordal tissue on the posteromedial half of the valve has become slightly thicker than normal, therefore the thickness of those elements were increased by 20%. We assumed that any changes that occurred on the anterolateral half were more severe and therefore were excised. The diseased tissue elements were then replaced with hemi-homograft elements (refer to Figure 5.1), which have normal tissue thickness and stiffness.

Papillary muscle contraction and annular contraction

In all models, papillary muscle contraction was simulated by progressively moving the papillary muscle nodes a total of 1 mm away from the annular plane in a perpendicular direction. This movement represents a 10% shortening of the papillary muscle.[28–31] Annular contraction was simulated by forces on the posterior annular nodes directed toward the centre of the annulus, perpendicular to the local curvature. The total decrease in posterior annular length was 8%.[18,32,33]

Pressure loading

The loading was intended to simulate the pressure that the valve is exposed to during isovolumic contraction (IVC) and rapid ventricular ejection. These pressures were applied to the ventricular surface of the leaflet elements incrementally, in 186 'load steps' (LS). During pressure loading, the ANSYS finite element software used a non-linear, transient, dynamic solution method (ANSYS method KAN = 4) to solve the finite element governing equations. However, the rate of loading was decreased by three orders of magnitude from actual cardiac rates in order to allow full numeric convergence, effectively making the analysis quasi-static.

Output parameters

During the solution of the model, the output variables (deformation, strain and stress) were recorded at the first load step, and at multiple load steps thereafter. At each of these load steps, both leaflet stress and coaptation were recorded. For stress results, the maximum principal stresses in the leaflets were plotted as colour contours superimposed on the deformed valve. From these plots, locations and values of stress concentrations and peak stress areas were identified. The extent and symmetry of coaptation was also observed in these plots. Finally, axial stresses in the chordae were examined.

Results

Leaflet stresses and coaptation

At early IVC, the stress levels were very low for both the anterior and posterior leaflet (Figure 5.2). Even at this early stage, the posterior leaflet was beginning to undergo compression, and the distribution of these stresses was slightly asymmetrical. At end IVC, this asymmetry was even more pronounced. The stress levels in the native tissue were slightly lower than in the homograft tissue, reflective of the increased thickness. As a secondary result of the increased thickness, the mobility of the leaflet is restricted, and the prominent 'folding' or 'natural redundancy' of the posterior leaflet is not seen in the native tissue, as compared to the homograft, and coaptation is significantly reduced in the native tissue. This is even more evident at peak loading, where the restricted motion prevents coaptation. The result is to prevent stress sharing between the leaflets, resulting in an increased stress concentration at the posteromedial commissure.

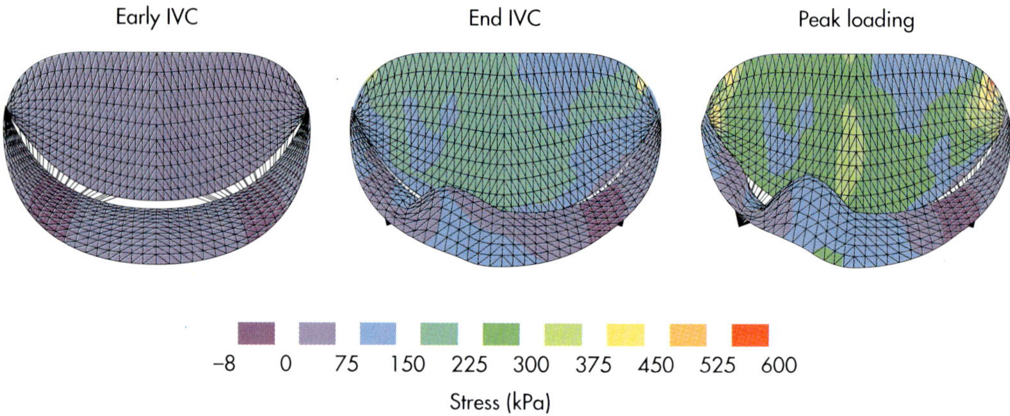

Figure 5.2 Maximum principal leaflet stress contours at peak ventricular pressure. The colour contours represent the stress values in kPa. Note the asymmetrical stress distribution and gap evident near the posteromedial commissure, allowing regurgitation.

Chordal stresses

These stress differences between the homograft (anterolateral) and native (posteromedial) halves of the valves are transmitted through the chordae, and the results are complementary. At the same three time points (early IVC, end IVC and peak loading), the stress in both the anterior marginal and anterior basal chords is reduced in most of the native chords, except those just at the commissure (Figure 5.3). The results are even more striking in the posterior marginal and posterior basal chords, where again the stress levels were slightly lower in most of the native chords, but greatly increased at the commissure (Figure 5.4).

Discussion

In our hemi-homograft model, the 20% difference in thickness between the remaining diseased native tissue versus the normal homograft tissue resulted in very noticeable changes in the system. First, the stress distribution in the repaired valve structure is no longer symmetrical about the midline. This is due to the difference in thickness between the remaining diseased tissue and the new homograft tissue. An increase in thickness under the same applied pressure will, by definition, reduce the calculated stress. However, as a result of these tissue differences, the amount of coaptation also differs between the two halves of the repaired valve. Coaptation is returned near to

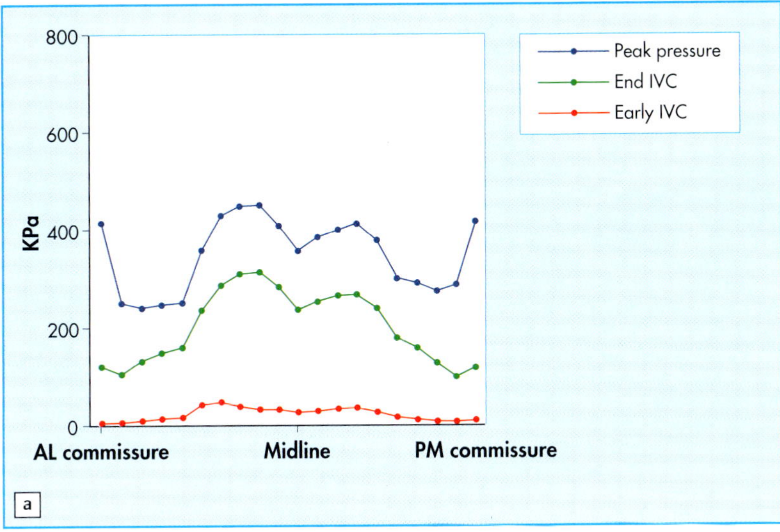

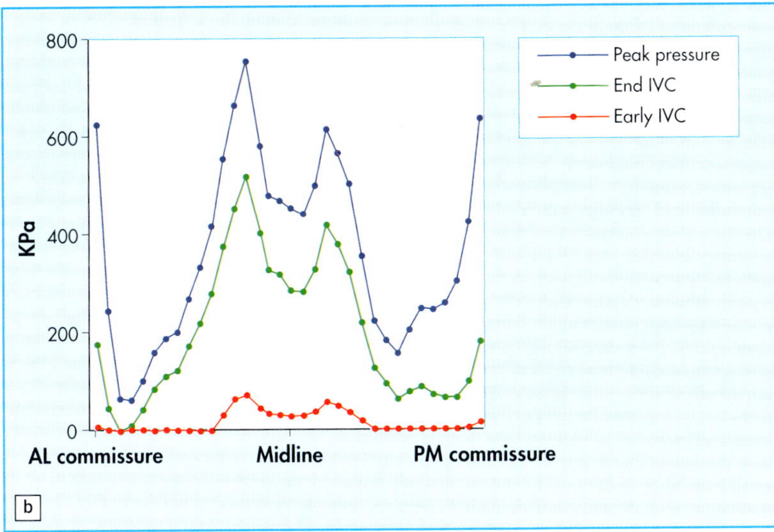

Figure 5.3 Chordal stresses at peak ventricular pressure: (a) anterior basal chordae; (b) anterior marginal chordae.

normal by the hemi-homograft tissue, but remains reduced in the thicker native tissue. Finally, due to this reduction in coaptation, the amount of stress that is normally shared between the leaflets by means of mutual support is now transferred to some of the chordae instead. This increase in chordal stress is located at a potentially vulnerable area of the valve, which is the commissure.

Conclusions

Although this is just the first of several studies we have planned regarding full and partial homograft replacement, there are a few conclusions that we can draw from this one study. Firstly, it would seem that partial replacement is ideal for acute bacterial endocarditis. As the remaining tissue is relatively unaffected by the disease process, the tissue should have near-normal properties, and thus be mechanically compatible with the homograft tissue. Secondly, other indications should consider the degree of tissue alteration that has taken place. By this study, we have shown that even a relatively minor degree of tissue alteration (20% increase in thickness) did have significant effects in terms of coaptation, as well as leaflet and chordal stress.

One caveat that this study points out is that annuloplasty becomes critical in partial replacement techniques. An annuloplasty ring is not presently included in the reported

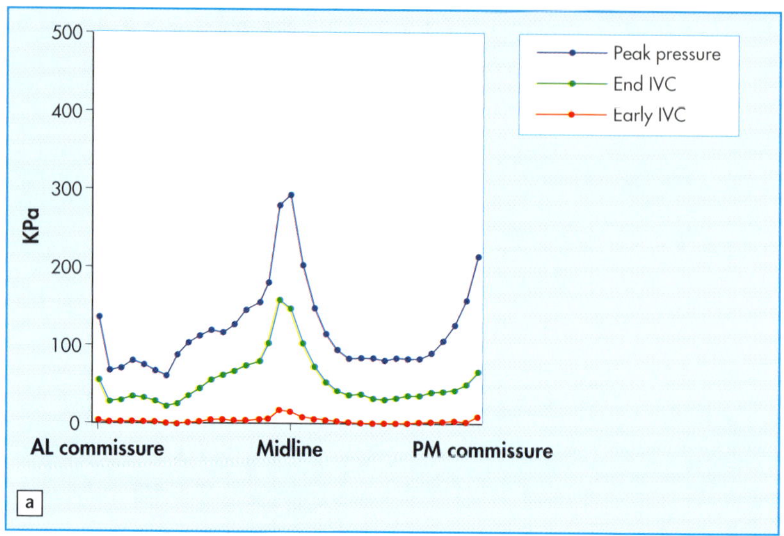

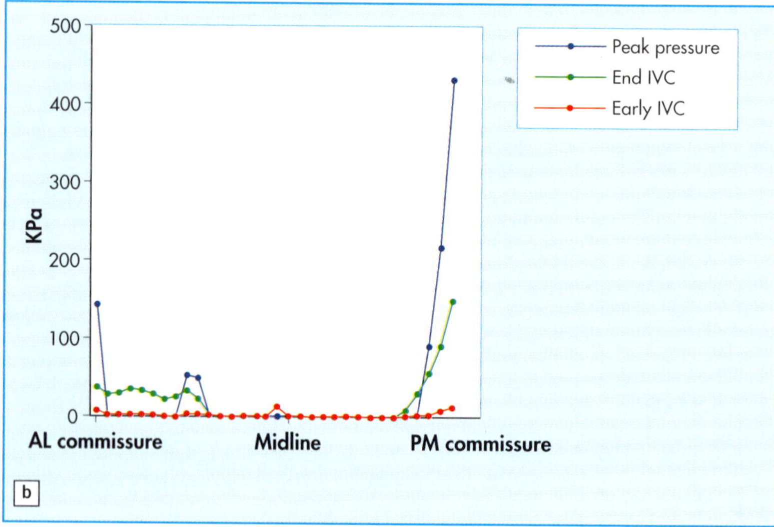

Figure 5.4
Chordal stresses at peak ventricular pressure: (a) posterior basal chordae; (b) posterior marginal chordae.

model, but is generally undertaken clinically with partial homograft replacement. It would seem that it is necessary to compensate for tissue changes, in order to re-establish coaptation. However, even annuloplasty is unlikely to be able to compensate for severe tissue changes, and greater alterations may obligate total homograft replacement. This must be remembered when undertaking repair of diseased valves and partial replacement with 'normal' homograft tissue. It is crucial in repairing or partially replacing thickened tissue that normal geometry and physiology be restored.

References

1. Deac R F, Simonescu D, Deac D 1995 New evolution in mitral physiology and surgery: mitral stentless pericardial valve. Ann Thorac Surg 60: S433–S438
2. Mickleborough L L, Ovil Y, Wilson G J *et al* 1989 A simplified concept for a bileaflet atrioventricular valve that maintains annular–papillary muscle continuity. J Card Surg 4: 58–68
3. Sussman M, Middlemost S, Frater R W, Barlow J 1997 The Quadrileaflet Mitral Valve (QMV): the start of the pilot trial. In: Huijsmans H, David T E, Westaby S (eds) Stentless bioprostheses. 2nd edn. Isis Medical Media Ltd, Oxford, UK pp 34–39
4. Vrandecic M, Gontijo BF, Fantini FA *et al* 1994 Porcine stentless mitral valve heart substitute: short term clinical data. J Cardiovasc Surg Torino 35: 41–45

5. Vrandecic M, Gontijo B F, Fantini F A *et al* 1992 Anatomically complete heterograft mitral valve substitute: surgical technique and immediate results. J Heart Valve Disease 1: 254–259
6. Morea M, DePaulis R, Galloni M, Gastaldi L, diSumma M 1994 Mitral valve replacement with the Biocor stentless mitral valve: early results. J Heart Valve Dis 3: 476–482
7. Vrandecic M O, Fantini F A, Gontijo B F *et al* 1995 Surgical technique of implanting stentless porcine mitral valve. Ann Thorac Surg 60: S349–S352
8. Cachera J P, Salvatore L, Hermant J, Herbinet B 1964 Reconstructions plastiques de l'appareil mitral chez le chien au moyen de valves mitrale homologues conservées. Ann Chir Thorac Cardiovasc 3: 459–474
9. Rastelli G C, Berghuis J, Swan H J C 1965 Evaluation of function of mitral valve after homotransplantation in the dog. J Thorac Cardiovasc Surg 49: 459–474
10. Vliet P D, Titus J L, Berghuis J *et al* 1965 Morphologic features of homotransplanted canine mitral valves. J Thorac Cardiovasc Surg 49: 504–510
11. Acar C, Farge A, Ramsheyi A *et al* 1994 Mitral valve replacement using a cryopreserved mitral homograft. Ann Thorac Surg 57: 746–748
12. Acar C, Gaer J, Chauvaud S, Carpentier A 1995 Technique of homograft replacement of the mitral valve. J Heart Valve Dis 4: 31–34
13. Acar C, Tolan M, Berrebi A *et al* 1996 Homograft replacement of the mitral valve. Graft selection, technique of implantation, and results in forty-three patients. J Thorac Cardiovasc Surg 111: 367–378
14. Revuelta J M, Bernal J M, Rabasa J M 1996 Transvalvular technique for implantation of a mitral valve homograft. J Thorac Cardiovasc Surg 111: 281–282
15. Revuelta J M, Cagigas J C, Bernal J M, Val F, Rabasa J M, Lequerica M A 1992 Partial replacement of mitral valve by homograft. An experimental study. J Thorac Cardiovasc Surg 104: 1274–1279
16. Revuelta J M, Bernal J M, Rabasa J M 1994 Partial homograft replacement of mitral valve. Lancet 344: 514
17. Acar C, Berrebi A, Tolan M, Chachqu'es J C 1995 Partial mitral homograft: a new technique for mitral valve repair. J Heart Valve Dis 4: 665–667
18. Kunzelman K S, Cochran R P, Chuong C, Ring W S, Verrier E D, Eberhart R D 1993 Finite element analysis of the mitral valve. J Heart Valve Dis 2: 326–340
19. Kunzelman K S, Cochran R P, Verrier E D, Chuong C J, Ring W S, Eberhart RC 1993 Finite element analysis of mitral valve pathology. J Long Term Effects Med Impl 3: 161–179
20. Kunzelman K S, Reimink M S, Cochran R P 1997 Annular dilatation increases stress in the mitral valve and delays coaptation: a finite element computer model. J Cardiovasc Surg 5: 427–434
21. Kunzelman K S, Reimink M S, Verrier E D, Cochran R P 1996 Replacement of mitral valve posterior chordae tendineae with expanded polytetrafluoroethylene suture: a finite element study. J Card Surg 11: 136–145
22. Reimink M S, Kunzelman K S, Verrier E D, Cochran R P 1995 The effect of anterior chordal replacement on mitral valve function and stresses. A finite element study. ASAIO J 41: M754–M762
23. Reimink M S, Kunzelman K S, Cochran RP 1996 The effect of chordal replacement suture length on function and stresses in repaired mitral valves: a finite element study. J Heart Valve Dis 5: 365–375
24. Kunzelman K S, Cochran R P, Verrier E D, Eberhart R C 1994 Anatomic basis for mitral valve modeling. J Heart Valve Dis 3: 491–496
25. van Rijk Zwikker G L, Delemarre B J, Huysmans H A 1994 Mitral valve anatomy and morphology: relevance to mitral valve replacement and valve reconstruction. J Card Surg 9: 255–261
26. Acar D, Deloche A 1985 Anatomie et physiologie des valves mitrales et tricuspides. In: Acar J (ed) Cardiopathies valvulaires acquises. Flammarion, Paris; pp 3–20
27. Kunzelman K S, Cochran R P, Murphree S S, Ring W S, Verrier E D, Eberhart R C 1993 Differential collagen distribution in the mitral valve and its influence on biomechanical behaviour. J Heart Valve Dis 2: 236–244
28. Burch G E, DePasquale N P 1965 Time course of tension in papillary muscles of the heart. JAMA 192: 701–704
29. Grimm A F, Lendrum B O, Lin H L 1975 Papillary muscle shortening in the intact dog; a cineradiographic study of tranquilized dogs in the upright position. Circ Res 36: 49–57
30. Hirakawa S, Sasayama S, Tomoike H *et al* 1977 In situ measurement of papillary muscle dynamics in the dog left ventricle. Am J Physiol 233: H384–H391
31. Huntsman L L, Day S R, Stewart D K 1977 Nonuniform contraction in the isolated cat papillary muscle. Am J Physiol 233: H613–H616

32. Glasson J R, Komeda M K, Daughters G T *et al* 1996 Three-dimensional regional dynamics of the normal mitral annulus during left ventricular ejection. J Thorac Cardiovasc Surg 111: 574–585

33. Gorman R C, McCaughan J S, Ratcliffe M B *et al* 1995 Pathogenesis of acute ischemic mitral regurgitation in three dimensions. J Thorac Cardiovasc Surg 109: 684–693

CHAPTER 6

The Quadrileaflet Mitral Valve: the start of the pilot trial

M. Sussman, S. Middlemost, J. Barlow and R. W. M. Frater

The Quadrileaflet Mitral Valve (QMV) is a stentless chordally supported mitral bioprosthesis with a post-aldehyde tanning treatment that retards calcification and encourages spontaneous host endothelial coverage. By virtue of its chordal support it automatically re-establishes annular–papillary connection. The design and its validation have been described previously.[1–4]

The premises of the design were several:

1. Aldehyde tanning effectively minimizes the antigenicity of xenograft collagen-based tissues; however, residual unbound aldehydes are associated with a marked tendency to calcification and a level of bioincompatibility that inhibits endothelial growth.
2. The earlier xenograft tissues are tanned after harvesting; the lower the bioburden, the less the autodigestion, the greater the breaking strength and the less the tendency to calcification after implantation.
3. Mounting biological tissues on stents results in increased flexion stresses as well as increased stresses in parts of the closed valve.
4. Each natural valve has the variability of a fingerprint and matching irregular anatomy to irregular anatomy makes harvested xenograft or homograft valves difficult to use.
5. The natural valve is susceptible to quite modest changes in ventricular dimension: an artificial valve needs to be less susceptible to such changes than the natural valve, should fit the wide variety of annular–papillary distances encountered in patients with pathological mitral valves, and should stay competent with the shrinkage of left ventricular dimensions that accompanies the correction of insufficiency.
6. The natural leaflet tissue has measurable breaking strength and strain properties, collagen fibres that run between annulus and papillary muscle, and a covering of endothelium that probably provides natural resistance to thromboembolism, infection and calcification; the ideal replacement device would mimic these features.
7. It is essential that the valve be easy to insert, with consistent results.
8. Finally, the cost of making the valve should be as low as possible since the majority of patients around the world who need mitral valve replacement are poor.

The Quadrileaflet valve

These design requirements were met by making a valve of bovine pericardium with one large anterior leaflet and a posterior leaflet consisting of three scallops. In closure the three posterior scallops meet one another and the anterior leaflet. The leaflets open and close without folds or crimps and move through no more that 30° between systole and diastole. The chordal support is brought together into left and right papillary flaps which are stitched to the invariably substantial *anterior* parts of the papillary muscles on each side. The depth of the papillary holding sutures is varied so that the valve, after insertion, is in a natural resting position that ensures competence. The length of the leaflets is such that they stay competent over a wide range of depths of insertion: in fact, the papillary attachment to annular distance may be varied over 1.5 cm without incurring incompetence. This feature removes completely the problem of normal variability in papillary anatomy and the potential for postoperative changes in ventricular dimension and papillary position to interfere with late function. The valve is stentless and made entirely of pericardium. Its parts are aligned with sutures which are not load bearing. The ring is strong enough to act as an annuloplasty device.

The material is bovine pericardium selected for strength, thickness, flexibility and fibre direction. The strength requirement is significantly in excess of the strength of the natural mitral valve. The fibre direction imitates the papillary muscle to annulus direction of fibres found in the natural valve. The thickness and flexibility requirements produce the properties that aid haemodynamic performance. The tanning of the pericardium starts at the abattoir to minimize bacterial growth and autodigestion. The tanning produces stable collagen cross-linking and reduces antigenicity. The tendency to calcification is handled by 'capping' the residual aldehydes with a polyol treatment. The effectiveness of this treatment has been tested in subcutaneous implants in weanling rats and whole-valve implants in weanling sheep. In addition to the anticalcification effect, the polyol treatment removes all residual antigenicity, and allows spontaneous endothelial growth on the surface of the implanted tissue in aortic patches in dogs, arterial grafts in baboons, the atrial wall in weanling sheep and whole stentless mitral valves in weanling sheep.[5]

Pilot trial

A pilot trial was started to determine:

1. the ease of insertion;
2. the usefulness of the insertion tools;
3. the obstruction to forward flow and the susceptibility to incompetence;
4. the occurrence of unforeseen problems.

Material

Five patients have had insertion of the QMV. Their clinical features are shown in Table 6.1.

Operative methods

Operations were conducted at mild hypothermia with cold crystalloid cardioplegic arrest. The valve was approached via the interatrial groove. It was excised using a

Table 6.1 QMV pilot: clinical features

Sex/age	F30	F23	F48	F36	F55
NYHA class	IV	III	III	III	III
Lesion	MS/MI	MS/MI	MS/MI	MS/MI	MS/MI
Prior Rx	Med	Balloon	MV surg	MV surg	Att. rep.
Rhythm	Sinus	Sinus	Sinus	AF	Sinus

Abbreviations: MS/MI, mixed mitral stenosis and mitral insufficiency; Med, medical treatment (Rx); MV surg, previous mitral valve surgery; Att. rep., attempted repair which, at the same operation, was converted to valve replacement.

straight cut across the base of the anterior leaflet, and leaving a short tag of the main chorda on each side to help expose the papillary muscles. The choice of small, medium or large valve was made by finding the Sizer/Suture Guide that best fitted the intertrigonal distance. Notches on the Sizer/Suture Guide show where the sutures are to be placed at the trigones, and in the middle and on each side the posterior or mural annulus. Two pledgetted mattress sutures are placed side by side, from posterior to anterior through the main anterior part of each papillary muscle. These sutures are placed below the tips of the muscles. The distance from the annulus to the point of emergence of the suture from the anterior surface of the papillary muscle is measured using the Chordal Depth Gauge. Knowing this distance, there is a corresponding place on the papillary flap where the suture must be placed to maintain the valve in a neutral closed form. The range of distance from the sewing ring that is available on each papillary flap is 25–35 mm for the small size, 30–40 mm for the medium size, and 35–40 mm for the large size. In fact, the valve will stay competent over a range of depths of 1.5 cm around the resting neutral position. After the papillary sutures are tied down, the annular sutures are then placed in the sewing ring using guiding grooves in the removable valve holder that correspond to the grooves in the Sizer/Suture Guide.

The annular attachment is completed by running the sutures to one another (Figures 6.1 and 6.2).

Results

The sizes of valves used, the early clinical NYHA class and the echocardiographic results are shown in Table 6.2. Two patients restudied at 3 months had maintained their early status. Table 6.3 shows three patients with three+ regurgitation preoperatively, whose ventricular dimensions shrank postoperatively without the development of insufficiency. Note that the designation +/– for mitral regurgitation is

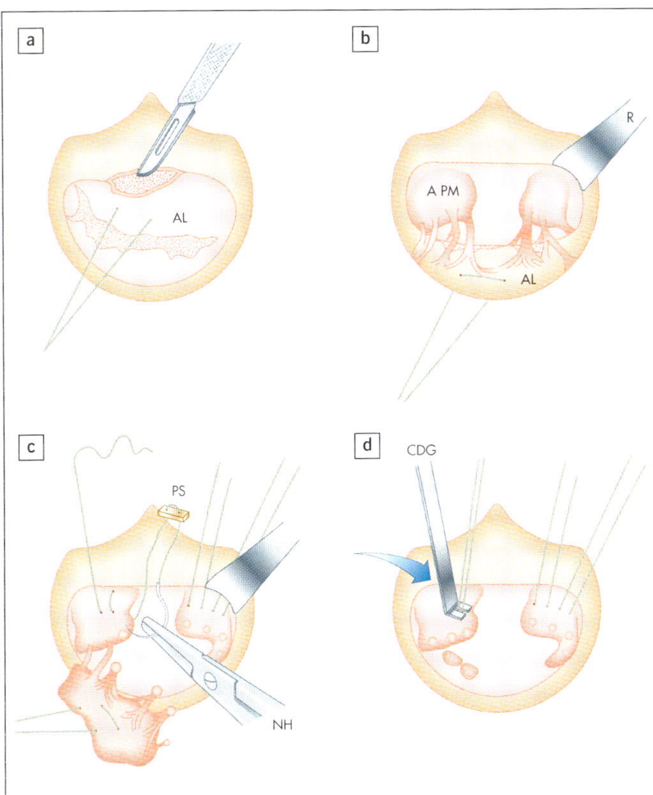

Figure 6.1 (a) The anterior leaflet is incised in a straight line from trigone to trigone. The incision is continued around the posterior leaflet. AL, anterior leaflet. (b) With the valve completely detached from the annulus it is retracted backwards, putting the chordae and papillary muscles on tension. AL, ventricular surface of the anterior leaflet; APM, anterior papillary muscle; R, retractor exposing the posterior papillary muscle. (c) The posterior papillary muscle has had two papillary sutures inserted from posterior to anterior in the anterior half of the posterior papillary muscle. Maintaining tension on the chordae still attached to the anterior papillary muscle, another pledgetted papillary suture (PS) is inserted from posterior to anterior in the anterior half of the anterior papillary muscle. NH, needle holder. (d) The Chordal Depth Gauge (CDG) has been slid down to the point where a papillary suture comes through the papillary muscle and the distance from there to the annulus is being measured (arrow).

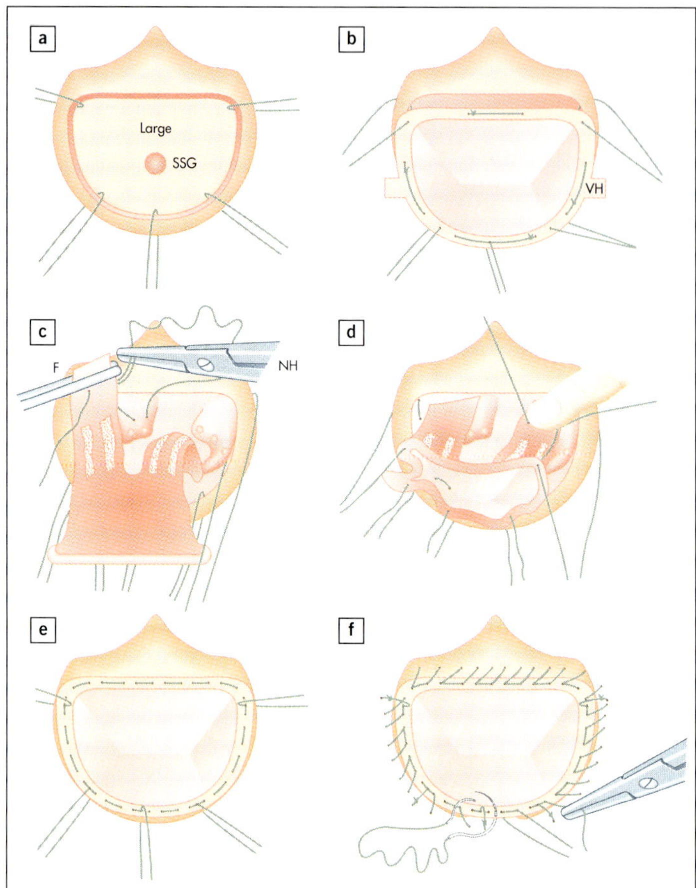

Figure 6.2 (a) The Sizer/Suture Guide (SSG) is in the orifice. Annular sutures have been placed in the annulus following the guide marks. (b) The QMV still with its holder (VH) attached is brought into the field and the annular sutures are placed in the sewing ring following the guide notches in the holder. (c) A forceps (F) holds one papillary flap so that a papillary suture can be passed through it at the mark that is correct for the depth previously measured (NH = needle holder). (d) The two anterior papillary sutures have been tied. A posterior papillary suture is being tied. (e) The sewing ring and annulus have been brought in contact. (f) The sewing ring and annulus are being sutured together.

used to describe the very small puff of regurgitation often seen in natural valves, stented three-leaflet biological valves, and this valve, during the process of leaflet opposition. This is the obligatory regurgitant volume that is needed to close any valve.

There were no technical difficulties with the operations. Reoperations after failed repairs did not present a problem of exposure.

First impressions were:

1. Insertion is not difficult.
2. The insertion tools help.
3. Three sizes are so far adequate.
4. Haemodynamics are satisfactory.

Table 6.2 QMV pilot: valve sizes, NYHA classes and echocardiographic results

	F30	F23	F48	F36	F55
Size	M	S	M	M	L
NYHA class (1 week)	I	I	I	I	I
EOA (cont. eq.)	2.9	3.5	2.8	2.26	2.0
MR	+	0	+	+/–	+/–
3 Month	I	I			
	2.8	4.1			
	+	0			

Abbreviations: EOA (cont. eq.), effective orifice area (continuity equation); MR, mitral regurgitation; M, medium; S, small; L, large.

Table 6.3 QMV pilot: regurgitation data

	F23	F36	F55
Preop MR	+++	+++	+++
LVEDD	5.1	5.4	5.2
LVESD	3.2	3.3	3.8
Postop MR	0	+/–	+/–
LVEDD	4.7	4.7	3.7
LVESD	2.7	3.8	3.0

Abbreviations: MR, mitral regurgitation; LVEDD, left ventricular end-diastolic dimension; LVESD, left ventricular end-systolic dimension.

Acknowledgement

The Quadrileaflet Mitral Valve is made by Glycar Pty Ltd, of Irene, South Africa, a company in which Dr Frater has an interest.

References

1. Frater R W M, Liao K, Selfter E 1994 Stentless chordally supported mitral bioprosthetic valve. In: Gabbay S, Frater R W M (eds) New horizons and the future of heart valve bioprostheses. Silent Partners Inc., Austin, TX, USA, pp 103–116
2. Frater R W M, Liao K, Wasserman F 1993 In vitro hemodynamics and durability of stentless chordally supported quadrileaflet mitral bioprosthesis. In: The Proceedings of the Cardiovascular Science and Technology Conference, AAMI and the National Heart Lung and Blood Institute, Washington DC, p 91
3. Frater R W M, Liao K, Hoffman D, Gancfhi D, Nguyen K, Gong G 1993 Stentless, chordally supported quadricusp mitral bioprosthesis. Poster Presentation, 29th Annual Meeting of the Society of Thoracic Surgeons, San Antonio, Texas
4. Liao K, Wu J-J, Frater R W M 1993 Intraoperative echo/Doppler evaluation of stentless chordally supported mitral valve prosthesis. Proceedings ASAIO, Vol. 39, p 28
5. Frater R W M, Scifter E, Liao K, Wasserman F 1997 Anticalcification, proendothelial, and antiinflammatory effect of post aldehyde polyol Rx of bioprosthetic material. In: Gabbay S, Wheatley D J (eds) Advances in anticalcific and antidegenerative treatment of heart valve bioprostheses. Silent Partners Inc., Austin, TX, USA, pp. 105–114

III Clinical Outcomes (I)

CHAPTER 7

Aortic valve replacement with the stentless bovine pericardial valve: early experience with the Sorin valve

J. E. Rubay, G. El Khoury and M. Buche

Since the first valve replacement by Starr and Edwards[1] and Harken *et al.* [2] in 1960, none of the currently available prosthetic heart valves approaches the normal human valve in terms of haemodynamic function or freedom from valve-related complications. Mechanical valves are thrombogenic and long-term anticoagulation is associated with the risk of bleeding. Structural degeneration of the xenograft valves limits their durability.

Simultaneous with the advances made in the design of prosthetic valves, good long-term function and lack of major valve-related morbidity of 'freehand' aortic allografts in the subcoronary position have been reported[3,4] and their superiority over stented aortic allografts has been demonstrated.[5] An important limitation of this type of valve is their limited availability.

The stent and the sewing ring of stented xenografts cause some degree of obstruction to blood flow, thereby impairing the haemodynamic performance of the valve. Fatigue tests suggest that the best stent for a valve is the native aortic root.[6] The lack of a sewing ring and the use of the aortic wall as a natural stent should improve durability.

Finally, there is a renewed interest in pericardial xenografts.[7] We have reviewed our early experience with the Sorin bovine pericardial stentless valve.

Materials and methods

The valve (Figure 7.1) is manufactured by Sorin Biomedica, Saluggia, Italy. It is made of two separate sheets of glutaraldehyde-treated bovine pericardium. The first sheet is shaped to form the three leaflets by means of a process of atraumatic tissue fixation without the use of moulds (Figure 7.2). It is then sutured to the second sheet using a pyrolite carbon-coated suture. The suture line is especially designed to dampen the mechanical stress at the level of the commissures. This valve is not designed for intraluminal cylinder or root replacement.

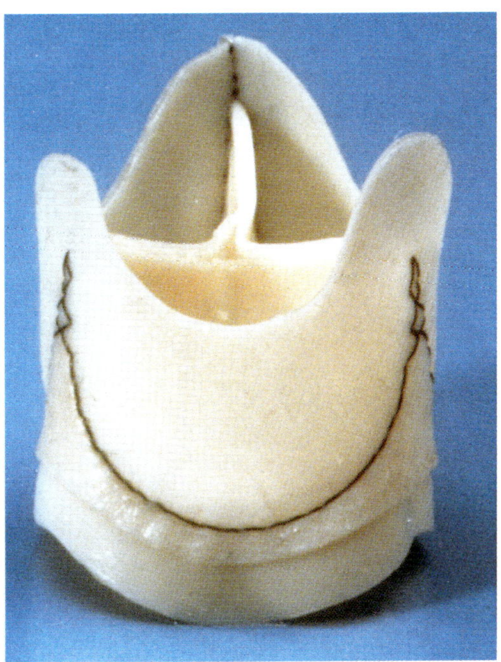

Figure 7.1 The stentless bovine pericardial valve.

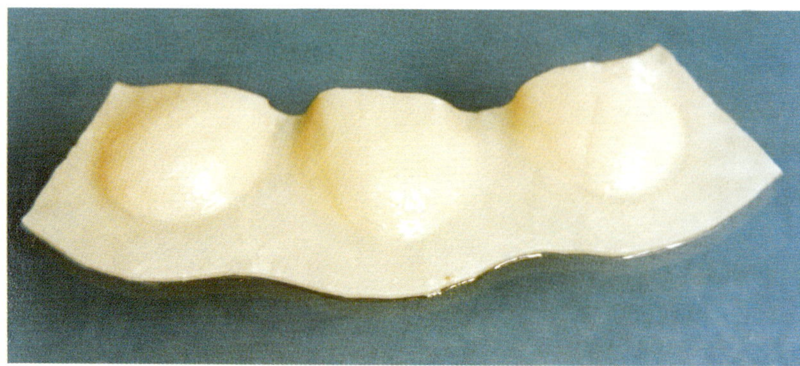

Figure 7.2 The first sheet of pericardium is shaped to form the three leaflets by an atraumatic process of fixation.

Patients

Thirty-seven consecutive patients have been operated upon for aortic valve replacement in our institution between March 1992 and November 1996. Ages ranged between 64 and 75 years (mean 71 years). There were 17 male and 20 female patients. Aortic stenosis was the main reason for operation in 35 patients. Two patients had aortic incompetence. At surgery, 37 stentless valves were implanted with a technique similar to that used for allografts in the subcoronary position. The diameter of the xenograft valves ranged between 21 and 29 mm (mean 25 mm). The patient's aortic wall was exposed by a longitudinal incision ending at the upper level of the commissures (sinotubular level) in the non-coronary sinus. The lower suture line was performed in a horizontal plane using interrupted 3/0 braided material for the majority of the patients, the valve being inverted into the left ventricular cavity. The three commissures were suspended above the level of the native commissures and the second layer was anastomosed with continuous 4/0 polypropylene suture (Figure 7.3). Tailoring the external layer of the xenograft to match with the coronary ostia is possible (Figure 7.4) but not mandatory. All patients had perioperative transoesophageal echocardiography.

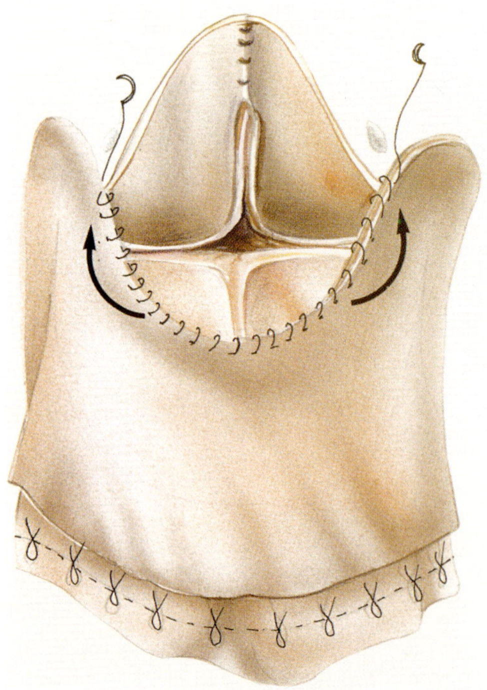

Figure 7.3 The valve is secured at annular level by interrupted sutures and in a subcoronary position by continuous sutures.

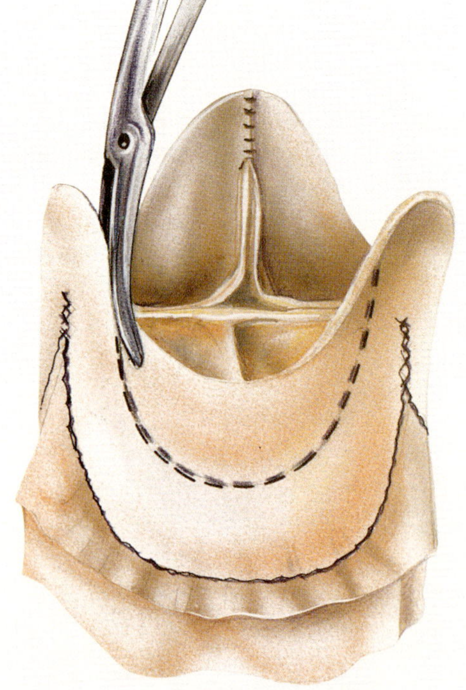

Figure 7.4 The external pericardial layer is tailored to match the coronary ostia.

All patients had postoperative transthoracic echocardiography using continuous waveform and colour-flow Doppler on a regular schedule at 1 week, 1 month, 3 months, 6 months and every year thereafter.

Aortic incompetence was classified as 0 (absent), grade 1 (trivial), grade 2 (mild), grade 3 (moderate) and grade 4 (severe).

Results

There were no early deaths. The aortic cross-clamp time ranged from 78 min to 129 min (mean 105 min). Peroperative transoesophageal echocardiography was normal in all but six patients. Four patients had trivial incompetence and two patients had grade 1–2 incompetence. One patient had a grade 3 mitral incompetence. He was known to have preoperative moderate mitral insufficiency and it may have been worsened by temporary dysfunction of one papillary muscle. He had a concomitant mitral valve replacement with a mechanical valve.

One patient had his xenograft valve taken down at surgery. He developed delayed ECG changes in the right coronary territory which were believed but not demonstrated to be due to valve dysfunction. The valve was replaced by a mechanical prosthesis; the xenograft valve, however, seemed to be normal. Thirty-six patients were followed up from 5 months to 60 months (mean 37 months). There were four late deaths. One was due to lung cancer, 18 months after surgery, and another one to bleeding from oesophageal varices. Two deaths were from cardiac causes: one from cardiac failure and one from endocarditis 3 months after surgery.

All but two patients are in functional class I of the NYHA. There was one thromboembolic event, in a 70-year-old female patient who developed a transient ischaemic attack with left hemiparesis 4 months after surgery. None of the surviving patients had to be reoperated. At later echocardiographic studies (Figure 7.5) average peak systolic gradient was 22.7 ± 9 mmHg and the mean gradient was 12 ± 5.5 mmHg. Aortic incompetence was absent in 25 patients. Four patients had trivial and three patients had mild incompetence.

Discussion

After promising experimental results using a stentless porcine valve in sheep,[8] David and colleagues started a clinical trial[9] (with excellent results) many years after the pioneering experiences of Binet[10] and O'Brien.[11]

The concept of the stentless valve is similar to that of the aortic allograft but does not have its limited availability. Moreover, the two are complementary as stentless xenografts

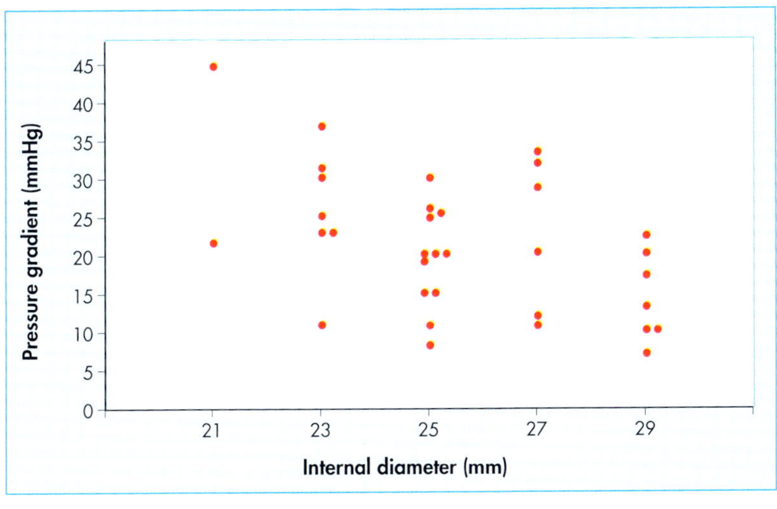

Figure 7.5 Transvalvular peak systolic pressure gradients related to the internal diameter of the pericardial xenograft.

are dedicated to the end of the age spectrum, whereas allografts and auto-grafts target young patients and paedi-atric age groups.

The superiority of pericardial valves has been established haemodynamically[12] as well as for their long-term low rate of valve-related events.[7,12]

The Sorin valve is made of two sheets of glutaraldehyde-treated bovine pericardium. As no additional foreign material is added, in particular no Dacron is used to reinforce the valve, it can be considered as the only true stentless valve available. The shape of the valve is designed in such a way that only subcoronary implantation is allowed. Even if this results in a more difficult procedure than inserting a stented valve or a cylinder, it will obviously avoid the risk of calcification of the sinus walls when xenografts are implanted as an intraluminal cylinder.

Eliminating any rigid component will result in improved haemodynamic performance[13] and may contribute to longer durability by lowering mechanical stresses, known to be an important determinant in xenograft valve failure.[14]

Clinical experience with aortic valve allografts[3–5] has supported the concept of the native aortic root as the ideal stent for an aortic valve.[9] Dilatation of the aortic annulus and calcification or dilatation of the ascending aorta are contraindications for use of the Sorin valve.

Even though there is increasing evidence of the superiority of cylinder or root implantation for allografts,[15] a perfectly aligned and resuspended subcoronary xenograft valve might offer similar results in terms of aortic competence and do away with the risk of degeneration of the prosthetic sinuses and potential narrowing of the reimplanted coronary ostia by growing calcifications. When compared to the former techniques, according to David,[9] we believe that, as with aortic allografts, there is a learning curve. At the time of surgery, six of our patients had evidence of trivial or mild incompetence reflecting inappropriate coaptation of the leaflets due to incorrect alignment of the commissures or inadequate tissue to cover the aortic orifice. We support David's recommendation that oversizing the xenograft will usually correct this problem. Our early results suggest that the valve may be implanted safely with good early clinical results. The long-term morbidity should be comparable to that of aortic allografts.[3–5] Further investigations are needed to confirm these promising results.

References

1. Starr A, Edwards M L 1961 Mitral replacement. Clinical experience with ball-valve prosthesis. Ann Surg 154: 726–740
2. Harken D E, Soroff H S, Taylor W *et al* 1960 Partial and complete prostheses in aortic insufficiency. J Thorac Cardiovasc Surg 40: 744–762
3. O'Brien M F, McGiffin D, Stafford E G *et al* 1991 Allograft aortic valve replacement. Analysis of the viable cryopreserved and antibiotic 4°C stored valves. J Card Surg 6(Suppl): 534–543
4. Kirklin J K, Smith D, Novick W *et al* 1993 Long term function of cryopreserved aortic homografts. A ten year study. J Thorac Cardiovasc Surg 106: 154–166
5. Angell W W, Angell J D, Oury J H *et al* 1987 Long term follow-up of viable frozen aortic homografts. A viable homograft bank. J Thorac Cardiovasc Surg 93: 815–822
6. Drury P J, Dobrin J, Bodnar E *et al* 1986 Distribution of flexibility in the porcine aortic root and in cardiac support frames. In: Bodnar E, Yacoub M (eds) Biological bioprosthetic valves. Yorke Medical Books, New York, p 580
7. Aupart M, Neville P, Dreyfus X *et al* 1994 The Carpentier–Edwards pericardial aortic valve: intermediate results in 420 patients. Eur J Cardiothorac Surg 8: 277–280
8. David T E, Ropchan G C, Butany J W 1988 Aortic valve replacement with stentless porcine bioprostheses. J Card Surg 3: 501–505
9. David T E, Pollick C, Bos J 1990 Aortic valve replacement with stentless porcine aortic bioprosthesis. J Thorac Cardiovasc Surg 99: 113–118
10. Binet J P, Duran C G, Carpentier A, Langlois J 1965 Heterologous aortic valve transplantation. Lancet 2: 1275

11. O'Brien M F, Clareborough J K 1967 Heterograft aortic valve replacement . Lancet 7: 929–930
12. Cosgrove D M, Lyte B W, Gill C C *et al* 1985 In vivo hemodynamic comparison of porcine and pericardial valves. J Thorac Cardiovasc Surg 89: 358–368
13. Thubrikar M J, Skinner J R, Aouad J, Finkelmeir B, Nolan S P 1982 Analysis of the design and dynamics of aortic valvular prosthesis in vivo. J Thorac Cardiovasc Surg 84: 282–290
14. Thubrikar M, Deck J D, Aouad J, Nolan S P 1983 Role of mechanical stress in calcification of aortic bioprosthetic valves. J Thorac Cardiovasc Surg 86: 115–126
15. Knott-Craig C J, Elkins R C, Stelzer P L *et al* 1994 Homograft replacement of the aortic valve and root as a functional unit. Ann Thorac Surg 57: 1501–1506

CHAPTER 8

Clinical results with the use of the SJM Biocor stentless aortic valve at 7 years

M. P. Vrandecic, B. Gontijo, F. A. Fantini, O. C. de Oliveira, I. C. Martins Jr, M. Hermeto, J. T. Barbosa, J. A. de Paula e Silva, M. F. de Castro, E. Vrandecic and E. Vrandecic

In the normal aortic valve, resulting blood flow eddies promote proper valve closure and lessen leaflet impact during opening. An ideal aortic valve substitute should therefore incorporate the aortic sinuses to achieve this physiological haemodynamic performance. Homografts and the stentless aortic valve are the present substitutes that respect this important principle.

Stentless aortic valves have been used in clinical practice with increasing frequency in the last 10 years. Haemodynamic benefits already demonstrated by several authors, and a possible better durability due to a more physiological design, are the main advantages of the stentless valve over the classical stented bioprosthesis. The large amount of experience with biological tissues acquired in the last 20 years in heart surgery in our country has led to the development of an aortic stentless valve with the following main features:

1. it is a totally biological valve;
2. it has a composite design with three selected porcine leaflets;
3. it has a unique design that is easily adapted to any kind of aortic root, and
4. it is also an easily available and low-cost product.

The laboratory tests showed excellent haemodynamic performance in fatigue testing up to 300 million by cycles.

In 1990 we started the clinical trial with the SJM Biocor valve, with very good early results. This report reflects the 7 years of experience with this valve at our institution.

Materials and methods

Patients

From June 1990 until December 1996, 164 patients underwent aortic valve replacement with the SJM Biocor valve. Their ages ranged from 1 to 76 years (mean 38.16 ± 17.24). There was a predominance of male patients (73.2%). Most patients were functional classes III and IV (Table 8.1). The main aetiological indications are shown in Table 8.2; primary rheumatic aortic valvulopathy was the main factor (43.9%). Aortic insufficiency was the predominant haemodynamic lesion in the group (46.3%). The stentless valve was used in 49 patients (29.8%) who had a previous aortic valve replacement. In these patients the indication was due to prosthetic malfunction in 35 or to prosthetic endocarditis in 14. There were nine other patients with native aortic valve endocarditis; therefore, the total number of patients operated upon with active infection was 23.

Table 8.1 SJM Biocor valve: period June 1990–December 1996

Number of patients: 164
Clinical data
Age: 1–76 years (m = 38.1 ± 17.2)
Sex:
Male = 120 (73.2%)
Female = 44 (26.8%)
Functional class III/IV = 140 (85.3%)
II = 24 (14.7%)

Table 8.2 SJM Biocor valve: aetiology of aortic lesion

	No.	(%)
Primary rheumatic valve disease	72	(43.9)
Aortic prosthetic dysfunction	35	(21.3)
Congenital	21	(12.8)
Prosthetic endocarditis	14	(8.5)
Native valve endocarditis	9	(5.5)
Senile calcification	7	(4.3)
Myxomatous degeneration	6	(3.7)

Material

The SJM Biocor valve is a tricomposite porcine leaflet mounted on a slightly conical pericardial tube. There are two pericardial rims of approximately 3 mm for lower and upper sutures. The non-commissural height (related to the coronary ostiae) is approximately 5 mm. The fresh porcine tissue is readily fixated in glutaraldehyde under low pressure.

Surgical technique

The surgical procedure has been described in previous reports.[1,2] Basically, all patients underwent cardiopulmonary bypass under moderate hypothermia with myocardial protection achieved by intracoronary infusion of cold crystalloid cardioplegia (St Thomas). Aortotomy was either transverse or longitudinal in an italic 's' fashion towards the non-coronary sinus. This choice was usually based on the aortic root shape and the sinotubular junction. If the ascending aorta was small with a narrow sinotubular junction, we preferred the longitudinal incision, which was usually widened with a pericardial patch for its closure (32.9% of the cases). The SJM Biocor valve was chosen according to the annulus size and was used irrespective of the kind of sinotubular junction. The SJM Biocor valve sizes used in the patients are shown in Table 8.3. All implants but two were performed with the freehand technique. In patients with acute endocarditis extensive debridement was accomplished and all cavitations were excluded from the circulation by the SJM Biocor valve pericardial wall, avoiding the use of separate patches. Epicardial peroperation echocardiography was performed in the first 50 patients to evaluate the valve perfomance but it was discontinued in view of the consistency of the results. Associated procedures were

Table 8.3 SJM Biocor valve: sizes used

Valve size (mm)	Frequency	(%)
19	2	(1.2)
21	16	(9.8)
23	51	(31.1)
25	48	(29.3)
27	41	(25.0)
29	6	(3.7)

required in 18 patients, the majority of them (12 patients) related to concomitant mitral valve disease.

Myocardial revascularization was required in five patients and one child underwent a Konno procedure.

Results

Hospital mortality

There were eight (4.9%) postoperative deaths in the first month after surgery. Two patients died with sudden ventricular arrhythmias; two patients died from complications secondary to cerebrovascular accidents (CVA). One of them had acute endocarditis and preoperative CVA worsening after operation. One patient with ischaemic cardiopathy developed acute myocardial infarction in the sixth postoperative day. There was one death due to mediastinitis and another to coagulation disturbance. The last patient died with AV block and had acute dysfunction of a temporary pacemaker in the seventh postoperative day. No death was related to the SJM Biocor valve.

Hospital morbidity

Permanent AV block occurred in nine patients and all underwent pacemaker implantation before hospital discharge. Reoperation for haemostasis revision was undertaken in five patients. One patient developed pulmonary thromboembolism with prolonged respiratory ventilation. One patient developed partial dehiscence of the lower suture line, requiring reoperation. This was a patient with acute endocarditis and a running suture was used in the lower rim. After this case, interrupted buttressed sutures were employed in all patients with weakened aortic annulus.

Postoperative follow-up

Follow-up was achieved in 141 (90.4%) of the hospital survivors; 94.3% of the patients were in functional class I and II. There were 11 late deaths and the causes are shown in Table 8.4. No death was related to structural failure of the SJM Biocor valve. The actuarial survival curve (Figure 8.1) shows an 86.4% probability of survival at 78 months postoperatively. Reoperations were necessary in nine patients.

Although the major cause of late reoperation was endocarditis (four patients) that always occurred later than 1 year postoperatively, there was a 95.5% chance of freedom from endocarditis after 78 months (Figure 8.2). Two of these patients required root replacement by a valved conduit and in the other two, a regular bioprosthesis was implanted since only the leaflets were involved by the disease. Paravalvular leak was the reason for reoperation in two patients. In one patient the stentless valve was preserved and the other patient received a regular bioprosthesis.Three patients were reoperated for structural failure (all under 15 years of age). Two patients developed moderate to severe aortic insufficiency caused by prolapse of one aortic leaflet. The last reoperation was performed in a 14-year-old boy who developed accelerated degeneration of the prosthesis 3 years after the operation. There was no mortality in the reoperated patients. At 78 months postoperatively 92.3% of the patients were free from reoperations (Figure 8.3) and 96.6% were free from structural failure (Figure 8.4).

Table 8.4 SJM Biocor valve: late mortality

Late mortality: 11 patients	
Causes	
Cancer	2
Pulmonary embolism	2
Unknown	2
AV block	1
GI bleeding	1
Ventricular arrhythmia	1
Candida superinfection	1
Progressive heart failure	1

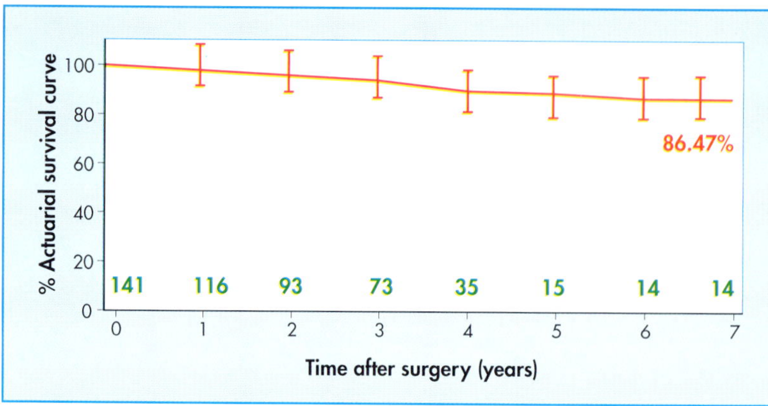

Figure 8.1 Aortic stentless valve – actuarial survival curve. (Hospital mortality excluded.)

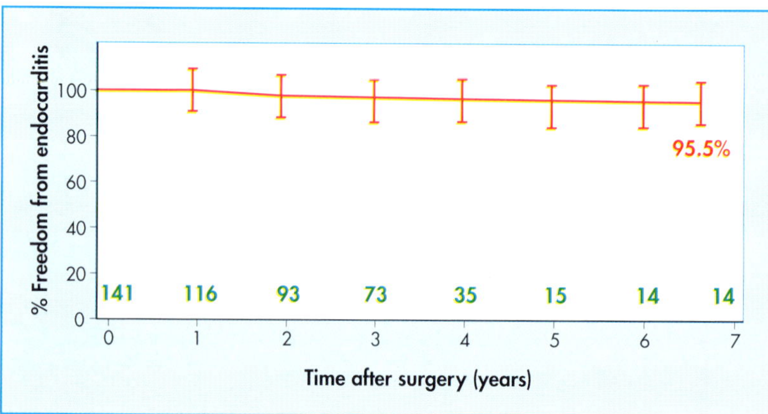

Figure 8.2 Aortic stentless valve – freedom from endocarditis.

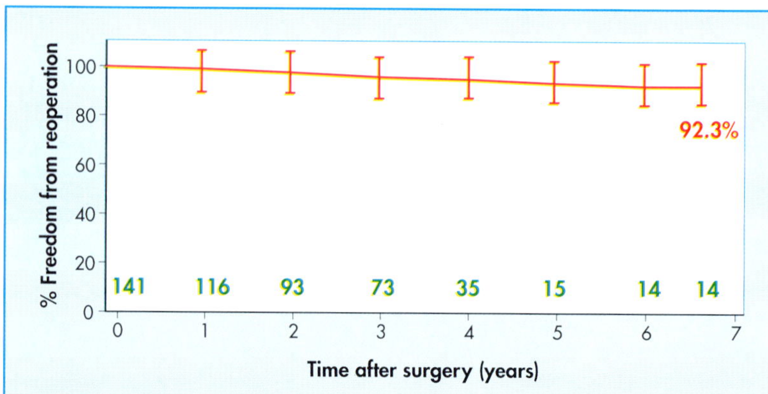

Figure 8.3 Aortic stentless valve – freedom from reoperation.

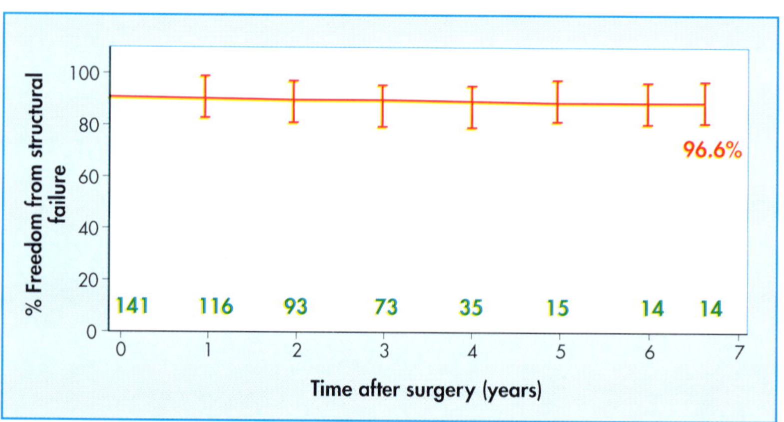

Figure 8.4 Aortic stentless valve – freedom from structural failure.

Echocardiographic data

All patients underwent Doppler-echocardiography analysis and information for effective orifice area, peak gradient, mean gradient and peak velocity was recorded. There was a clear superiority of the stentless valve, particularly the smaller size, which has already been stressed in our previous publications.[1,2]

Mild stable aortic regurgitation was recorded in nine patients (6.4%) with no evidence of progression. All other patients showed a competent valve (93.6%).

Discussion

Although the use of a stentless aortic valve dates back to 1962 with Ross[3] and to 1964 with Barratt-Boyes,[4] renewed enthusiasm for this kind of substitute has occurred in the last 10 years and has led to all major heart valve manufacturers developing their own version of a stentless valve.

When analysing initial and mid-term results with the stentless aortic valve we must not overlook the long experience with aortic homografts reported by many important centres, because even though major differences concerning tissue selection, composition and storage are evident, they were the first stentless product used as aortic substitutes.

One of the major drawbacks with aortic homografts has been the development of postoperative aortic insufficiency. This problem can be related to the technique of implantation and to the homograft preservation method. There is much evidence indicating that homograft implantation is most important in predicting early and late results. Since, in the normal aortic valve, leaflet coaptation is so naturally perfect, small malalignments in the suture line can lead to early or late progressive aortic insufficiency. In the classical freehand implant a perfect match must be achieved between aortic annulus and homograft to avoid rotation of any leaflet which will affect coaptation. No less important, in the upper suture line, absolutely equidistant commissural points are essential to avoid leaflet prolapse. These facts make the freehand implant particularly vulnerable to complications and it demands an absolutely precise technique.

Kirklin[5] reported that most allografts showed mild asymptomatic aortic insufficiency after 5 years, even though these valves were totally competent in the immediate postoperative period. Daicoff[6] reported progressive aortic insufficiency in all patients operated upon with the freehand technique. For this reason, the freehand technique has been abandoned by some surgeons in favour of the mini-root procedure.[7] Although the early reports with the mini-root technique showed improved results, the problem of progressive aortic regurgitation has not been completely eliminated and Daicoff reported mild regurgitation in approximately 21% of the patients. Analysis of most stentless aortic valves presently available for clinical use will show that they all originate from one complete porcine aortic valve and so the same problems reported with the homografts are expected to occur with these substitutes.

The stentless aortic valve referred to in this report, although implanted with the freehand technique in all but two patients, has eliminated these technical pitfalls because of its particular design.

The slight conical shape of the SJM Biocor valve ensures a good accommodation of the valve to any kind of aortic root. In some patients, widening of the aortotomy with a patch, usually placed at the non-coronary sinus, is required to precisely adapt the commissural post. The other important point is that the SJM Biocor valve is a composite valve, and the three selected porcine leaflets are sutured in a way to assure a wider margin of coaptation, providing a much safer implant not affected by minor rotations at the suture line.

The composite design of the SJM Biocor valve also eliminates the septal porcine leaflet, which has been shown to be a major drawback in the long-term run of the stented bioprosthesis. Actually, aortic regurgitation has not been a major problem with the SJM Biocor valve. Only one patient needed reoperation in the immediate postoperative period and it was due to suture dehiscence on a weak aortic annulus. At long-term follow-up, only two patients required reoperation because of a prolapsed cusp which resulted in a moderate to severe aortic incompetence. The other reoperations were either caused by endocarditis or suture line problems. It is important to emphasize that no patient with mild aortic insufficiency has shown any evidence of progression during this period of observation.

Other reports have already stressed the clear haemodynamic benefits of the stentless aortic valve.[8] Some of these benefits are actually best noticed some months after the operation, with a progressive decrease of the transaortic gradient. In a comparative study performed in our institution between the SJM Biocor valve and regular bioprostheses, there was a significant advantage to the stentless design, particularly in the smaller sizes, which can decrease the need for annular enlargement.

The high number of patients with previous aortic valve replacement and acute aortic endocarditis (total of 58 patients) makes this series very different from other stentless valve reports. It is well known that there is a much higher incidence of postoperative complications in this group of patients.[9] We previously reported the excellent results obtained with the SJM Biocor valve in this situation.[10] There was a low incidence of suture leak (2/58) and no reinfection in cases of endocarditis, which makes the SJM Biocor valve the substitute of choice for these patients.

Conclusion

The 7-year results obtained with the SJM Biocor valve demonstrate the excellent performance of the valve and confirm its definitive place in our surgical armamentarium.

References

1. Gontijo F B, Vrandecic M O, Morea M *et al* 1992 Nova bioprótese aórtica sem suporte: resultados clínicos. Rev Bras Cir Cardiovasc 7: 208–214
2. Vrandecic M P, Gontijo B F, Fantini F A *et al* 1992 Clinical use of a new stentless porcine aortic bioprosthesis: a multicentric study. In: Grossi A, Donatelli F, Corno A, Brodman R (eds) Cardiology and cardiac surgery; current topics. Futura Publishing Co., Inc., Mount Kisco, NY, pp 223–234
3. Ross D N 1962 Homograft replacement of the aortic valve. Lancet: 2: 487–488
4. Barratt-Boyes B G 1964 Homograft aortic valve replacement in aortic incompetence and stenosis. Thorax 19: 131–150
5. Kirklin J K, Smith D, Novick W *et al* 1993 Long term function of cryopreserved aortic homografts: a ten year study. J Thorac Cardiovasc Surg 106: 154–166
6. Daicoff G R, Botero L M, Quintessenza J A 1993 Allograft replacement of the aortic valve versus the miniroot and valve. Ann Thorac Surg 55: 855–859
7. Jones E L, Shah V B, Shanewise J S *et al* 1995 Should the freehand allograft be abandoned as a reliable alternative for aortic valve replacement? Ann Thorac Surg 59: 1397–1440
8. Mohr F W, Walther T, Baryalei M *et al* 1995 The Toronto SPV bioprosthesis: one year results in 100 patients. Ann Thorac Surg 60: 171–175
9. Husebuge D J, Oluth J R, Pichleer J M *et al* 1983 Reoperation on prosthetic heart valves; an analysis of risk factors in 552 patients. J Thorac Cardiovasc Surg 86: 543–552
10. Gontijo F B, Vrandecic M, Fantini F A *et al* 1995 Porcine stentless aortic valve in re-replacements and acute aortic endocarditis. J Heart Valve Dis 4: 171–175

CHAPTER 9

Aortic valve replacement in elderly patients with the Unique Suture Line stentless porcine valve

J. A. Navia, R. Pizarro, E. Weinschelbaum and C. Nojek

Murray,[1] in 1956, reported the use of a semilunar aortic valve as valve transplant in the descending thoracic aorta, for patients with aortic incompetence; in July 1962, Ross,[2,3] in London, reported the first orthotopic insertion of a homograft valve using a double suture line technique, followed by Barratt-Boyes[4] in New Zealand (August 1962). Since then, other types of biological valves have been used.

The first stent-mounted porcine aortic valves were fixed, sterilized and preserved in a special formaldehyde solution. They were first implanted by Paul Binet[5] in France in 1965, with unsatisfactory results.

The glutaraldehyde-fixed and preserved, stent-mounted, porcine valve was introduced by Carpentier[6] in France in 1968. Bovine pericardium stent-mounted valves, glutaraldehyde-fixed and formaldehyde-preserved, were introduced by Ionescu in Leeds, England, in 1971.[7]

The decades of the 1970s and 1980s were occupied by the stented biological porcine and pericardial valves, indicated mainly in elderly patients given the possibility of avoiding anticoagulation treatments and their complications, leading to a better quality of life. With the development of glutaraldehyde tissue fixation and the commercial availability of stented tissue valves, simple to implant, the interest in stentless porcine valves dwindled until recently.

Valve design

The stentless Unique Suture Line (U.S.L.), BioSud S.A., Buenos Aires, Argentina, is a porcine bioprosthesis, low-pressure glutaraldehyde-fixed and preserved. It was developed at the Italian Hospital, Buenos Aires, Argentina, by one of us[8] in the mid 1980s, after a large experience in tissue valves acquired with the stented porcine low profile bioprostheses, previously developed at our institution, for which haemodynamic characteristics, surgical technique and long-term follow-up were described in previous publications.[9–12]

The development of the stentless U.S.L. aortic porcine valve was supported by the following advantages:

1. The aortic stentless tissue valve and the aortic root constitute a functional unit.
2. The main objective was the preservation of the outstanding physiology of both the aortic valve and the aortic root (Figure 9.1).[13]
3. Lower or decreased stresses in the valve tissue, especially at commissural level, due to the direct suturing of the porcine tissue on the soft and elastic tissue of the host's aortic annulus and root, give the bioprosthesis the possibility of following the physiological movements of the natural semilunar valve during the cardiac cycle.

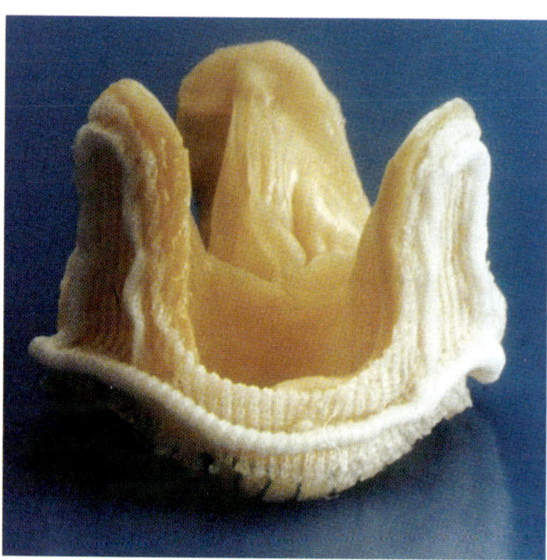

Figure 9.1 The stentless U.S.L. bioprosthesis.

4. A better orifice to tissue annulus ratio leads to larger effective orifice areas (EOA), and consequently to better haemodynamic characteristics than other valves of equivalent size, either mechanical or biological stented.
5. It is possible to implant a Stentless U.S.L. valve size matching the patient's aortic valve size.

The stentless U.S.L. valve has a Dacron cloth, covering the outer part of it, from the inflow edge and muscle bar to the entire height of the valve commissures. A tiny suture ring (Figure 9.2) is conformed as part of that Dacron cloth, allowing for a well-defined site to position the sutures.

The 'scalloped' design of the valve and the wavy shape of its tiny suture ring allow for implant of the bioprosthesis using a single suture line, either interrupted or continuous according to the patient native ring size. The suture line is done using the same technique as for a regular stented valve (Figure 9.3). The commissural posts are then fixed with interrupted single mattress sutures across the aortic wall, with Teflon pledgets placed outside.

The single suture line implantation technique avoids the longer and more complicated double suture line, at inflow and outflow edges, usually used for homografts, freehand, or other stentless valve designs.

A simple suture line at the tiny Dacron ring and fixation of the commissural posts with interrupted single mattress suture with Teflon pledgets across the aortic wall make the surgical technique simpler (Figure 9.4).

The implantation technique of the stentless U.S.L. has a special advantage in the small calcified aortic annulus, where the freehand technique is difficult and sometimes dangerous when coronary ostia are close to the calcified aortic ring. Special sizers were developed matching the scalloped design of the U.S.L. valve (Figures 9.5, 9.6a and 9.6b).

The implantation of the valve is performed after a meticulous decalcification is carried out. The aortic annulus is carefully sized with the sizer probe, and the valve is secured in the subcoronary position with 4/0 interrupted braided polyethylene sutures. We do not believe that the diameter of the sinotubular junction is more important than the diameter of the aortic annulus, and the stentless U.S.L. valve is implanted following the strict measurement of the native ring, avoiding oversize and leaflet plications.

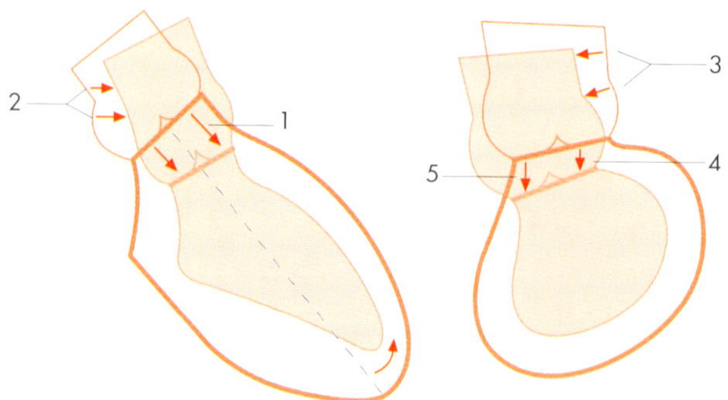

Figure 9.2 Normal physiological movement of the aortic valve and aortic root.

Materials and methods

We report our experience from November 1993 through to January 1997; 84 patients underwent aortic valve replacement (AVR). The patients were evaluated by age group, sex, preoperative symptoms, NYHA functional class, haemodynamic parameters, transvalvular gradients, effective orifice area, rhythm, etc.

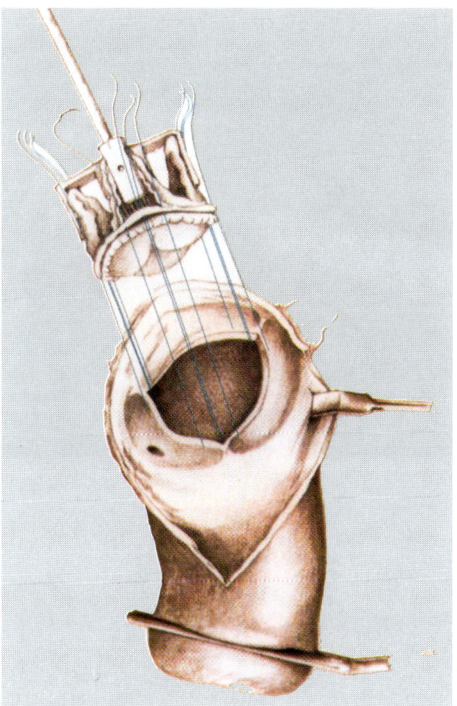

Figure 9.3 Single suture line of interrupted figure-of-eight stitches between native annulus and the tiny Dacron suture ring.

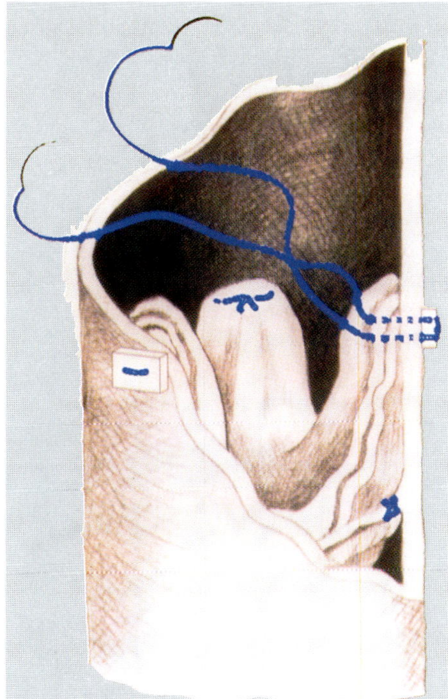

Figure 9.4 Fixation of the commissural valvular post with a single horizontal mattress stitch across the aortic wall tied over Teflon pledget.

The selection of the valve size was based on the exact size of the valve annulus measured with the anatomical sizer probe. These probes allow us to visualize the ring size and the commissural position simultaneously.

Patients were monitored by Doppler echocardiography preoperatively, before discharge from hospital, 3–6 months after discharge and yearly thereafter. Long-term follow-up was performed, and actuarial curves were constructed using the Kaplan–Meier method.

Table 9.1 summarizes the preoperative clinical data.

Operative clinical data

Hospital mortality was 5/84 patients (6.0%) none of whose deaths was valve related. One patient died due to pneumonia, one developed acute renal failure, one developed acute left ventricular failure, one had postoperative bleeding, and there was one sudden death.

Of the 84 patients, 30 had concomitant procedures; 28 had coronary artery bypass graft (CABG), one had a mitral valve repair, and one had a patent ductus arteriosus (Figure 9.7).

The valve size distribution is shown in Figure 9.8. More than 85% of the elderly patients had small calcific annulus sizes between 19 and 23 mm.

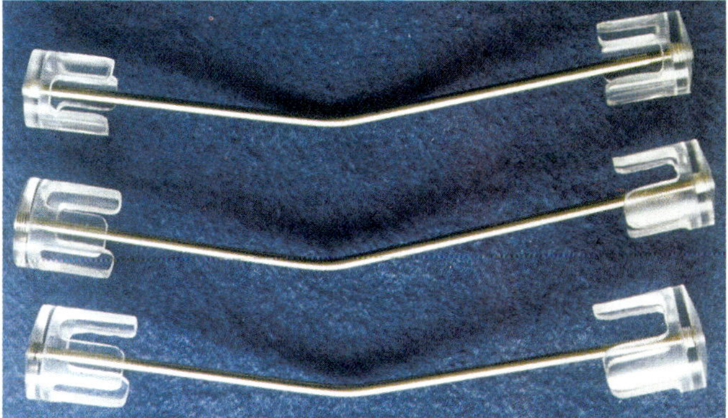

Figure 9.5 Examples of sizer probes.

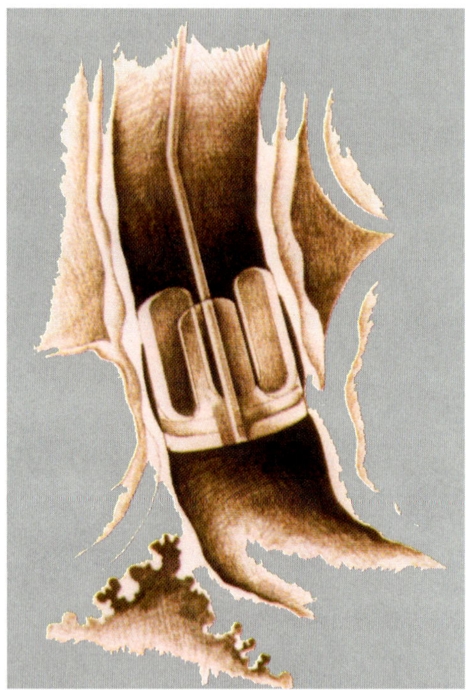

Figure 9.6 (a) The aortic annulus is carefully sized with the sizer probe.

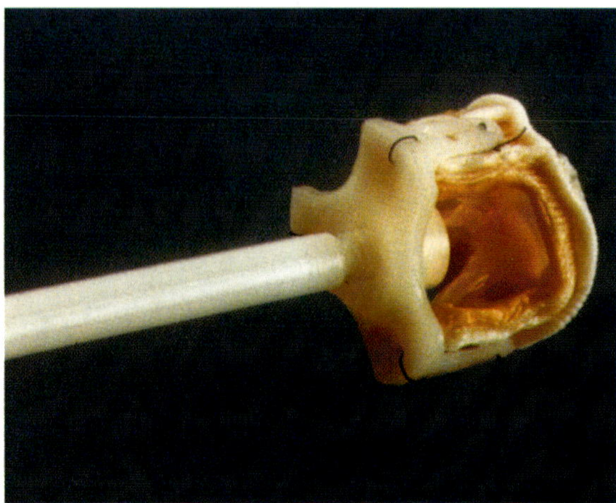

Figure 9.6 (b) The stentless U.S.L. bioprosthesis with holder.

Early postoperative evaluation

A comparative performance of the stentless U.S.L. vs stented biological valves was performed[14] using pre-, intra- and post-operative transoesophageal echocardiography. Recording of intracardiac pressure together with cardiac output measurement by thermodilution were performed just before cardiopulmonary bypass and 18 hours after surgery. Clinical and surgical variables – age, sex, combined surgery, pump time, ischaemic time, haemodynamic and valvular performance – were considered (Table 9.2).

Data 18 hours after valve implantation showed significant improvements in favour of the stentless U.S.L. valve performance over stented valve in: peak LVP, peak LV stress, valve pressure drop, valve energy lost, LV stroke work, work index and d*P*/d*T*/DP (%).

Late results

All patients showed improvements in their NYHA classification after surgery, evolving postoperatively to: 96% in Class I, 5% in Class II, and 1% in Class III. Preoperative and postoperative functional classes are presented in Figure 9.9.

Haemodynamic assessment by Doppler echocardiography

Doppler assessment of preoperative and postoperative peak and mean (average) gradients are shown in Figure 9.10. Correlation of EOA and size of valve implanted, preoperatively and postoperatively, are shown in Figure 9.11.

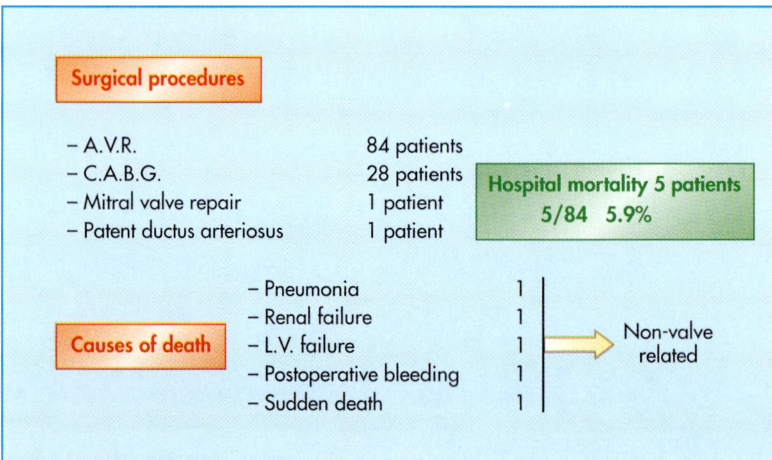

Figure 9.7 Operative clinical data.

Table 9.1 Preoperative clinical data

	No. of patients	(%)
Number of patients: 84		
Age (years)		
Mean 76		
Range 61–86		
Sex		
Male	33	(39.3)
Female	51	(60.7)
Principal symptoms*		
Syncope	14	(16.7)
Dizziness	7	(8.3)
Dyspnoea	36	(42.9)
Angina	24	(28.6)
Acute pulmonary oedema	12	(14.3)
ECG		
Sinus rhythm	65	(77.4)
Atrial fibrillation	14	(16.7)
Heart block	5	(6)
Functional class NYHA		
Class I	0	(0)
Class II	13	(15.5)
Class III	35	(41.7)
Class IV	36	(42.9)
Aortic valve lesions		
Senile calcific aortic stenosis	75	(89.3)
Rheumatic	6	(7.1)
Infective endocarditis	3	(3.6)

* Most of the patients had combined symptoms.

Table 9.2 Comparison of valve performance

	Stentless U.S.L. $n = 26$ (U.S.L. valve)	Stented valves $n = 16$ (low profile stented valve)	p-Value
Age	74 ± 6	72 ± 4	ns
Sex: male/female	14 / 12	9 / 7	ns
Cardiopulmonary time	121 ± 30	104 ± 22	$p < 0.02$
Ischaemic time*	100 ± 26	76 ± 16	$p < 0.02$
Peak LVP (mmHg)	99 ± 10	120 ± 18	$p < 0.01$
Peak LVS (g/cm^2)	132 ± 36	153 ± 42	$p < 0.001$
Valve pressure drop (mmHg)	12 ± 4	21 ± 12	$p < 0.02$
Valve energy lost (% of LVSWI)	7 ± 7	20 ± 12	$p < 0.02$
LVSWI	0.34 ± 0.08	0.39 ± 0.09	$p < 0.03$
dP/dT/ DP (%)	13.7 ± 2.5	10.6 ± 1.7	$p < 0.002$

* 17 patients underwent combined procedures (AVR + CABG).

DP, developed pressure; LVP, left ventricular pressure; LVS, left ventricular wall stress; LVSWI, left ventricular stroke work index.

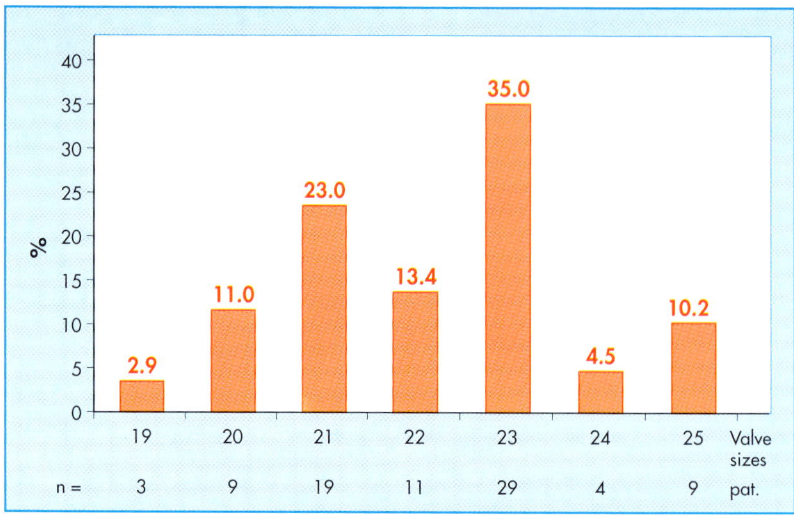

Figure 9.8 Valve size distribution.

All patients underwent echocardiographic assessment, with transthoracic echocardiography or transoesophageal echocardiography.

The presence of aortic regurgitation was specifically sought, using colour-flow Doppler.

Only five patients (6.3%) of the entire group presented aortic insufficiency after implantation: in two it was trivial, in one mild, in one moderate and in one patient it was severe (this patient later underwent reoperation); the regurgitation was due to erroneous indication in a dilated aortic root.

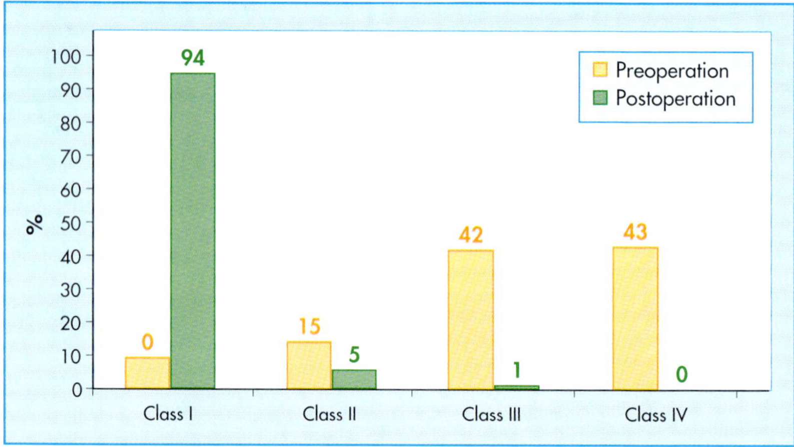

Figure 9.9 Pre- and postoperative functional class.

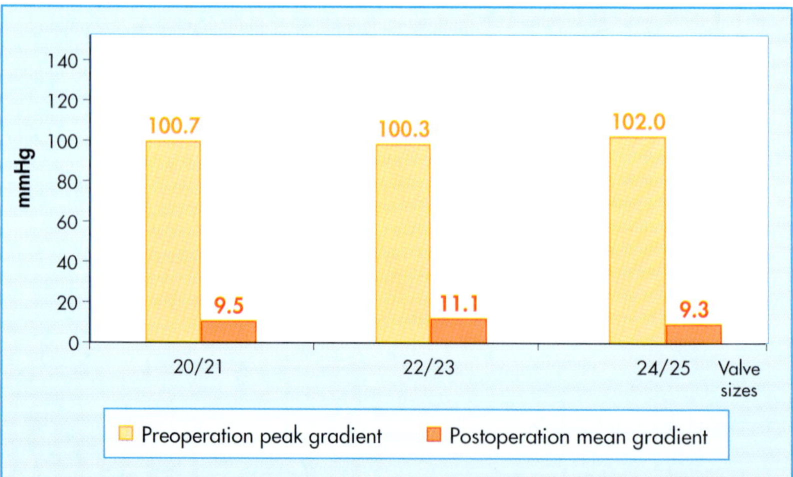

Figure 9.10 Doppler assessment of pre- and postoperative peak and mean (average) valvular gradients.

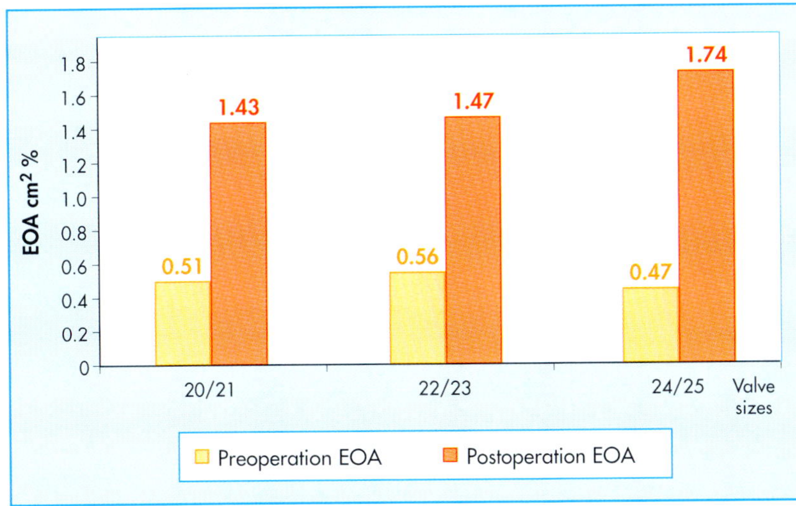

Figure 9.11 Correlation of pre- and postoperative effective orifice area (EOA) and valvular size.

Late follow-up

Late follow-up data were obtained by contacting each patient or his/her primary physician. A comprehensive questionnaire assessing the clinical status was completed, and these data were subjected to computer-assisted analysis.

Actuarial curves were constructed using the Kaplan–Meier method. Of 79 patients, 72 (91%) were followed during a mean follow-up of 13.3 months (range 1–41 months).

The actuarial survival curve is shown in Figure 9.12. Three patients died during the late follow-up: one (81 years old) died 24 months after surgery due to pneumonia, one (88 years old) died at 26 months of acute pulmonary embolus and one (76 years old) died 3 months after operation due to sudden death.

Actuarial freedom from thromboembolic events was 100% (Figure 9.13); freedom from structural valve deterioration was 100% (Figure 9.14).

Actuarial freedom from infective endocarditis was 98.6%: one patient developed infective endocarditis 2 months after AVR due to the insertion of a pacemaker catheter (Figure 9.15).

Discussion

In a previously published paper Westaby and Piwnica emphasize: 'The only conceivable argument against the use of stentless as opposed to stented xenografts is an element of difficulty in the surgical techniques ... the stentless xenograft has been linked to an aortic homograft, which requires a certain amount of judgement during implantation.'[15]

Wong *et al.* stated: 'Homografts offer distinct advantages in aortic valve replacement including good haemodynamics, low valve related complications and

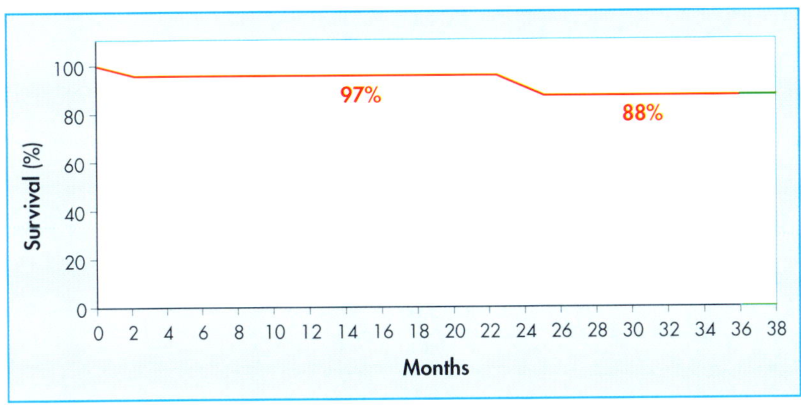

Figure 9.12 Actuarial survival curve.

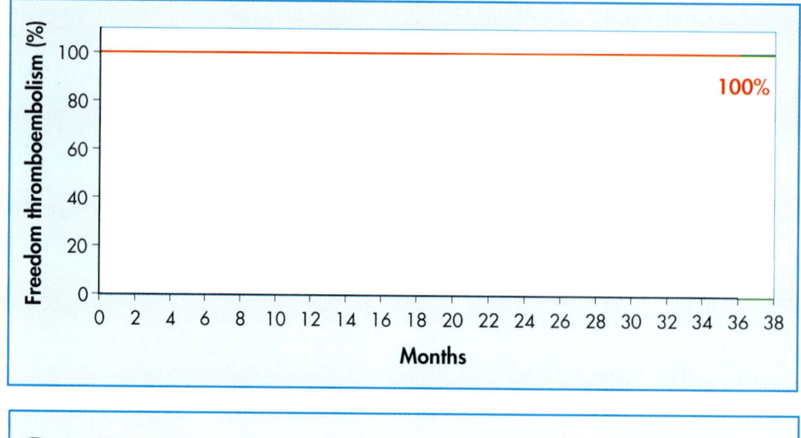

Figure 9.13 Freedom from thromboembolic events.

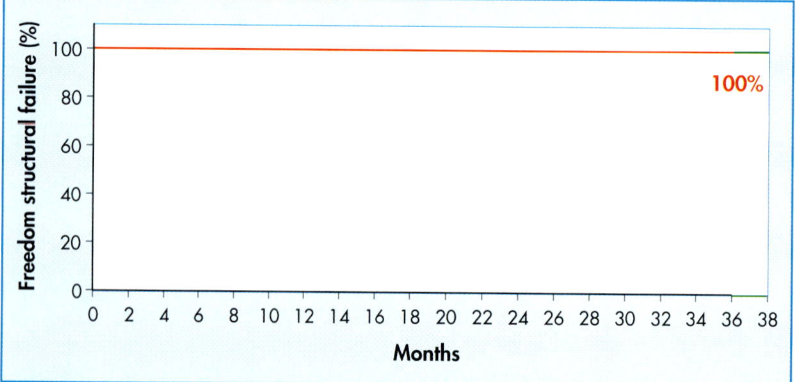

Figure 9.14 Freedom from structural valve deterioration.

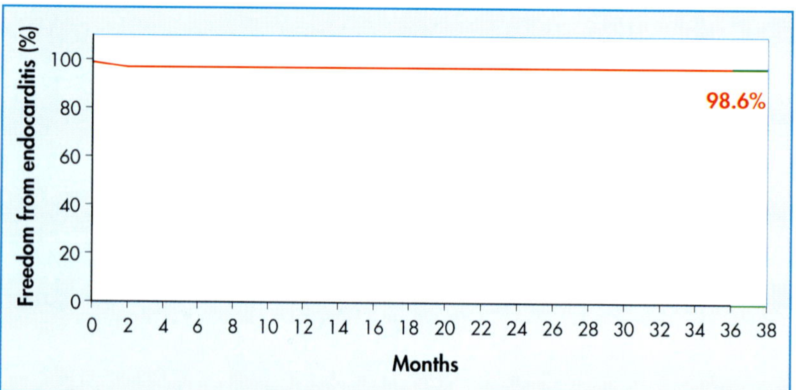

Figure 9.15 Freedom from infective endocarditis.

longer durability than bioprosthetic valves. Their advantages in the setting of endocarditis and aortic valve reoperations have also been demonstrated.'[16]

The main disadvantage of homografts is their limited availability, and stentless porcine valves may bridge this 'gap'.

The surgical implant technique of these valves is similar to that used with the homograft, and may be technically more demanding for surgeons with limited experience in this field.[16]

The 'scalloped' design of the stentless U.S.L. valve and the wavy shape of its tiny suture ring allow for a single suture line of simple interrupted or figure-of-eight stitches, using 4/0 braided polyethylene suture, in the small calcific aortic stenosis ring. The fixation of the commissural posts, using interrupted single mattress sutures with Teflon pledgets, across the aortic wall makes the surgical technique as simple as the implant of a regular stented valve, decreasing the technical demand for surgeons who have limited availability of homografts and consequently little experience in the freehand or mini-root techniques.

The implant technique of the stentless U.S.L. valve has great advantages, especially in the small aortic calcified annulus, in elderly patients, where the freehand technique is difficult and sometimes the second suture line can be dangerous, i.e. when coronary ostia are near the aortic ring or the aortic wall is calcified.

Another advantage is the ease of implant, making it simple to tie the knots, even when the aortic annulus is small. In our experience, more than 85% of the elderly patients had aortic valves sized between 19 and 23 mm.

The transvalvular gradients and effective orifice areas measured are very encouraging.

The comparison of valve performance 18 hours after valve implant showed significant improvements in favour of the stentless U.S.L. valve vs stented valve. These results are compatible with the hypothesis that the ventricle undergoes remodelling over time once the obstruction is relieved. In conclusion, early results suggest that the stentless U.S.L. valve provides excellent haemodynamics, easier implant than other stentless designs, and low incidence of valve complications, in elderly patients with truly small calcific annulus.

References

1. Murray G 1956 Homologous aortic valve segment transplant as surgical treatment for aortic and mitral insufficiency. Angiology 7: 466
2. Ross D N 1962 Homograft replacement of the aortic valve. Lancet 2: 487–488
3. Duran G G, Gunning A J 1962 A method for placing a total homologous aortic valve in the subcoronary position. Lancet 2: 488
4. Barratt-Boyes B G 1964 Homograft aortic valve replacement in aortic incompetence and stenosis. Thorax 19: 131–150
5. Binet J P, Duran C G, Carpentier A, Langlois J 1965 Heterologous aortic valve transplantation. Lancet 2: 1275
6. Carpentier A, Lemaigre G, Robert L, Carpentier S, Dubost C 1969 Biological factors affecting long-term results of valvular heterografts. J Thorac Cardiovasc Surg 58: 467
7. Ionescu M I, Tandon A P 1979 The Ionescu–Shiley pericardial xenograft heart valve. In: Ionescu M I (ed) Tissue heart valves. London, Butterworth, pp 199–213
8. Navia J A 1989 Valvular surgery: presentation of the stentless porcine valve design. Symposium of the Cleveland Clinic Foundation during the XIII Inter-American Congress of Cardiology, Rio de Janeiro, Brasil July 23–28
9. Navia J A, Gimenez O, Pujadas G, Tamashiro A, Vulcano N, Liotta D 1980 Low profile bioprosthesis for cardiac valve replacement. VIII European Congress of Cardiology. Paris, June
10. Navia J A, Liotta D 1980 Site and frequency of infection in porcine valve bioprosthesis. Am J Cardiol 46: 137–138
11. Navia J A, Swanson W, Jordana J, Liotta D 1982 Steady and pulsatile flow test of low profile bioprosthesis. International Symposium on Cardiac Bioprosthesis , Rome, Italy
12. Navia J A, Meletti J, Belzitti C, Franck L, Liotta D 1986 Low profile bioprosthesis, a highly flexible stent: late follow-up. X World Congress of Cardiology, Washington, DC
13. Del Río M, Liotta D, Pettinari M *et al* 1985 Angiographic evaluation of the aortic root (Part I–II). Rev Argentina Cardiol 53(5): 87
14. Pizarro R, Navia J A 1997 Stented vs stentless aortic valve: an early postoperative evaluation. (Abstract) Submitted to VII International Symposium on Cardiac Bioprostheses, Spain
15. Westaby S, Piwnica A 1995 Why stentless valves? In: Piwnica A, Westaby S (eds) Stentless bioprostheses. Isis Medical Media, Oxford, pp 3–15
16. Wong K, Brecker S, Khaghani A, Yacoub M H, Peper J R 1995 Early experience with the Toronto stentless porcine valve in aortic valve replacement. In: Piwnica A, Westaby S (eds) Stentless bioprostheses. Isis Medical Media, Oxford, pp 146–153

CHAPTER 10

The stentless CryoLife–O'Brien porcine valve in small aortic roots: 5-year results

U. Hvass and M. O'Brien

The number of elderly patients operated on for calcification of their aortic valve has increased over the last decade and reflects the satisfactory outlook for most operative survivors. However, in elderly patients, a small aortic root is not an unusual feature, and those with a body surface area (BSA) > 1.70 m^2 are at risk of replacement device mismatch, leading to suboptimal haemodynamic performance with higher residual postoperative rest and exercise gradients.[1]

Since August 1991, 410 stentless CryoLife–O'Brien aortic porcine valves have been implanted (CryoLife International, Marietta, GA, USA). Among these, 106 (25.8%) were used in patients with a measured aortic annulus of 19 or 21 mm.

Materials and methods

Patient population

The study population includes patients operated on in two institutions: the Bichat Hospital in Paris, France and the Prince Charles Hospital in Brisbane, Queensland, Australia. Both institutions are reference centres for the CryoLife–O'Brien stentless prosthesis.

Patient demographics are listed in Table 10.1. The study group is essentially represented by elderly females with symptomatic senescent calcified aortic valves. Concomitant procedures were not a criterion for exclusion.

The study valve

The CryoLife–O'Brien stentless porcine aortic prosthesis is manufactured by CryoLife International, Marietta, GA, USA. This stentless valve is of a composite design, constructed with non-coronary leaflets obtained from three porcine valves. Leaflets are carefully excised from valves already fixed in glutaraldehyde under very low or near zero pressure. Individual non-coronary leaflets are matched for size and symmetry to assure synchronous opening and to promote maximum leaflet coaptation. The matched set of leaflets is sutured together along the free edges of the aortic wall at the leaflet commissures. The base of the valve is finished with a blanket stitch to assure its integrity. There is no Dacron reinforcement, a significant difference when compared to other stentless valves (Figure 10.1).

The surgical technique is simple and safe, and needs only one running suture line as previously reported.[2,3] The replacement valve is placed in a supra-annular position, a 21 mm valve being used for the 19 mm annulus and a 23 mm valve for the 21 mm annulus.

Haemodynamic evaluation

All patients underwent preoperative transthoracic echocardiography. All survivors were followed-up with serial transthoracic echocardiograms, the first before discharge,

Table 10.1 Preoperative clinical data

No. of patients	**106 (with aortic annulus of 19 or 21 mm)**
Age (years)	
Mean ± SD	74 ± 5.6
Range	61–90
Sex	
Men	29 (27%)
Women	77 (73%)
ECG	
Sinus rhythm	81 (76%)
Atrial fibrillation	27 (25.4%)
Complete heart block	8 (7.5%)
NYHA class	
Class I–II	16 (15%)
Class III–IV	90 (85%)
Aortic valve lesion	
Stenosis	101 (95%)
Insufficiency	5 (5%)
Coronary artery disease	22 (20%)
Mitral valve disease	17 (16%)

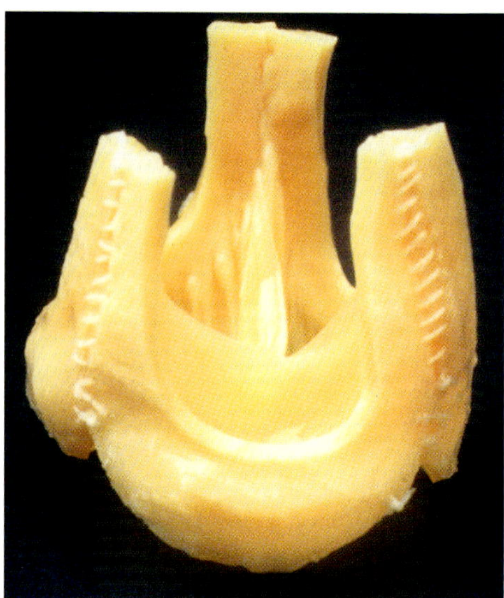

Figure 10.1 The CryoLife–O'Brien stentless porcine aortic prosthesis.

and then annually by the referring cardiologist. Transthoracic echocardiographic analysis of the leaflets, the left ventricular outflow tract and continuous-wave and colour Doppler studies were performed at each examination to assess valve function, mean aortic valve gradient and effective orifice area (EOA) (calculated by the continuity equation).

Complication rates for primary and secondary events

Operative and long-term mortality and morbidity were collected during the 5-year follow-up period using the Edmunds guidelines for reporting morbidity and mortality after cardiac valvular operations.[4] Discrete variables are presented as counts and percentages. Continuous variables are presented as means ± standard deviation. For complication rates, both the simple percentage of patients with early events (<30 days) and linearized rates for late events (>30 days) are reported. Linearized rates (in percentage per patient-year) were calculated by dividing the number of events by patient-years of follow-up and multiplying by 100%. Survival was determined by the Kaplan–Meier product limit method.

Results

Operative data are listed in Table 10.2. The size of the aortic annulus was 19 mm in 22 cases (21%) and 21 mm in 84 cases (79%). BSA was respectively 1.49 ± 0.34 m^2 (range 1.25–1.74) for patients with a 19 mm annulus and 1.78 ± 0.45 m^2 (range 1.37–2.10) for patients with a 21 mm annulus.

Table 10.2 Operative data

Aortic valve disease	
Degenerative calcific	88 (83%)
Congenital bicuspid	4 (3.77%)
Failed bioprosthesis	10 (9.4%)
Size of the aortic annulus	
19 mm	22 (21%)
21 mm	84 (79%)
BSA (m^2) for patients with a	
19 mm annulus	1.49 ± 0.34
21 mm annulus	1.78 ± 0.45
Coronary artery bypass grafts	
Single vessel	15 (14%)
Double vessel	7 (6.6%)
Other procedures	
Mitral valve repair	5 (4.7%)
Mitral valve replacement	12 (11%)
Subaortic muscle resection	8 (7.5%)
Aortic cross-clamp time (min)	
Isolated procedures	47 ± 16
Combined procedures	78 ± 25
Redo operations	96 ± 32

The hospital mortality (up to 3 months) was 3.7%. Two patients had reoperations performed on an emergency basis and the patients died from multi-organ failure; one patient died from sepsis and another patient from mitral annular disruption. All patients were anticoagulated over a period of 2–3 months. Anticoagulation was only maintained thereafter in the presence of atrial fibrillation.

Echocardiographic results at discharge and after 1 year are displayed in Table 10.3. During the first year, improved haemodynamics could be demonstrated in some patients. Over the 5-year follow-up, the results were stable. Regurgitation was absent or minimal. None of the patients underwent cardiac catheterization.

Complication rates for secondary events are listed in Table 10.4. At the time of this report, 86 patients have reached the 2-year follow-up interval, 54 have reached the 3-year mark, 27 the 4-year mark and 12 the 5-year mark. During the 5-year follow-up period, one patient (aged 86 years), died 3 years after surgery of stroke. Two others died from malignancy. Two patients have experienced non-fatal myocardial infarctions in the second and fourth postoperative years, respectively. Two patients, aged 84 and 79, in atrial fibrillation experienced femoral artery embolism 1 year postoperatively,

Table 10.3 Echocardiographic results

Aortic annulus diameter (mm)	19	21
Mean postoperative gradient (mean ± SD, mmHg)		
< 1 month	12 ± 4.2	10.5 ± 2
> 12 months	9 ± 2	6 ±1.7
Effective orifice area (cm^2)		
< 1 month	1.25 ± 0.1	1.58 ± 0.6
> 12 months	1.45 ± 0.3	1.72 ± 0.4

Table 10.4 Complication rates for secondary events

Event	No.	Linearized rate (patient-years × 100%)
Structural valve deterioration	0	0
Non-structural dysfunction	0	0
Valve thrombosis	0	0
Embolism	2	0.8 ± 0.2
Anticoagulant-related bleeding	0	0
Operated valvular endocarditis	1	0.4 ± 0.2
Reoperation	1	0.4 ± 0.2
Non-fatal cardiac events (myocardial infarction)	2	0.8 ± 0.2
Valve-related mortality	1	0.4 ± 0.2
Cardiac deaths	0	0
Total deaths	5	2.11 ± 0.3

requiring vascular surgery in both cases, amputation in one. Although we have explanted stentless valves due to technical errors in the early phase of our experience with stentless valves, none of the reoperations affected this subgroup of patients with small aortic roots. There have been no instances of structural valve deterioration. The Kaplan–Meier freedom from death at 5 years is 85 ± 3%.

Discussion

In the present study, we encountered a small aortic annulus in 30% of the patients over 70 years of age. In patients over 80, the percentage reaches 40%.

The superior haemodynamics of stentless valves are attractive for patients with small aortic roots and are expected to allow valve replacement without having to enlarge the aortic annulus.[5]

Most studies agree that stentless valves demonstrate excellent haemodynamics,[6–8] superior to those encountered with stented models, and that valves constructed with bovine pericardium show no significant improvement compared to porcine valves in respect of transvalvular gradients and EOA in the small sizes.[9] Allografts would be an ideal valve substitute[10] but their availability is already problematic for younger patients in most institutions.

The low transprosthetic gradients obtained in the study group met with our expectations and ruled out the need to take into consideration the individual patient's BSA and the anticipated physical activity. As with all stentless valves, correct sizing is important. Respecting simple rules and understanding that with the supra-annular implantation technique, the interior diameter of the valve must match the measured aortic outflow tract at the level of the annulus, the surgeon can be confident of obtaining excellent haemodynamic results.

Lower residual gradients and larger EOAs with a substantial regression of left ventricular hypertrophy,[11,12] a major determinant of left ventricular function and possibly of long-term clinical status.

Finally, the gradients recorded with the unstented valves selected for a 19 or a 21 mm aortic annulus are lower[13] than those reported for 19 or 21 mm mechanical valves (Table 10.5). Therefore, mechanical valves should no longer be considered as an alternative to annular enlargement in elderly patients with small aortic roots and all surgeons should become familiar with the unstented porcine valves.

Table 10.5 Haemodynamic data of four valves used for a 19 mm or a 21 mm aortic annulus (mean gradients mmHg ± SD)

Aortic annulus	19 mm	21 mm
CryoLife–O'Brien*	12 ± 4.2	9 ± 2
CE pericardial†	26.3 ± 9.4	22.6 ± 9.7
Med Hall**	17 ± 5	8 ± 4
SJM***	22 ± 7	12 ± 5

CE, Carpentier–Edwards; Med Hall, Medtronic Hall; SJM, St Jude Medical.

* Present study.

† MacDonald *et al.*[9]

** Manufacturers' data.

*** Panidis *et al.*[13]

The early haemodynamic results obtained in patients with a small aortic root and the low 5-year complication rates for secondary events are comparable to those of patients with a normal aortic root, and tend to prove that the CryoLife–O'Brien stentless valve is suitable in all valve sizes.

Conclusion

The excellent haemodynamics obtained in patients with a 19 or a 21 mm aortic annulus indicate that replacement device mismatch has been successfully addressed with the CryoLife–O'Brien stentless valve in patients with small aortic roots.

References

1. Kirklin J W, Barratt-Boyes B G 1993 Aortic valve disease. In: Kirklin J W, Barratt-Boyes B G. Cardiac surgery 2nd edn. Churchill Livingstone, New York, pp 536–538
2. O'Brien M F, Clarebrough J K 1966 Heterograft aortic valve transplantation for human valve disease. Med J Aust 2: 228–230
3. Hvass U, Chatel D, Assayag P *et al* 1995 The O'Brien–Angell stentless porcine valve. Early results with 150 implants. Ann Thorac Surg 60: S414–S417
4. Edmunds L H, Clark R E, Cohn L H, Miller D C, Weisel R D 1988 Guidelines for reporting morbidity and mortality after cardiac valvular operations. Ann Thorac Surg 46: 257–259
5. Kitamura M, Satoh M, Hachida M *et al* 1996 Aortic valve replacement in small aortic annulus with or without annular enlargement. J Heart Valve Dis 5 (Suppl III): S284–S288
6. Westaby S, Amarasena N, Ormerod 0, Amarasena C, Pillai R 1995 Aortic valve replacement with the freestyle stentless xenograft. Ann Thorac Surg 60: S422–S427
7. David T E, Feindel C M, Bos J, Sun Z, Scully H E, Rakowski H 1994 Aortic valve replacement with a stentless porcine aortic valve. A six year experience. J Thorac Cardiovasc Surg 108: 1030–1036
8. Sintek C F, Fletcher A D, Khonsari S 1995 Stentless porcine aortic root: valve of choice for the elderly patient with small aortic root? J Thorac Cardiovasc Surg 109: 871–876
9. MacDonald M L, Daly R C, Schaff H V *et al* 1997 Hemodynamic performance of small aortic valve bioprostheses: is there a difference? Ann Thorac Surg 63: 362–366
10. O'Brien M F, Stafford E G, Gardner M A H *et al* 1995 Allograft aortic valve replacement: long term follow-up. Ann Thorac Surg 60: S65–S70
11. Jin X Y, Zhang Z, Gibson D G, Yacoub M H, Pepper J R 1996 Changes in left ventricular function and hypertrophy following aortic valve replacement using aortic homografts, stentless or stented valves. Ann Thorac Surg 62: 683–690
12. Gonzales-Juanatey J R, Garcia-Acuna J M, Fernandez M V *et al* 1996 Influence of the size of aortic valve prostheses on hemodynamics and change in left ventricular mass: implications for the surgical management of aortic stenosis. J Thorac Cardiovasc Surg 112(3): 273–280
13. Panidis I P, Ross J Jr and Mintz G S 1986 Normal and abnormal prosthetic valve function as assessed by Doppler echocardiography. J Am Coll Cardiol 8: 317–326

CHAPTER 11

Intermediate results of aortic valve replacement with the Toronto SPV valve

B. S. Goldman, D. F. Del Rizzo, G. T. Christakis, C. Joyner, J. Sever and S. E. Fremes

There has been considerable interest in aortic valve replacement (AVR) with stentless bioprostheses due to the low gradients observed and the evidence for regression of left ventricular (LV) mass and hypertrophy.[1–3] We implanted 127 stentless porcine bioprostheses between March 1992 and March 1997; the initial 88 patients were part of an international, multicentre, phase II FDA prospective clinical trial which was reported earlier.[2] This chapter presents our continued clinical experience and documents the haemodynamic benefits of the stentless porcine aortic valve in 116 patients during intermediate term follow-up (3–48 months, mean 18 months).

Clinical trial

The 116 patients were unselected and operated upon consecutively. We used only the Toronto SPV valve (St Jude Medical Inc.). The indications for a stentless porcine valve (SPV) implant were:

1. patient and/or physician preference for tissue valve, and
2. no abnormalities of the ascending aorta requiring repair.

During the same time interval, 265 other patients received stented aortic valves (mechanical 106, bioprosthetic 159). The mean age of the SPV patients was 62.6 years ± 11.7 (range 33–82 years) and 66.4% were male. The preoperative pathology was dominant aortic stenosis in 61.2%, aortic insufficiency in 16.4% and mixed disease in 22.4%; heavy calcification or a bicuspid valve was present in 81.9%; 32.8% had concomitant coronary artery disease. Only five patients (4.3%) had undergone prior aortic valve surgery.

Operative details

Despite a large proportion of patients with aortic stenosis, 87.9% of patients received valve sizes 25 mm, 27 mm or 29 mm (Figure 11.1). The average aortic occlusion time was 118 ± 19.4 (range 79–176) min for isolated AVR and 148.4 ± 30.6 (range 102–225) min for patients with concomitant procedures. Coronary artery bypass graft surgery was performed in 32.8% of patients.

Results

Preoperatively the majority of patients (65.5%) were in class III or IV, while at last follow-up, 82.1% were in class I (Figure 11.2).

There were two perioperative deaths: one patient died within 24 hours from right ventricular infarction after injury to a small and non-dominant right coronary artery

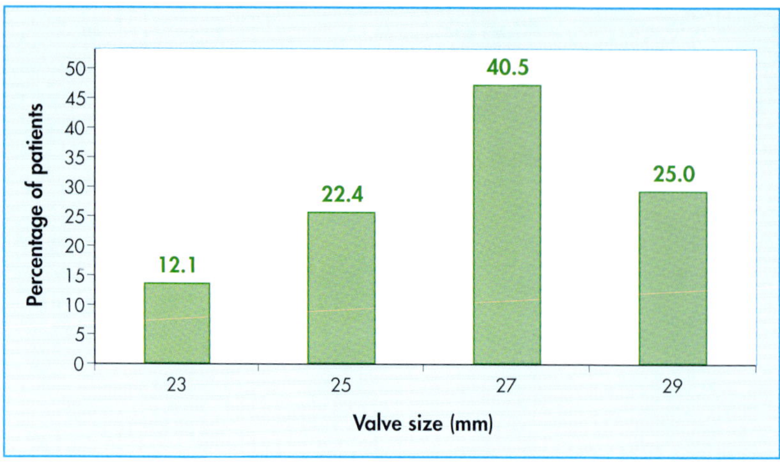

Figure 11.1 Stentless porcine valve sizes implanted.

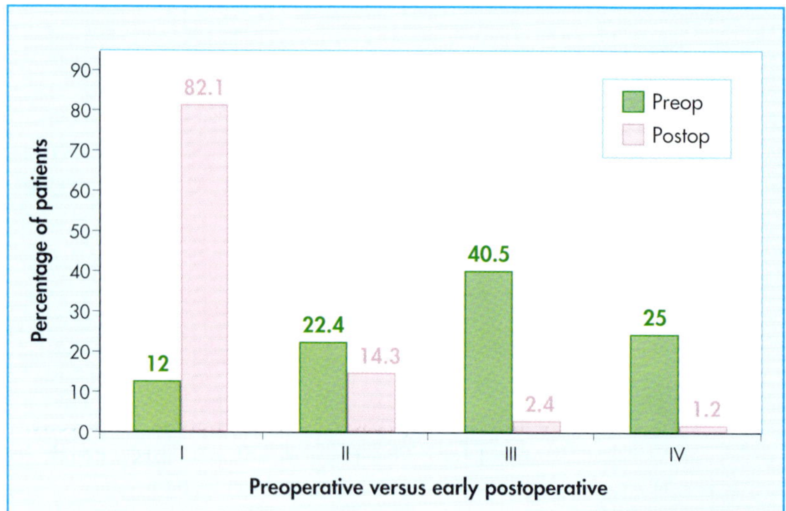

Figure 11.2 Preoperative and postoperative functional status, NYHA classification.

during valve implant, and another with preoperative epilepsy died a neurological death in status epilepticus. One patient required immediate mitral valve replacement due to ruptured chordae in the early hours following AVR (4 hours postoperatively). There were four reoperations for postoperative bleeding. There was one neurological event, presumably thromboembolic, with a persistent deficit. All patients were discharged on enteric coated aspirin, except for three who were given coumadin (24 patients in total had atrial fibrillation).

Late complications (after 30 days) occurred in 11 patients and included four deaths: one unrecognized endocarditis from *Staphylococcus aureus* presented with septic embolism, valve thrombosis and destruction (at 6 weeks); acute myocardial infarction in a patient with old unrecognized atherosclerotic proximal coronary disease (at 4 months); and cerebral haemorrhage in a hypertensive patient on anticoagulants (at 21 months). One other patient died of multiple myeloma (at 4 months). Two other patients had clinical evidence of endocarditis without valvular sequelae. In one, *Streptococcus viridans* (at 2 months) was treated by systemic antibiotics and in the other, a diagnosis of Q-fever endocarditis was made at 24 months, with probable inoculation by a farm animal 7 years prior to AVR. There is no evidence of valve deterioration in either patient. Neurological events (transient ischaemic attacks) occurred in four patients during follow-up. Complication rates for early and late events are shown in Table 11.1.

Six patients developed new (four patients) or recurrent (two patients) angina pectoris, 3–7 months postoperatively and three have undergone reoperation for

Table 11.1 Complication rates (n = 116 patients) for early and late events

	Early events (30 days)		Late events (>30 days)	
	n	%	*n*	%
Endocarditis	0	0	3	2.5
Anticoagulant-related haemorrhage	0	0	1	0.9
Myocardial infarction	1	0.9	1	0.9
Thromboembolism	1	0.9	5	4.3
Thrombosis	0	0	1	0.9
Death (all causes)	2	1.7	4	3.4

revascularization. The influence of coronary artery injury from either coronary perfusion, accelerated atherosclerosis, the stentless valve or the implant procedure is discussed in a separate chapter.[4]

Echocardiography was used to assess both the clinical performance of the valve and its early and subsequent haemodynamics. In the early postoperative period, 95% of patients showed no or trivial aortic insufficiency and this has been reasonably sustained through 36 months of follow-up (Figure 11.3). Early postoperative results were compared with those of follow-up visits at 3–6 months and at 1, 2 and 3 years (Table 11.2). An increase in the effective orifice area (EOA), and a decrease in the mean transvalvular gradient were observed over time (Figures 11.4, 11.5). The changes noted at 3–6 months continued: on average, there was a 2.7 mmHg decrease in mean systolic gradient from the early to the 24-month postoperative visit (n = 23) (Figure 11.6) and an increase of 0.20 cm^2 in EOA from the early to the 24-month visit (n = 23) (Figure 11.7). The data for changes in LV mass are presented elsewhere in this text.[5] Actuarial patient survival is shown in Figure 11.8. The number of patients at risk is shown along the x-axis. At 4 years after operation, survival was 93.3% (Figure 11.8).

Discussion

We continue to be satisfied with the clinical and haemodynamic results of aortic valve replacement with the Toronto SPV valve, despite the somewhat longer implant times required. We have previously stated that larger valve sizes can be implanted, 2.4 valve sizes larger than a conventional stented valve.[6,7] However, consideration of internal diameters (which are 4 mm < external diameter, and the external diameter is the designated valve size) and the differences in manufacturers' labelling may necessitate modification of this claim.[8] We have chosen the valve size for a Toronto SPV valve

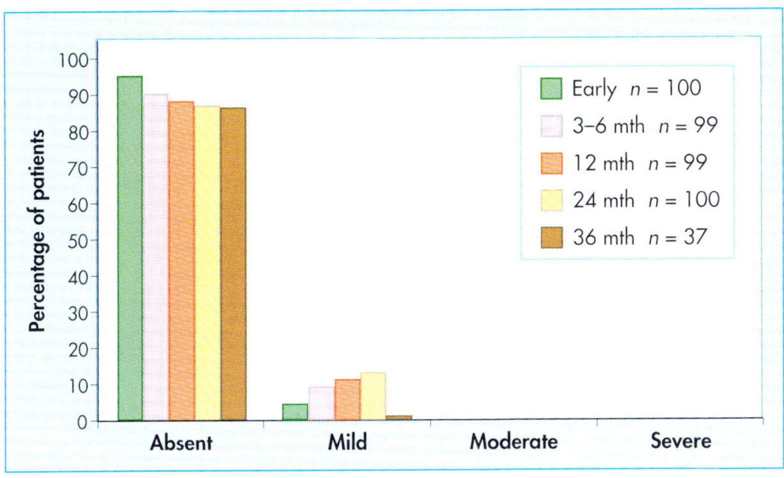

Figure 11.3 Echocardiographic assessment of post-operative aortic insufficiency.

Table 11.2 Mean gradient and effective orifice area (EOA) by postoperative visit

Valve size (mm)	Postoperative visit (months)	Mean gradient (mmHg)		EOA (cm^2)	
		n	Mean±SD	*n*	Mean±SD
23	Early	12	10.7±3.6	11	1.22±0.35
	3–6	12	7.9±3.3	12	1.39±0.44
	12	8	8.0±2.6	8	1.38±0.43
	24	4	7.1±3.4	4	1.48±0.33
	36	1	7.7	1	1.48
25	Early	19	8.0±3.9	18	1.55±0.41
	3–6	19	8.1±2.5	17	1.48±0.24
	12	14	7.7±1.9	13	1.51±0.16
	24	4	8.6±4.2	4	1.53±0.50
	36	3	7.8±3.3	3	1.54±0.35
27	Early	32	8.1±2.6	30	1.87±0.45
	3–6	31	5.4±2.1	30	2.08±0.54
	12	23	5.6±1.9	21	1.95±0.43
	24	10	4.6±1.4	10	1.99±0.47
	36	6	4.7±1.2	6	2.13±0.33
29	Early	23	6.9±2.6	22	2.20±0.59
	3–6	22	5.4±2.1	22	2.46±0.70
	12	17	4.0±1.7	16	2.59±0.62
	24	5	2.9±0.9	5	2.89±0.63
	36	3	2.5±1.4	3	2.91±0.83
All	Early	86	8.1±3.2	81	1.80±0.57
	3–6	84	6.2±2.8	81	1.96±0.67
	12	62	6.0±2.4	58	1.95±0.63
	24	23	5.4±3.0	23	2.04±0.65
	36	13	5.1±2.4	13	2.12±0.67

Data are presented as mean ± 1 standard deviation.

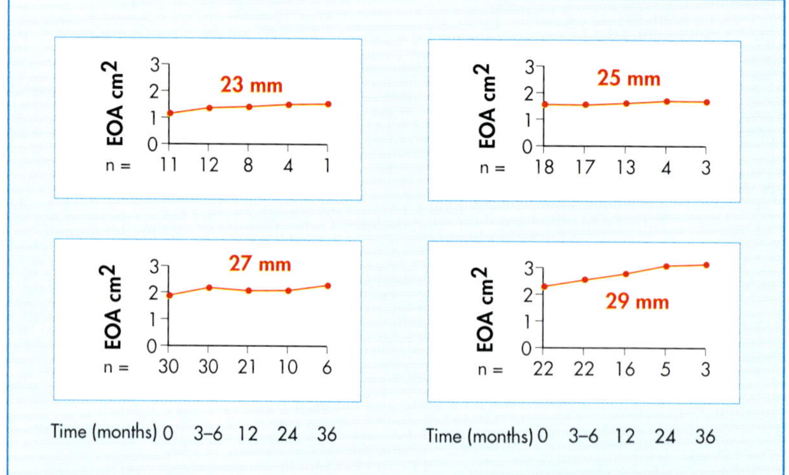

Figure 11.4 Effective orifice area (cm^2) by valve size and post-operative visit.

implant based on measurement of the sinotubular junction, rather than the native aortic annulus, thus oversizing to produce a large coaptation surface. This is reflected in the minimal evidence of aortic insufficiency, and more than 85% of patients continue to have no evidence of postoperative valvular regurgitation throughout the follow-up interval.

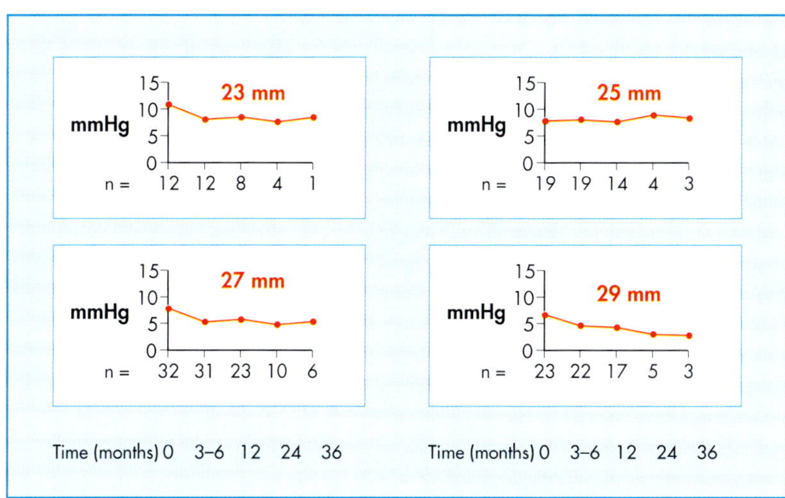

Figure 11.5 Mean gradients (mmHg) by valve size and post-operative visit.

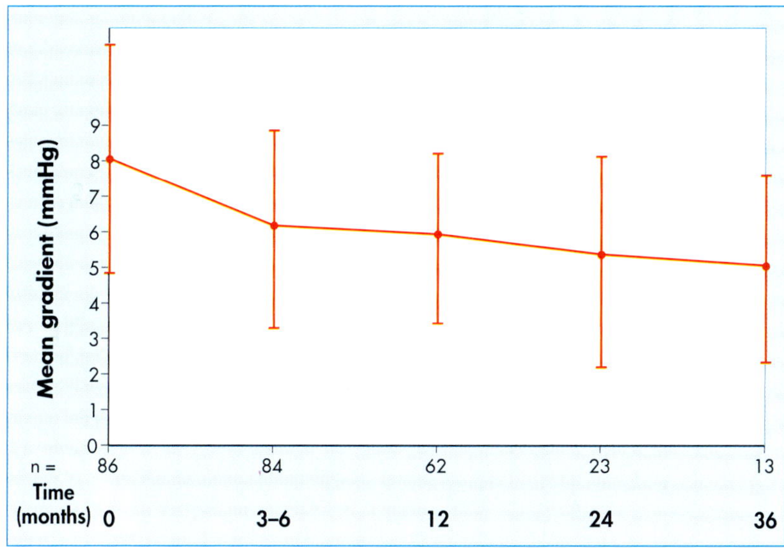

Figure 11.6 Overall mean gradients (mmHg) postoperative.

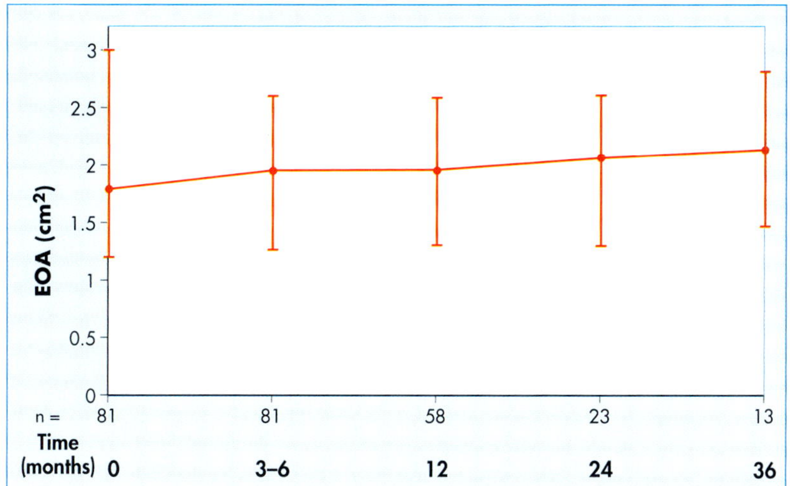

Figure 11.7 Overall change in effective orifice area (cm^2) post-operative.

The stentless porcine aortic valve has superior haemodynamic performance in the sizes implanted when compared to stented bioprostheses and this has been well documented by numerous authors.[2,9–12] There has been no evidence of tissue valve failure during this intermediate term follow-up but admittedly, long-term durability remains unknown. The lack of valve destruction in two patients with documented and

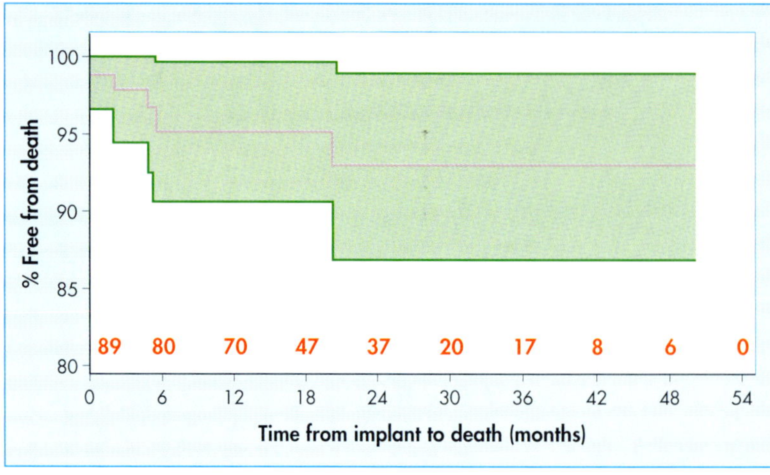

Figure 11.8 Actuarial survival determined by the Kaplan–Meier method. The number of patients at risk is shown along the *x* axis. At 4 years after operation, survival was 93.3% (data through January 31, 1997.)

treated endocarditis is hopefully suggestive of an increased resistance to injury due to central flow, biological tissue and little visible foreign material.

We and others have suggested that the progressive decrease in mean postoperative systolic gradient observed, accompanied by an increase in the effective valvular orifice and a consistent decrease in LV mass, is due in part to implanting a larger valve without a rigid obstructive stent or sewing ring, with leaflets that can open more fully since the commissural areas are pulled apart during systole. The early improvement in clinical status may be related to a significant increase in the velocity of circumferential fibre shortening, when compared to stented valves.[13,14] The beneficial haemodynamic changes are well maintained throughout the follow-up period and are accompanied by a low incidence of postoperative valve-related events. The haemodynamic benefits may ultimately be translated into an improvement of left ventricular function. This could be of significant benefit for those younger patients who receive an SPV valve and who might ultimately require a reoperation. However, the prime candidate for a stentless bioprosthesis at this time is the older patient (>65 years) with severe left ventricular hypertrophy from marked valvular obstruction.

References

1. Del Rizzo D F, Goldman B S, David T E 1995 Canadian investigators of Toronto SPV valve trial. Aortic valve replacement with a stentless porcine bioprosthesis: multicentre trial. Can J Cardiol 11: 597–603
2. Del Rizzo D F, Goldman B S, Christakis G T, David TE 1996 Hemodynamic benefits of the Toronto stentless valve. J Thorac Cardiovasc Surg 112: 1431–1446
3. Jin X Y, Zhang Z, Gibson D G, Yacoub M H, Pepper JR 1996 Changes in left ventricular function and hypertrophy following aortic valve replacement using aortic homograft, stentless, or stented valve. Ann Thorac Surg 62: 683–690
4. Goldman B S, Schampaert E, Christakis G T, Sever J, Fremes S E 1997 Coronary stenosis following AVR with a stentless bioprosthesis: complication or coincidence. Presented at the Second International Symposium on Stentless Valves. April 11–12, 1997, Noordwijk, The Netherlands
5. Del Rizzo D F, Sever J, Christakis G T, Fremes S E, Goldman B S1997 LV remodeling following AVR with the Toronto SPV valve. Presented at the Second International Symposium on Stentless Valves, April 11–12, 1997, Noordwijk, The Netherlands
6. Del Rizzo D F, Goldman B S, Joyner C P, Sever J, Fremes S E, Christakis G T 1994 Initial clinical experience with the Toronto stentless porcine valve. J Cardiac Surg 9: 379–385
7. Goldman B S, David T E, Del Rizzo D F, Sever J, Bos J 1994 Stentless porcine bioprosthesis for aortic valve replacement. J Cardiovasc Surg 35(Suppl 1–6): 105–110
8. Cochran R P, Kunzelman K S 1996 Discrepancies between labeled and actual dimensions of prosthetic valves and sizers. J Card Surg 11: 318–324
9. Wong Kit, Shad Sujay, Waterworth P D, Khaghani A, Pepper J R, Yacoub M H 1995 Early experience with the Toronto stentless porcine valve. Ann Thorac Surg 60: S402–S405

10. Westaby S, Amarasena N, Long V *et al* 1995 Time–related hemodynamic changes after aortic replacement with the Freestyle stentless xenograft. Ann Thorac Surg 60: 1633–1639
11. Mohr F W, Walther T, Baryalei M *et al* 1995 The Toronto SPV bioprosthesis: one year results in 100 patients. Ann Thorac Surg 60: 171–175
12. Sintek C F, Fletcher A D, Khonsari S 1995 Stentless porcine aortic root: valve of choice for the elderly patient with small aortic root? J Thorac Cardiovasc Surg 109: 871–876
13. Christakis G T, Joyner C, Morgan C D *et al* 1996 Left ventricular mass regression early following aortic valve replacement. Ann Thorac Surg 62: 1084–1089
14. Cohen G, Christakis G T, Buth K J *et al* 1996 Are stentless aortic valves hemodynamically superior to stented valves? Presented at the 69th Scientific Sessions of the American Heart Association, New Orleans, LA, November 10–14

CHAPTER 12

Early experience and results with the Toronto SPV valve and freehand insertion of Freestyle bioprostheses: comparative results at 1 year

A. Prat, V. Doisy, A. Vincentelli, G. Shaaban, J. Saez de Ibarra, D. Moreau and C. Stankowiak

Over the last 10 years[1,2] increasing interest has developed in stentless aortic porcine bioprostheses. These valves are designed to mimic the function of the aortic homograft and their potential advantages over conventional stented bioprostheses are increased durability and better haemodynamics.

Patients and methods

Our institution is one of the study centres in France for the Toronto SPV valve (St Jude Medical, Inc.) and the Medtronic Freestyle bioprosthesis. A clinical trial was initiated in December 1992, but actually developed since February 1994, to evaluate the Toronto SPV valve. Another clinical trial was initiated in October 1993 to evaluate the Freestyle valve. Written informed consent was obtained from all patients and these studies were approved by the hospital's ethics committee. The aim of our study was to compare the clinical and haemodynamic results with subcoronary implantation of Toronto SPV valve and Freestyle bioprosthesis. From December 1992 through December 1996, 125 patients underwent aortic valve replacement (AVR), with or without coronary artery bypass grafting (CABG), by subcoronary implantation of either the Toronto SPV valve (Group I = 75 patients) or Freestyle (Group II = 50 patients) bioprosthesis. The choice of prosthesis was not randomized but based upon surgeon preference. Two senior surgeons (A.P., C.S) performed 95% of these implantations.

Prospective clinical and transthoracic echo-Doppler studies were performed at the time of hospital discharge and 3–6 months and 11–14 months after operation. From the echocardiogram (Vingmed CFM 800) performed by two examiners only, mean aortic valve gradient, cardiac output (CO), effective orifice area (EOA) and degree of aortic regurgitation were determined.

Patient demographics, clinical parameters, and size of implanted valve are listed in Tables 12.1, 12.2 and 12.3, respectively.

There were no differences in sex, age, age groups, aortic lesion, valve pathology, preoperative condition and size of implanted valve between the two groups (Tables 12.1–12.3). In younger patients (under 65 years of age) the choice for a bioprosthesis was determined by patient preference or contraindication to oral anticoagulation or lack of aortic homograft. A significantly higher incidence of concomitant CABG was

Table 12.1 Patient demographics

	Group I	Group II	*p*-Value
Total patients	75	50	
Female (%)	43 (57%)	26 (52%)	ns
Age (years)			
Mean	68	68	ns
Range	47–84	49–82	
Patient age groups (years)			ns
< 50	3 (4%)	1 (2%)	
51–65	20 (27%)	14 (28%)	
66–75	40 (53%)	31 (62%)	
> 75	12 (16%)	4 (8%)	

Table 12.2 Clinical parameters

	Group I	Group II	*p*-Value
Aortic lesion, no. (%)			ns
Predominant AS	68 (90%)	45 (90%)	
Predominant AI	7 (10%)	5 (10%)	
Aortic valve pathology, no. (%)			
Senile calcific degeneration	54 (72%)	34 (68%)	
Rheumatic	9 (12%)	6 (12%)	
Congenital	7 (9.3%)	4 (8%)	
Failed prosthesis	3 (4%)	3 (6%)	
Healed endocarditis	2 (2.6%)	1 (2%)	
Dystrophic	0	2 (4%)	
NYHA Class III – IV, no. (%)	65 (86%)	38 (76%)	ns
Mean valve size (mm)	24.9	25.6	ns
Body surface area (m^2	1.81	1.78	ns
Redo surgery, no. (%)	3 (4%)	3 (6%)	ns
Concomitant CABG, no. (%)	4 (5.6%)	9 (18%)	0.05
Average cross-clamp time, min (range)			
Isolated AVR	73 (45–99)	87 (61–135)	0.01
With CABG	109 (83–130)	110 (92–153)	ns
Follow-up time (months)			
Median	17	13	ns
Range	3–51	3–41	

AVR, aortic valve replacement; CABG, coronary artery bypass graft; ns, not significant.

Table 12.3 Size of implanted valve

Valve size (mm)	Group I (no.)	Group II (no.)
21	4	1
23	18	6
25	34	19
27	16	24
29	3	–

noted in the Freestyle group (18% vs 5.6%; $p = 0.05$; Table 12.2). A significantly shorter mean aortic cross-clamp time was noted in the Toronto SPV valve group (73 min vs 87 min; $p = 0.01$; Table 12.2). This difference only occurred for isolated AVR. The follow-up was similar.

Operative technique

Whereas the Toronto SPV valve, with all three sinuses scalloped, can be inserted only by subcoronary implantation, the total root design of the Freestyle valve allows the surgeon to choose among all techniques described for allograft insertion (full root replacement, root inclusion, complete or modified, non-coronary sinus retained, subcoronary implantation). In this comparative study only patients with subcoronary implantation of a Freestyle valve have been included.

The implantation technique in group I and group II was exactly the same as for freehand insertion of an aortic homograft without inversion in the left ventricle. A transverse aortotomy was used in all patients to expose the aortic valve. The selection of the size of the stentless valve implanted was based on the diameter of the sinotubular junction, according to the technique described by David and associates.[2] If the sinotubular diameter exceeded that of the annulus by more than 10%, freehand insertion of a stentless bioprosthesis was contraindicated and another implantation technique was used, as outward stretching of the commissures will lead to aortic insufficiency. The proximal suture line was constructed with interrupted 3/0 Ti-Cron (Sherwood Medical, St. Louis, USA) stitches in a horizontal plane. The distal suture line was constructed with running 4/0 polypropylene suture. Myocardial protection was achieved through cold blood antegrade cardioplegia.

Clinical results

The 30-day operative mortality, non-valve-related, was similar in the two groups, being 4% in the Toronto SPV valve group and 6% in the Freestyle group. The six hospital deaths were due to multiorgan failure (two), left ventricular failure (two), small bowel infarction (one), cerebral haemorrhage (one). All the deaths occurred in patients aged over 70 years. Four patients required pacemaker implantation for complete heart block after extensive decalcification of annulus and septum. Clinical results are shown in Table 12.4.

There were four late non-valve-related deaths, due to myocardial infarction (three) and cerebral haemorrhage (one) in a patient who did not receive anticoagulation or antiplatelet therapy. One patient, in the Toronto SPV valve group, developed an infective endocarditis 6 months after implantation. This patient was referred to our hospital in so poor a condition that reoperation was postponed. A Gram-negative organism was isolated from blood cultures and left leg ulcer. Echo-Doppler study

Table 12.4 Clinical results

Event	Group I *n* (%)	Group II *n* (%)	p-Value
30-day mortality	3 (4)	3 (6)	ns
Pacemaker implantation	3 (4)	1 (2)	ns
Late mortality	3 (4)	1 (2)	ns
Late endocarditis	1 (1.3)	0	
Thromboembolic complication	0	1 (2)	
Explantation	0	0	

showed a small paraprosthetic collection in the absence of valvular dysfunction. Medical treatment alone was efficient and serial echocardiograms demonstrated resorption of paraprosthetic collection. Unfortunately the patient died suddenly 7 months later at home and a postmortem examination was not performed.

Of the 115 long-term survivors, 67 have completed the 1-year control study. All surviving patients were improved after surgery and are in NYHA class I or II.

Echo-Doppler results

No patient of either group had significant aortic regurgitation. Trivial or mild transvalvular regurgitation was noted in 6% of patients in the Toronto SPV valve group and 4% in the Freestyle group. No progression of regurgitation was noted during follow-up. A paraprosthetic leak was never encountered in either group.

The baseline average mean systolic gradient (Table 12.5) and mean EOA (Table 12.6) at discharge were excellent in all patients and there were no significant differences between the two groups. Transvalvular gradients decreased progressively during follow-up in the two groups and were similar (Table 12.7). EOA was consistently superior to 2 cm^2, except for 21 mm valves, with no difference between the two groups (Table 12.8).

Discussion

The durability of porcine bioprostheses is greatly influenced by mechanical and biological factors. Minimization of the mechanical stress on leaflets and commissures by elimination of the stent should increase durability.[3] Furthermore, recent data[4] have reported the superior durability of non-stented, as opposed to stented, allografts. By extrapolation of these results to xenografts one can anticipate that the durability of stentless bioprostheses will be longer than that of stented bioprostheses. Bioprostheses

Table 12.5 Baseline average mean systolic gradient in 115 patients at discharge

Valve size		Group I		Group II	*p*-Value
(mm)	*n*	Mean grad (mmHg)	*n*	Mean grad (mmHg)	
21	4	11.0	1	7.5	ns
23	16	7.5	5	7.5	ns
25	32	5.5	17	5.1	ns
27	15	3.6	22	4.5	ns
29	3	3.0	–	–	
Total	70		45		

Table 12.6 Baseline average effective orifice area (EOA) in 115 patients at discharge

Valve size		Group I		Group II	*p*-Value
(mm)	*n*	EOA (cm^2)	*n*	EOA (cm^2)	
21	4	1.5	1	1.4	ns
23	16	2.0	5	1.6	ns
25	32	2.0	17	2.2	ns
27	15	2.3	22	2.4	ns
29	3	2.7	–	–	
Total	70		45		

Table 12.7 Baseline average mean systolic gradient at follow-up for 67 patients followed for 1 year

Valve size (mm)		Group I Mean gradient (mmHg)				Group II Mean gradient (mmHg)			p-Value
	n	Discharge	6 mths	1 year	*n*	Discharge	6 mths	1 year	
21	2	9	4.5	4.0	0	–	–	–	
23	9	6.4	4.6	5.1	2	8.2	3.0	3.0	ns
25	21	5.3	5.5	5.3	7	3.6	3.2	2.6	ns
27	9	3.3	2.5	4.0	14	2.4	2.6	2.6	ns
29	3	3.0	1.6	3.3	0	–	–	–	
Total	44				23				

Table 12.8 Baseline average effective orifice area (EOA) at follow-up for 67 patients followed for 1 year

Valve size (mm)		Group I EOA (cm^2)				Group II EOA (cm^2)			p-Value
	n	Discharge	6 mths	1 year	*n*	Discharge	6 mths	1 year	
21	2	1.5	1.5	1.5	0	–	–	–	
23	9	2.2	2.0	1.9	2	1.8	2.2	2.1	ns
25	21	2.1	2.2	2.2	7	2.2	2.4	2.6	ns
27	9	2.2	2.2	2.2	14	2.4	2.6	2.5	ns
29	3	2.7	2.8	2.7	0	–	–	–	
Total	44				23				

deteriorate more slowly in elderly patients. Jamieson and associates[5] recently reported a 94% freedom from structural failure at 12 years and 82% at 15 and 17 years for the age group 65–69 years, and 96% freedom at 12 years for the age group 70 years and older for the Carpentier–Edwards standard porcine bioprosthesis. Given these excellent results, the potential advantage of prolonged durability of stentless bioprostheses is therefore questionable, as aortic bioprostheses are mostly implanted in patients over 65 years of age. If long-term follow-up of the stentless bioprostheses results in a lower tissue failure rate than that of stented bioprostheses, the use of stentless xenografts may eventually be extended to younger age groups.

The superior haemodynamic performance of stentless porcine valves has been demonstrated by several authors for Toronto SPV valves[6–8] and Freestyle[9,10] bioprostheses. Lower transvalvular gradients result in more extensive regression of ventricular hypertrophy and greater improvement of left ventricular function than occurs with stented bioprostheses.[11,12] The influence of superior heart valve haemodynamics is not yet clear in the absence of long-term studies but one can anticipate that effects on functional result and long-term survival will be beneficial.[13,14]

Discussion still goes on regarding the ideal method of stentless valve implantation. Total root replacement is the technique of choice for homograft and autograft aortic valve replacement.[15] Kon and associates[16] have compared the advantages of a partial scallop inclusion technique (PSI) with those of a total root replacement (TRR) in 75 patients undergoing aortic valve replacement with a Freestyle bioprosthesis. Both techniques proved to be quite satisfactory. Specific advantages of the inclusion technique included shorter cross-clamp time, comparable with those noted when a stented bioprosthesis is implanted. Total root replacement needed longer cross-clamp time. Specific advantages of TRR were that it was applicable regardless of the aortic root pathology. These authors found a very low incidence of any discernible aortic regurgitation in patients who received a TRR (92% vs 58% at discharge, 100% vs 33% at 3–6 months). By 3–6 months they found no discernible differences in transvalvular gradients between the two implantation techniques. Subcoronary implantation carries the risk of valve distortion if one of the commissures of the xenograft is malpositioned and of cusp prolapse if the commissures of the xenograft are not inserted slightly above the commissures of the native aortic valve. The Toronto SPV valves and Freestyle valves, glutaraldehyde-fixed and polyester cloth-covered, are stiffer than homografts and autografts, and more forgiving. Mohr[8] reported a 7% incidence of minimal aortic valve insufficiency at discharge with no progression over follow-up in a series of 100 patients receiving a Toronto SPV valve. Our results are similar. In the modified subcoronary implantation technique, with a preserved non-coronary sinus, the risk of distortion is lower as only one commissure can be distorted. Sintek[10] reported a series of 64 Freestyle valves implanted with this technique and no patient had more than a trace of aortic insufficiency.

Sizing is crucial in the subcoronary implantation technique. Undersizing the stentless bioprosthesis can give rise to serious complications, such as early suture dehiscence, paraprosthetic leaks, and loss of central leaflet coaptation leading to valvular insufficiency. In 1992 David[7] reported the results of aortic valve replacement with the Toronto SPV valve in 53 patients. At discharge six patients had 1/4 insufficiency, after 3–6 months 11 patients had 1/4 insufficiency and one had 2/4 insufficiency, at 1 year postoperatively 13 patients had 1/4 insufficiency and two had 2/4 insufficiency. After 1 year no further changes had occurred (average follow-up 27 months, range 4–58 months). In all patients the cause of aortic insufficiency was undersizing of the prosthesis leading to central transvalvular regurgitation due to imperfect leaflet coaptation.

Oversizing bears the risk of wrinkling of the lower suture line that may cause either valve insufficiency due to leaflet buckling and asymmetric valve closure, or obstruction resulting in high systolic gradient.

Thus, in the subcoronary implantation technique, the size of the stentless valve implanted should be the same as the diameter of the sinotubular ridge. As the sinotubular diameter is larger than that of the annulus in almost all patients, the stentless bioprosthesis is slightly oversized, resulting in a rather large average valve size implanted. In our study an average 24.9 mm could be implanted in the Toronto SPV valve group and 25.6 mm in the Freestyle group. In their report, Mohr and associates[8] noted an average valve size implanted of 26.5 mm.

Conclusions

The subcoronary implantation provides good clinical results, despite slightly increased difficulty in insertion. Haemodynamic results are excellent at 1 year and similar for Toronto SPV valves and Freestyle valves.

To the best of our knowledge this study is the first comparative study evaluating the clinical and haemodynamic results of Toronto SPV valves and Freestyle bioprostheses. These findings encourage the use of these stentless valves in older patients requiring aortic valve replacement.

References

1. Sievers H H, Lange P E, Bernhard A 1985 Implantation of a xenogenic stentless aortic bioprosthesis – first experience. J Thorac Cardiovasc Surg 33: 225–226
2. David T E, Ropchan G C, Butany J W 1988 Aortic valve replacement with stentless porcine bioprostheses. J Card Surg 3: 501–505
3. Thrubikar M J, Deck JD, Aoad J, Nolan S P 1983 Role of mechanical stress in calcification of aortic bioprosthetic valves. J Thorac Cardiovasc Surg 86: 115–125

4. Angell W W, Pupello D F, Bessone L N, Hiro S P, Brock J C 1991 Effect of stent mounting on tissue valves for aortic valve replacement. J Cardiac Surg (Suppl 4): 595–599
5. Jamieson W R E, Munro A I, Miyagishima R T, Allen P, Burr L H, Tyers G F O 1995 Carpentier Edwards standard porcine bioprosthesis: clinical performance to seventeen years. Ann Thorac Surg 60: 999–1007
6. David T E, Pollick C, Bos J 1990 Aortic valve replacement with stentless porcine aortic bioprostheses. J Thorac Cardiovasc Surg 99: 113–118
7. David TE, Bos J, Rakowski H 1992 Aortic valve replacement with the Toronto SPV bioprosthesis. J Heart Valve Dis 1: 244–248
8. Mohr F W, Walther T, Baryalei M *et al* 1995 The Toronto SPV bioprosthesis : one year results in 100 patients. Ann Thorac Surg 60: 171–175
9. Westaby S, Amarasena N, Long V *et al* 1995 Time-related hemodynamic changes after aortic replacement with the Freestyle stentless xenograft. Ann Thorac Surg 60: 1633–1639
10. Sintek C F, Fletcher A D, Khonsari S 1995 Stentless porcine aortic root: valve of choice for the elderly patient with small aortic root? J Thorac Cardiovasc Surg 109: 871–876
11. Del Rizzo D F, Goldman B S, Christakis G T, David T E 1996 Hemodynamic benefits of the Toronto stentless valve. J Thorac Cardiovasc Surg 112: 1431–1446
12. Jin X J, Zhang Z M, Gibson D G, Yacoub M H, Pepper J R 1996 Effects of valve substitute on changes in left ventricular function and hypertrophy after aortic valve replacement. Ann Thorac Surg 62: 683–690
13. Levy D, Garrison R J, Savage D D, Kannel W B, Castelli W P 1990 Prognostic implications of echocardiographically determined left ventricular mass in the Framingham heart study. N Engl J Med 322: 1561–1566
14. Hoffmann A, Haefeli R, Weiss P *et al* 1992 Influence of different pressure gradients on later clinical outcome after aortic valve replacement. J Heart Valve Dis 1: 51–54
15. Prat A G, Doisy V C, Savoye C, Moreau D C, Monier E J, Stankowiak C 1995 Total aortic root replacement with pulmonary autografts: short term results in 45 consecutive patients. J Heart Valve Dis 4: 368–373
16. Kon N D, Westaby S A, Amarasena N, Pillai R, Cordell A R 1995 Comparison of implantation techniques using Freestyle stentless porcine aortic valve. Ann Thorac Surg 59: 857–862

IV Clinical Outcomes (II)

CHAPTER 13

Aortic valve replacement with the Medtronic Freestyle bioprosthesis

D. B. Doty, J. H. Flores and R. C. Millar

The porcine aortic valve was proposed for replacement of the aortic valve by Binet and associates[1] in 1965. Originally, they implanted the valve directly in the aortic root, but this technique gave way to the popular stent-mounted porcine heterograft valve. The stent-mounted device could be easily implanted and gave reproducible results. Unfortunately, it soon became apparent that stent-mounted porcine heterografts had less than desirable haemodynamic performance, especially in small sizes. Stent-mounted porcine heterografts also showed calcification and cusp rupture, especially in young patients. David and associates[2] came back to the idea of direct insertion of porcine heterografts into the aortic root. The Toronto valve was devised as a stentless valve derived from glutaraldehyde-preserved porcine aortic root with the sinus aorta removed and the exterior of the aorta covered with Dacron cloth for ease of implantation. The Medtronic Freestyle bioprosthesis was designed, tested, and approved for trial implantation in humans in 1992. While the device is similar to the Toronto SPV valve in that it is a glutaraldehyde-preserved porcine aortic root, there are some significant differences in preparation and implantation techniques. This chapter describes the initial trial experience at LDS Hospital in Salt Lake City, UT, USA.

Materials and methods

Eighty-five patients had replacement of the aortic valve with the Medtronic Freestyle bioprosthesis using a standard freehand subcoronary valve implant technique. The patients were treated in a common investigational protocol as part of a multi-institutional clinical trial under an investigational device exemption granted by the Food and Drug Administration of the USA. The protocol received prior approval of the Investigational Review Board of LDS Hospital, Salt Lake City, UT. All patients gave written informed consent before operation. The first implant was performed on January 10, 1994. This study includes implants until January 7, 1997 (3 years). Clinical follow-up is complete in all patients, with none lost to follow-up. Only occasional patients received anticoagulation with coumadin when there was atrial fibrillation which could not be converted to sinus rhythm. Some patients were given aspirin therapy according to surgeon preference when there was associated coronary artery disease. Echocardiography provided the main means of objective follow-up with studies obtained intraoperatively, at hospital discharge, 3–6 months, 12 months, and annually. The standardized echocardiographic protocol included calculation of transvalvular pressure gradient and effective valve orifice area.

Operative technique

All of the valves were implanted by two surgeons using a standard technique. Operations were performed on cardiopulmonary bypass, moderate hypothermia (28°C), with the aorta occluded and the myocardium protected by intermittent infusion of cold blood potassium cardioplegia through the coronary sinus (heart temperature 10–20°C). A transverse aortotomy was made, extending the incision into the non-coronary sinus of Valsalva. This provided optimum exposure of the aortic root and the coronary arteries. The aortic valve was excised and calcium deposits thoroughly debrided from the aortic root. The diameter of the aortic root was measured at the ventriculoaortic junction (valve annulus) and an equal size Medtronic Freestyle bioprosthesis chosen for implantation. Associated procedures were accomplished while the bioprosthesis was taken through the rinsing process to remove glutaraldehyde.

The sinus aorta was removed from the bioprosthesis in the right and the left coronary sinuses of Valsalva. In the right coronary sinus, the aorta was removed as close as possible from the cloth reinforcement without disrupting the cloth attachment. The non-coronary sinus aorta of the graft remained intact. The graft was implanted into the patient in anatomical position (without rotation). The cloth sewing rim of the graft was attached to the patient's aortic root at the dense fibrous tissue of the hinge point of the natural aortic valve (annulus). The suture line was kept at a level plane except in the region of the membranous septum where it had to follow the annulus to protect the conduction system from injury. Continuous stitches of 3/0 polypropylene suture were employed. The bioprosthesis was held away from the annulus during suture placement (Figure 13.1). A 2/0 silk suture loop (pulley string) was placed every

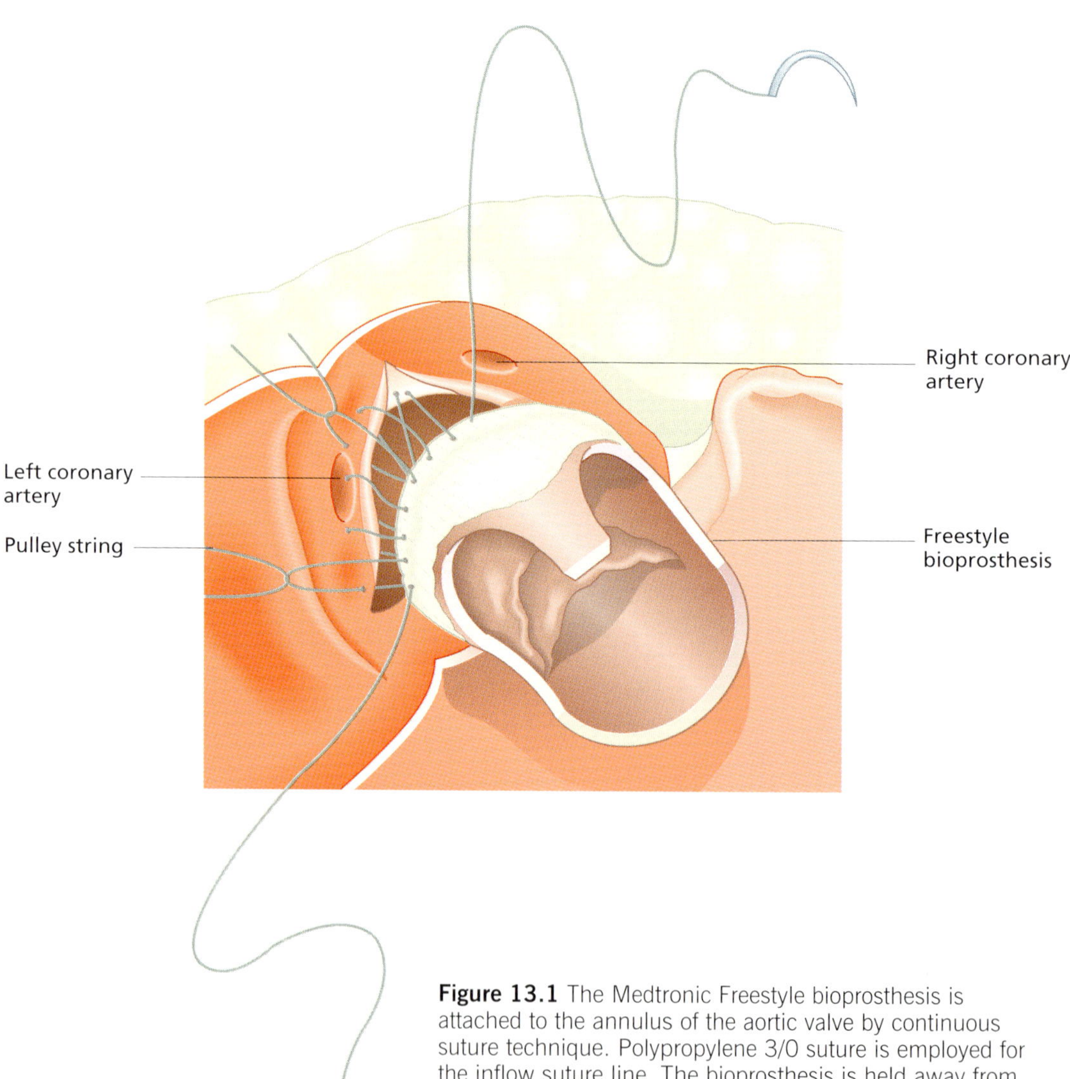

Figure 13.1 The Medtronic Freestyle bioprosthesis is attached to the annulus of the aortic valve by continuous suture technique. Polypropylene 3/0 suture is employed for the inflow suture line. The bioprosthesis is held away from the annulus as the sutures are placed. A 2/0 silk suture is placed around every third suture loop (pulley string) to aid in the adjustment of suture tension.

third stitch to aid in the adjustment of suture loop tension.[3] When all the suture loops were placed below the right and left coronary sinuses, the bioprosthesis was drawn into the aortic root. The non-coronary sinus suture loops were then placed and finally tension was adjusted to complete the proximal suture line. The sinus aorta of the right coronary sinus of the graft was then attached to the right coronary sinus aorta of the patient using continuous stitches of 4/0 polypropylene. Stitches were placed very close to the right coronary ostium so as not to buckle the graft below the artery. A similar technique was used to attach the left coronary sinus aorta (Figure 13.2). The position

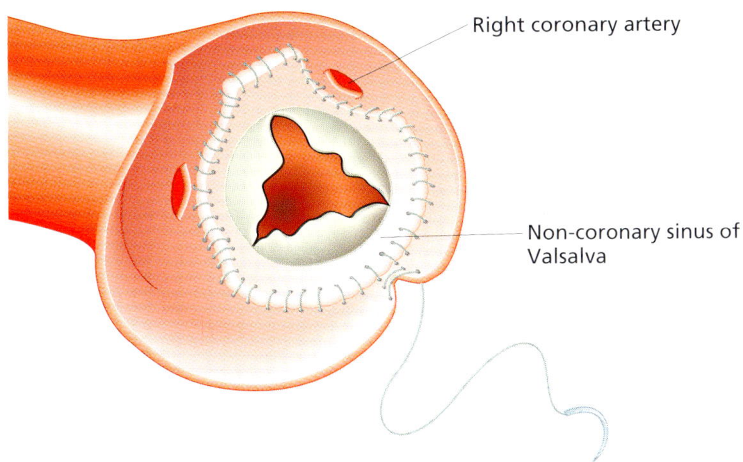

Figure 13.2 The outflow suture line is continuous stitches of 4/0 polypropylene. The stitches are placed close to the coronary ostia (especially the right) because the graft is quite stiff and stands up quite high due to the glutaraldehyde preservation process applied to the graft. The non-coronary sinus aorta is closed over the graft if the graft is contained within the sinus without distortion. The sinus rim of the graft is attached directly to the aorta.

and spatial relations of the commissures bordering the non-coronary sinus are fixed by leaving the non-coronary sinus intact. The surgeon need only properly locate the position of the commissure between the right and left sinuses of Valsalva to assure a competent valve implant. Proper location of this commissure is aided by the fixation characteristics of the graft aorta, which holds its shape quite nicely making undistorted approximation to the aorta very reproducible as suturing in the right and left coronary sinuses proceeds. The non-coronary sinus aorta of the patient may be closed over the graft as long as there is sufficient space to accommodate the graft without distortion (Figure 13.2). In this situation, the graft is trimmed above the sinotubular junction (sinus rim) and approximated to the closed aorta of the patient. If there is not enough room to accommodate the graft, the patient aorta is attached to the outside of the graft, leaving the graft to widen the aorta (Figure 13.3). Configuration and competence of the aortic reconstruction are always checked by intraoperative echocardiography prior to discontinuation of cardiopulmonary bypass.

Results

There were 46 males and 39 females in the series. The mean age was 75 years with ages ranging from 55 to 88 years. The maximum duration of follow-up was 3 years. The mean time for occlusion of the aorta for valve implantation was 72 min with times ranging from 56 to 100 min. There were 47 associated procedures performed, the most common of which was aortocoronary bypass grafts in 42. When associated procedures were performed, the mean aortic occlusion time was 123 min (range 57–195 min).

Four patients (4.7%) died within 30 days after operation. One patient died of a cause related to the valve. Dehiscence of the commissure between the right and left

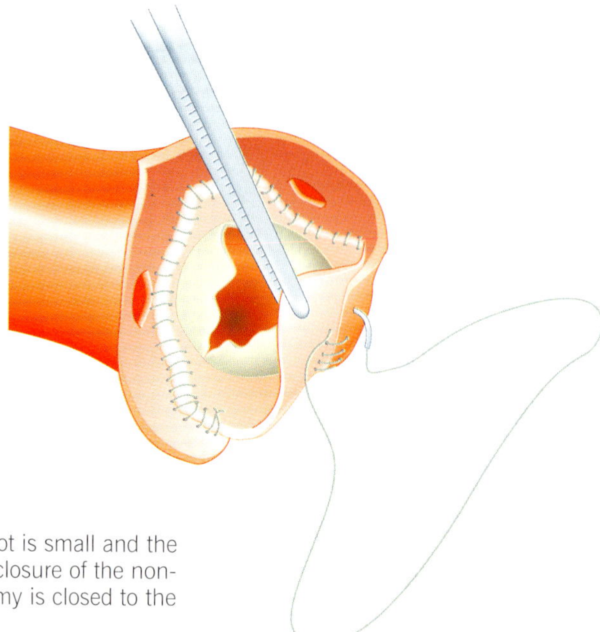

Figure 13.3 If the aortic root is small and the graft could be distorted by closure of the non-coronary sinus, the aortotomy is closed to the outside of the graft.

sinuses occurred, causing heart failure. The patient was admitted to another hospital where cardiac arrest and death occurred. Autopsy demonstrated the problem. Two patients died of cardiac causes. One patient with a markedly hypertrophied left ventricle had sudden ventricular fibrillation at operation during closure of the sternum. Ischaemic contracture of the ventricle resulted and the patient could not be resuscitated. Another patient with prior mediastinal radiation for breast carcinoma and severe coronary artery disease had low cardiac output syndrome requiring intra-aortic balloon pumping after operation. She lived for 8 days and finally died of intractable heart failure. One patient died 5 days postoperatively of multiorgan system failure following a family request to withdraw supportive care. The patient had suffered perioperative central nervous system injury as well. This death was considered a non-cardiac cause.

Five patients (6.2%) died more than 30 days after operation. One patient was considered to have a valve-related death. A paravalvular leak, presumed to be related to bacterial endocarditis, was diagnosed 14 days after operation. Blood cultures were positive for *Staphylococcus aureus* 24 days after operation. The patient deteriorated on medical management. Permission for reoperation was denied by the patient's family and supportive care was withdrawn 42 days after operation. There were two deaths related to cardiac causes. One patient died suddenly 3 months after operation of intractable ventricular tachycardia. This was considered a cardiac death. Three deaths were related to non-cardiac causes. One patient died of disseminated cancer of the prostate 16 months after operation. Another patient, who had been troubled by depression for several months, committed suicide 12 months after operation. One patient died 2 months after operation of uncontrolled sepsis related to wound infection, mediastinitis, and respiratory failure in spite of multiple operations to control the wound problem.

There were five significant thromboembolic or bleeding complications within 30 days of operation. One patient had a significant haemorrhage from the gastrointestinal tract, related to peptic ulcer disease, requiring transfusion of blood. This patient had been given aspirin after operation. Four patients had central nervous system events; two were transient and resolved almost immediately and two were permanent cerebrovascular accidents resulting in paresis. Of the permanent events, one patient developed left hemiparesis 3 days after operation which was thought to be embolic based on positive computerized axial tomography of the brain. The aortic valve was heavily calcified and extensive debridement was required at operation. The paresis improved markedly during hospitalization but significant residual disability remained. The other patient is included in the less than 30 day deaths described above. He failed to wake up after operation, suggesting perioperative neurological injury. Computerized axial tomography of the brain showed multiple cerebral infarcts, bilateral, probably secondary to atheroemboli. He died of multiorgan system failure.

There were two central nervous system events which occurred more than 30 days after operation. One patient had transient weakness of the right side of the body which occurred 7 months after operation. Transoesophageal echocardiography suggested that the non-coronary cusp of the porcine aortic valve was immobile. The significance of the finding was not clear. The patient was treated by anticoagulation with heparin and all neurological findings resolved. Aspirin was prescribed at hospital discharge. Transthoracic echocardiography 2 years after operation showed normal valve function and the patient had no further neurological symptoms. Another patient developed left hemiparesis symptoms 6 weeks after operation which were in addition to permanent left hemiparesis which the patient suffered 5 years prior to operation. A possible thromboembolic cardiac event occurred in one patient 6 months after operation. An acute myocardial infarction was the result of occlusion of a coronary artery which was normal angiographically prior to operation. This event was presumed to be embolic and the patient was treated with coumadin and aspirin.

Echocardiography at the time of discharge from the hospital is complete in 80 patients (Table 13.1). Mean gradient over the bioprosthesis and the estimated valve area are consistent with valve size. Smaller valve sizes are associated with higher gradient and lower valve area than the larger sizes. Pressure gradient over the valve had dropped and valve area had become larger for most of the valve sizes, especially the larger sizes, at the 3–6 months interval of follow-up (Table 13.2). Gradients continued to drop and valve area enlarged in the larger valves at the 1-year mark (Table 13.3). While numbers of patients presenting for examination at the 2-year mark were less, excellent haemodynamic parameters for the valve appeared to be sustained (Table 13.4). Aortic valve incompetence also appeared to follow a favourable trend (Table 13.5) so that by the 1-year mark 66% of patients had completely competent valves, 24% had trivial incompetence, and 10% had only mild incompetence. There were no patients having moderate or severe valve incompetence.

Discussion

The Medtronic Freestyle bioprosthesis appears to be an excellent substitute for the aortic valve which requires replacement due to disease or degeneration. The device is supplied as the intact porcine aortic root with the coronary arteries ligated. The surgeon is 'free' to choose the implant 'style', which may be subcoronary valve

Table 13.1 Freestyle bioprosthesis, echocardiogram: discharge

Valve size (mm)	*n*	Gradient (mmHg)	EOA (cm^2)
19	8	15 (8–23)	0.9 (0.5–1.2)
21	15	18 (8–35)	1.1 (0.8–2.2)
23	21	12 (8–20)	1.2 (0.6–1.7)
25	27	11 (2–22)	1.6 (0.8–3.0)
27	9	11 (7–17)	2.0 (1.6–2.6)

EOA, effective orifice area.

Table 13.2 Freestyle bioprosthesis, echocardiogram: 3–6 months

Valve size (mm)	*n*	Gradient (mmHg)	EOA (cm²)
19	8	14 (8–24)	1.1 (0.8–1.3)
21	11	15 (8–24)	1.2 (0.8–2.0)
23	16	13 (6–26)	1.4 (0.9–1.9)
25	19	8 (2–18)	1.7 (1.2–2.3)
27	6	7 (4–15)	1.9 (1.3–2.2)

EOA, effective orifice area.

Table 13.3 Freestyle bioprosthesis, echocardiogram: 1 year

Valve size (mm)	*n*	Gradient (mmHg)	EOA (cm²)
19	5	12 (6–17)	1.1 (0.9–1.4)
21	4	20 (8–26)	1.2 (0.8–1.4)
23	8	13 (6–23)	1.4 (0.8–2.0)
25	6	7 (5–11)	1.5 (1.0–1.9)
27	6	6 (5–11)	2.6 (1.6–3.3)

EOA, effective orifice area.

Table 13.4 Freestyle bioprosthesis, echocardiogram: 2 years

Valve size (mm)	*n*	Gradient (mmHg)	EOA (cm²)
19	4	11 (4–18)	1.1 (1.0–1.3)
21	1	22	1.1
23	5	13 (9–19)	1.5 (0.8–1.7)
25	3	6 (4–8)	2.1 (1.6–2.5)
27	3	11 (4–19)	1.7 (1.2–2.2)

EOA, effective orifice area.

Table 13.5 Freestyle bioprosthesis, valve insufficiency: 1 year

	n	(%)
None	19	(66)
Trivial	7	(24)
Mild	3	(10)
Moderate	0	(0)
Severe	0	(0)

replacement, inclusion root, or freestanding root replacement. Versatility is a feature which most surgeons desire so that a single bioprosthesis can be adapted to the clinical and anatomical situation which is presented at operation. These implant techniques have been thoroughly worked out by surgeons using cryopreserved or antibiotic-stored aortic homografts. There are some differences, however, in the tissue to be implanted comparing the Medtronic Freestyle bioprosthesis with an aortic homograft. The bioprosthetic device, being porcine aortic root fixed in glutaraldehyde, is thicker and stiffer so that it holds its shape and configuration even after extensive trimming or shaping of the aortic root. Thus, it is easier to work with the porcine tissue compared with an aortic homograft.

The subcoronary valve implantation technique was used exclusively in this series. The aortic root was trimmed extensively, removing the sinus aorta from the left and right coronary sinuses of Valsalva while leaving the non-coronary sinus intact. In spite of this alteration of the aortic root, the graft 'stood up' and retained its shape very well. The valve was implanted employing all continuous suture technique. The inflow suture line, placed in or below the aortic annulus, was performed by continuous suture with all suture loops placed before drawing the device tight to the annulus by adjusting the suture loop tension. Possible purse-string effect was eliminated by carefully adjusting only three suture loops at a time. The outflow suture line was also performed using the continuous suture technique. The sutures were placed close to the coronary ostia, both right and left. This is required not only because there is cloth covering extending up for some distance on the aortic wall, especially under the right coronary artery, but also because the glutaraldehyde tissues are stiff. This is a distinct difference from the homograft technique in which the flexibility of the tissue allows some folding and moulding so that sutures may be placed at a greater distance from the coronary arteries. The implant technique employed in this series has provided consistent competence of the aortic valve both early and later after operation.

Pressure gradient calculated over the bioprosthesis was low in all valve sizes although it was inversely correlated with the diameter of the bioprosthesis, with somewhat higher gradient in small (19 and 21 mm) sizes. Gradient and effective orifice area calculation in this series correlates with other reported series,[4–7] with higher gradients in the small sizes. The size of prosthesis chosen for implantation was determined by using the size calibrators provided by the manufacturer. Westaby and associates[5] have suggested that, with experience, there was a tendency to implant larger prostheses so that gradient was correspondingly lower. This 'up-sizing' usually means choosing a prosthesis 2 mm or more greater in diameter than the actual measured size of the left ventricular outflow tract at the ventriculoaortic junction. While it is generally agreed that the lowest possible gradient between the left ventricle and the aorta is desirable and that this is achieved by implanting the largest possible diameter of prosthesis, it is also recognized that smooth matching of the graft to the aortic contours is essential for proper function of the bioprosthesis. Forcing a large prosthesis into the aortic root is not recommended if the slightest distortion or buckling of the prosthesis is the result. Leaving edges of the aortotomy separated in the non-coronary sinus aorta of the patient, while closing the edges to the outside of the non-coronary sinus of the graft, allows the graft to remain undistorted and may allow a larger prosthesis to be implanted in a very small aortic root without compromising function.

Some technical enhancements have recently been employed during implantation of the Freestyle bioprosthesis, although these techniques were not used in this series of patients. The operation can be performed through a minimal incision. A ministernotomy is well suited for this operation. A lower-half sternotomy provides good exposure to the aortic root without compromise of the technical aspects of the operation. A 10–12 cm incision is made in the midline over the lower end of the sternum. The sternum is divided transversely at the third intercostal space, leaving the manubrium and part of the body of the sternum intact. The sternum is divided longitudinally from that point through the xiphoid process. A small sternal retractor separates the sternal edges and a modified Favolaro rake retractor is used to elevate the intact sternum. Additional exposure of the aortic root may be provided by dividing the ascending aorta. Illustrations of Westaby's technique,[8] in which a transverse aortotomy or two-thirds transection of the aorta is used, show only a short portion of the aorta posteriorly remaining intact. Continuing a transverse aortotomy to complete division of the aorta releases the aortic root, significantly enhancing exposure, and aids greatly in understanding proper dimensional relationships during valve implantation (Figure 13.4a,b).

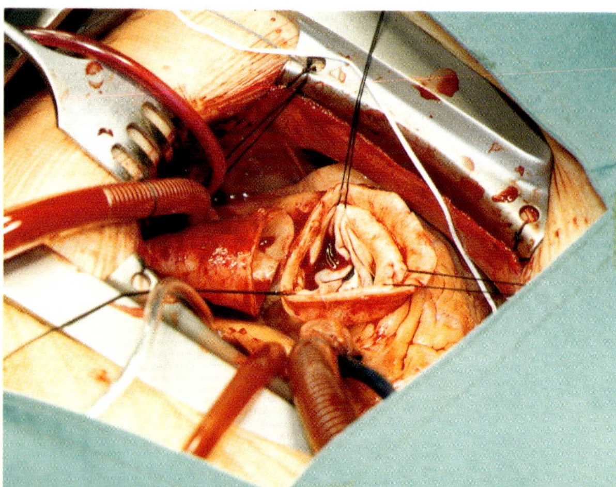

Figure 13.4 (a) When working through a ministernotomy, the aorta may be completely divided to enhance exposure of the aortic valve and improve understanding of spatial relationships during implantation of the Freestyle bioprosthesis.

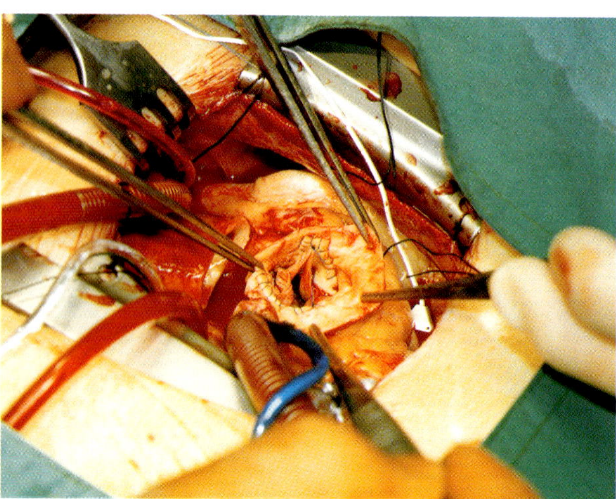

Figure 13.4 (b) The graft is shown here on completion of implantation.

Improving haemodynamic performance of the Freestyle bioprosthesis with passage of time was observed in this series and has been consistently observed by others.[4–7] The explanation of this phenomenon is unclear. Explanations which have been proposed include absorption of blood or thrombus in the aorta or between the aorta and the bioprosthesis[4] or more complete merging of the porcine graft with the native aorta.[7] The real explanation, however, is probably related to resolution of left ventricular hypertrophy and remodelling of the ventricle[9] and changing blood flow patterns over the left ventricular outflow tract.

Conclusions

The Medtronic Freestyle bioprosthesis has been shown to be an excellent device for replacement of the aortic valve. The device may be implanted by various techniques, making it applicable in a variety of clinical situations and for individual surgeon preference. Haemodynamic performance is excellent, and superior to stent-mounted bioprosthesis and mechanical valves in smaller aortic diameters. Complications related to the valve prosthesis appear to be infrequent. Durability issues are not resolved due to follow-up of less than 5 years. However, the early results with this bioprosthesis are encouraging.

References

1. Binet J P, Duran C G, Carpentier A, Langlois J 1965 Heterologous aortic valve transplantation. Lancet 2: 1275
2. David T E, Pollick C, Bos J 1990 Aortic valve replacement with stentless porcine aortic bioprosthesis. J Thorac Cardiovasc Surg 99: 113–118
3. Doty D B 1997 Cardiac surgery: operative technique. Mosby Inc., St Louis, MO
4. Sintek C F, Fletcher A D, Khonsari S 1995 Stentless porcine aortic root: valve of choice for the elderly patient with small aortic root? J Thorac Cardiovasc Surg 109: 871–876
5. Westaby S, Amarasena N, Long V *et al* 1996 Time-related hemodynamic changes after aortic replacement with the Freestyle stentless xenograft. Ann Thorac Surg 60: 1633–1639

6. Kon N D, Westaby S, Amarasena N, Pillai R, Cordell A R 1995 Comparison of implantation techniques using Freestyle stentless porcine aortic valve. Ann Thorac Surg 59: 857–862
7. Cartier P C, Metras J, Dusmesnil J G, Doyle D, Desaulniers D, Raymond G 1997 Clinical and hemodynamic performance of the Freestyle aortic root bioprosthesis. Abstract. Second International Symposium on Stentless Bioprostheses, April 11–12, Noordwijk, The Netherlands
8. Westaby S, Amarasena N, Ormerod O, Amarasena G A C, Pillai R 1995 Aortic valve replacement with the Freestyle stentless xenograft. Ann Thorac Surg 60: S422–S427
9. Walther T, Falk V, Diegeler A, Schilling L, Autschbach R, Mohr F W 1997 Left ventricular remodeling after stentless AVR. Abstract. Second International Symposium on Stentless Bioprostheses, April 11–12, Noordwijk, The Netherlands

CHAPTER 14

Aortic valve replacement with the Labcor stentless porcine bioprosthesis

R. C. Rabelo, G. G. Mota, C. H. Passerino and M. A. R. A. Coelho

Since the very beginning of cardiac surgery and extracorporeal circulation by Gibbon in 1953,[1] the search for the ideal valve substitute has been the major concern of those who deal with the art. The main commandments for a valve substitute should include:

1. free opening and competent closure;
2. prompt opening and closure in response to pressure changes;
3. biocompatible, non-thrombogenic, non-antigenic material that causes no damage to the blood elements;
4. durability for many years;
5. implantation technically feasible, and
6. maintenance of the patient's lifestyle.

Conventional biological and mechanical prostheses have important limitations with regard to the above characteristics, especially long-term durability. Stentless porcine aortic valves demonstrate superior performance when compared with their stented counterpart, and it is probable that the anatomy of the coronary sinuses, decreasing the stress on the aortic valve leaflets, makes this hand-sewn xenograft more durable than the stent-mounted one.

The good results obtained independently by Ross[2], and Barratt-Boyes[3] in the 1960s in replacing the aortic valve with allograft and homograft valves, using the technique described by Duran and Gunning,[4] encouraged many surgeons in the search for a stentless substitute for the aortic valve, although the technical considerations for its implantation may be demanding.

We report our experience with the Labcor stentless porcine bioprosthesis, made by Labcor Laboratories, Belo Horizonte-MG, Brazil.

The valve

Labcor Laboratories is a company located in Belo Horizonte, Brazil, which started prosthetic valve production in 1983. Since then more than 25 000 prostheses have been produced and implanted in many surgical centres in Brazil as well as in many other countries (Argentina, Uruguay, Portugal, Spain, France, Italy, Austria, Bulgaria, Israel, United Kingdom). The Labcor stentless porcine aortic valve is hand-sewn from three different leaflets (composite valve) selected from porcine aortic valves, from which all septal leaflets with a muscle shelf, or leaflets that present evidence of structural damage, as well as large areas of lipid infiltration are rejected (Figure 14.1). After passing inspection, the valves are individually sterilized and packed in 0.6% glutaraldehyde/20% ethanol solution, and stored in 0.2% glutaraldehyde solution, and are presented in dimensions corresponding to their internal diameters in millimetres,

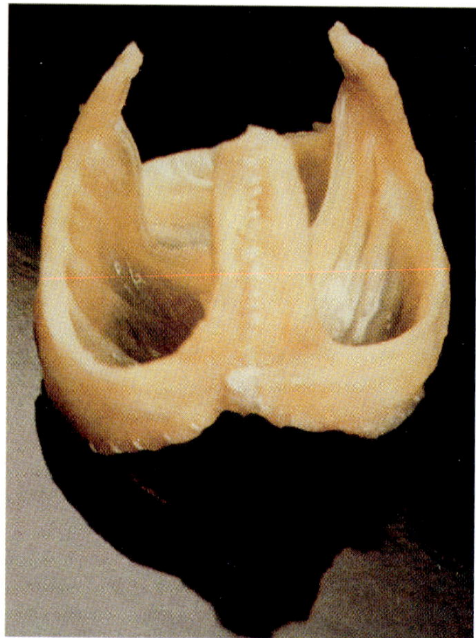

Figure 14.1 The Labcor stentless porcine bioprosthesis: a choice of three selected porcine leaflets, carefully hand-sewn.

which correspond to the sizers utilized during implantation.

Materials and methods

From April 1993 to November 1996, 61 patients have been submitted to aortic valve replacement employing the hand-sewn Labcor stentless bioprosthesis. In all patients a membrane oxygenator made by DMG Laboratories, Rio de Janeiro, Brazil, was used, and the operation was performed through a median sternotomy, under normothermic extracorporeal circulation, obtained by right atrio-aortic bypass, with retrograde continuous normothermic blood cardioplegia for myocardial protection. The aortic valve was exposed through an oblique aortotomy, coming down over the non-coronary sinus of Valsalva. After excision of the diseased aortic valve, the stentless prosthesis was implanted using the technique of double plane suture, the first with separated stitches of multifilamentary 2/0 polyester in the aortic annulus and a running suture with monofilamentary 4/0 polypropylene fixing the prosthesis to the aortic wall. Fifteen patients presented aortic stenosis, 34 insufficiency, nine stenosis plus insufficiency, and three dysfunction of an aortic prosthetic valve. There were 15 patients with associated pathologies: mitral valvopathy in seven, coronary insufficiency in six and aneurysm of the ascending aorta in two. Four patients had been submitted to previous cardiac operations: three cases of aortic valve replacement and one mitral valvoplasty. Associated operations were performed in 14 patients. The sizes of the valves implanted were: 21 mm (one patient), 23 mm (three patients), 25 mm (29 patients), 27 mm (16 patients) and 29 mm (12 patients).

Results

There was one (1.63%) perioperative death, due to low cardiac output syndrome in a reoperation of a thrombosed mechanical monoleaflet prosthesis. Two patients (3.27%) underwent emergency reoperation, both due to acute prosthetic regurgitation, one as a consequence of tearing a very fragile aortic wall and the other due to inadequacy of the size of the prosthesis to the aortic annulus, causing acute insufficiency. All the surviving patients were submitted to transthoracic echocardiogram at discharge and once at 6 months postoperatively. The echocardiogram identified a minimal regurgitation in most of the patients, which tended to disappear when an oversized prosthesis was implanted. The mean Doppler gradient for size was, respectively, 17.0 mmHg for size 21 mm, 14.8 mmHg for size 23 mm, 13.5 mmHg for size 25 mm, 12.0 mmHg for size 27 mm and 10.0 mmHg for size 29 mm, with a range of 4.0–20.0 mmHg and a mean gradient of 14.6 mmHg for all sizes. Five patients (8.19%) had been reoperated for prosthetic dysfunction: two due to pseudoaneurysm formation in the site of the second plane of suture on the aortic wall, two due to paravalvular leak caused by tunnel formation between the second and first planes of suture, and one consequent to infective endocarditis. All the surviving patients are doing well in follow-up, and are to be submitted to echo-Doppler cardiogram every 6 months.

Discussion

Although none of the now available bioprostheses meets all the criteria for acceptability, it is probable the anatomy of the coronary sinuses, reducing the stress on the leaflets of the porcine stentless valve, makes this prosthesis more durable than the stent-mounted ones. The first aortic valve replacement was reported by Ross in 1962,[2] followed by Barratt-Boyes in 1964.[3] Both used the technique of subcoronary implantation of an aortic valve homograft, as proposed by Duran and Gunning.[4] The first surgeon to describe the use of an aortic valve replacement with stentless heterologous aortic valve was Binet,[5] in 1965, and O'Brien,[6] in 1970 accumulated substantial experience with formaldehyde-preserved porcine stentless valves. The use of the stentless porcine valves was forgotten for many years, mainly as a consequence of failure of the homografts in many centres. Only recently, after the development of tissue fixation with glutaraldehyde and the good results obtained in the preservation of the stented porcine valves, has a renewed interest in the stentless porcine valves occurred in many countries, where all major heart valve manufacturers have developed their versions of stentless porcine aortic valves.

In our early experience, mild aortic valve insufficiency occurred frequently, a phenomenon that almost disappeared when an oversized prosthesis was implanted. Although mild, this regurgitation brought the concern of offering ideal conditions for infective endocarditis to develop and of precocious prosthetic failure due to increased mechanical failure. The claim that valve implantation using double plane suturing, a time-consuming procedure, is a more risky technique should not be taken into consideration, especially after the development of the continuous normothermic blood retroplegia, obtained by retrograde coronary sinus cannulation.

Another concern is the discrepancy between the aortic annulus and the aortic root in severe aortic insufficiency; this has been solved by some authors by suturing the valves in a supra-annular position, along with the non-coronary sinus, allowing the implantation of larger prostheses. We have some reservations about that procedure because two of our patients developed enormous pseudoaneurysms of the posterior aspect of the ascending aorta, close to the left coronary ostium, which resulted in an extremely serious complication, the correction of which involved many risks and difficulties. It is our major concern nowadays to put the stitches of the second plane of suture in the aortic wall very close to each other, in order to avoid any possibility of blood leaking between them. In addition, a pledget of bovine pericardium is used in the external aspect of the aorta, to reinforce the stitches used to hold the tops of the prostheses, before initiating the second plane of suture, in order to avoid tearing the aorta at those three points, with consequent penetration of the stitches inside the aortic lumen, as happened with some homografts implanted in our country in the early 1960s.

In spite of all these precautions we had two patients who developed paravalvular leak 3 years after original stentless porcine valve implantation in the aortic position. In both, the condition found at reoperation suggested a foreign-body reaction, and in one of them the supporting stitch came into the aortic lumen (Figure 14.2). This obliged us to send the explanted prostheses for meticulous anatomopathological studies, with the aim of discovering whether some delayed liberation of glutaraldehyde could have been the cause of failure in apposition and fixation between the prosthetic and the patient's tissues; the studies indicated no degeneration of the prostheses (Figure 14.3). It is surprising that this phenomenon appeared in late follow-up, the patients presenting absolutely competent prostheses in previous serial echo-Doppler cardiographic studies. None of the explanted valves showed any sign of degeneration, or tearing of cusps, or shrinkage of the leaflets, except in the case of infective endocarditis, in which one of the leaflets was perforated (Figure 14.4). We strongly suspect that the fragility of the

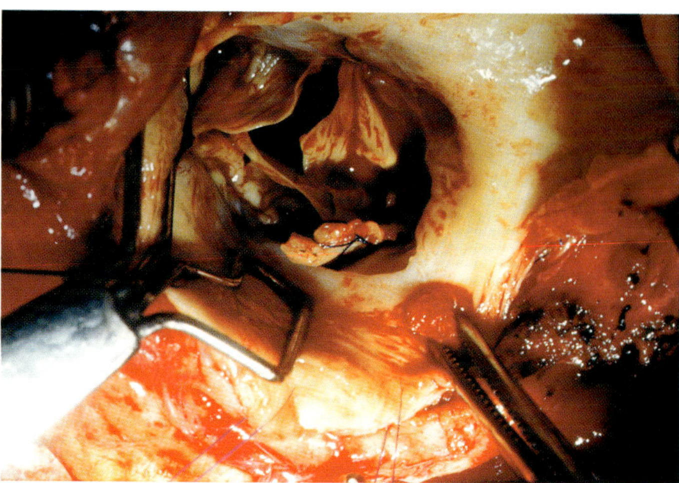

Figure 14.2 Labcor stentless porcine bioprosthesis in dysfunction in the aortic position: protrusion of one of the external holding stitches inside the aortic lumen.

ascending aorta should always be a major consideration when choosing the ideal aortic valve substitute. The stentless porcine bioprosthesis should not be considered in cases of degeneration of the ascending aorta, which would be, in the final analysis, the real stent of this bioprosthesis.

The indications for stentless porcine valve implantation are, in principle, the same as those for stented bioprostheses, but as longer durability is expected, younger patients should be considered as the main candidates. The Labcor stentless bioprosthesis is ideal for patients presenting severe aortic regurgitation in the presence of infective endocarditis, for no Dacron fabric is used in its manufacture, and the extreme flexibility of the porcine tissue allows the xenograft to fit perfectly over the irregularities of the destroyed aortic annulus which often present perivalvular abscesses. Another advantage of the stentless porcine bioprosthesis is the ease of its removal in cases of reoperation, when a very quick procedure must be performed.

Conclusions

The authors consider that the good early results with the Labcor stentless porcine aortic bioprosthesis indicate a promise of longer durability in comparison with stented prostheses. The early haemodynamic studies point to excellent long-term results, and Del Rizzo[7] reported remarkable reduction in the residual gradient and potential regression in left ventricular hypertrophy, a phenomenon that gives us the hope of progressive left ventricular remodelling more rapidly than if one implanted a stented prosthesis. Nevertheless, care must be taken and the criteria must be carefully evaluated when indicating this aortic substitute, avoiding its implantation in patients with very degenerated aortic walls. Despite the very demanding technique of implantation, our early results were encouraging, with few complications.

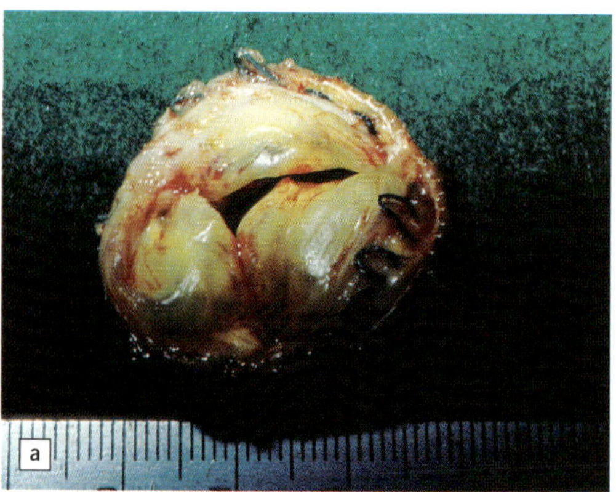

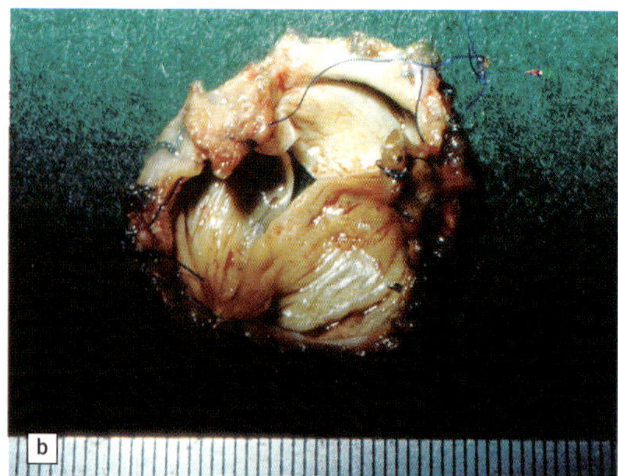

Figure 14.3 (a,b) Explanted Labcor stentless porcine bioprostheses in perfect aspect of conservation, without any sign of degeneration.

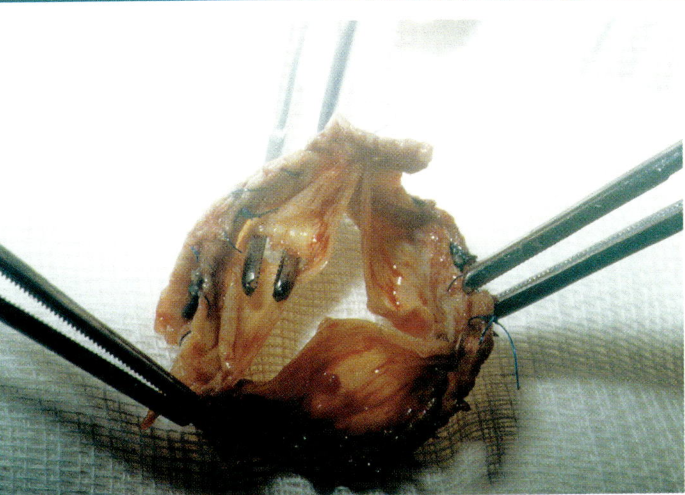

Figure 14.4 Perforation of one of the leaflets of a Labcor stentless porcine bioprosthesis in a case of infective endocarditis.

References

1. Gibbon J H Jr 1954 Application of mechanical heart and lung apparatus to cardiac surgery. Minn Med 37: 171–185
2. Ross D M 1964 Homotransplantation of aortic valve in subcoronary position. J Thorac Cardiovasc Surg 47: 713–719
3. Barratt-Boyes B G 1964 Homograft aortic valve replacement in aortic valve incompetence and stenosis. Thorax 19: 131–150
4. Duran C G, Gunning A J 1962 A method for placing a total homologous aortic valve in the subcoronary position. Lancet 2: 488–489
5. Binet J P, Duran C G, Carpentier A, Langloid J 1965 Heterologous valve transplantation. Lancet 2: 1275
6. O'Brien M F, Neilson G H, Galea E G *et al* 1970 Heterograft valves. Analysis of clinical results of valve replacement. Circulation 41(Suppl 5): 16–19
7. Del Rizzo D F, Goldman B S, Chritakis G T, David T E 1996 Hemodynamic benefits of the Toronto stentless valve. J Thorac Cardiovasc Surg 112(2): 1431–1446

CHAPTER 15

Haemodynamic performance and versatility of the porcine aortic root

S. Westaby and X. Y. Jin

Aortic valve disease in the elderly is dominated by calcific aortic stenosis. For worthwhile event-free survival in the very elderly it is important to achieve rapid improvement in ventricular mechanics, functional class and quality of life, without surgical or valve-related morbidity.[1,2] The type of valve prosthesis has an important bearing on postoperative left ventricular function, particularly in smaller sizes.[3] Comparisons between mechanical valves and bioprostheses tend to favour the bioprosthesis up to 5 years. After this time, tissue failure intervenes, so by 10 years the advantage is in favour of mechanical valves.[4]

Recently, it has become apparent that the non-physiological flow profile and residual pressure gradient across mechanical valves and stented bioprostheses are major determinants of event-free survival.[5] During normal activity (let alone physical exercise), Doppler-measured mean and peak pressure gradients increase from about 25 and 45 mmHg at rest to 40 and 70 mmHg, respectively (symptom-limited master two-step test).[6] Prosthesis-related left ventricular pressure increase is now emerging as the principal cause of incomplete regression of myocyte and ventricular hypertrophy, as well as the progression of interstitial fibrosis.[7] Residual gradients after valve replacement also result in impaired left ventricular diastolic function, irrespective of ejection fraction.[8] This has an important effect on late events, including the onset of fatal congestive heart failure.[9] Suboptimal left ventricular function impairs quality of life and increases mortality if aortic reoperation is required.

The role of stentless bioprostheses

Given that residual prosthetic pressure gradients are a late determinant of impaired left ventricular function, emerging stentless valve technology is of great importance. The objectives for the new stentless bioprostheses are improved haemodynamics, better durability and mitigation from early calcification through biochemical treatment. Though most surgeons avoid the use of homografts or autografts for routine aortic replacement, there is a resurgence of interest in their superlative haemodynamic performance in younger patients.[10,11] An understanding that these benefits need not be restricted to the young has prompted further evaluation of the stentless porcine xenografts first used by Binet in the 1960s.[12] For a specified external diameter, the effective orifice area is larger (and the pressure drop lower) than for stented valves.[13]

Accelerated fatigue tests show the valve stent to be obstructive and the major factor governing stress on the tissue component.[14] Stent mounting and tissue preservation methods lead to suboptimal valve geometry so that the durability of stented xenografts is less favourable than that of freehand sewn aortic homografts. Degeneration, calcification and cusp rupture occur earlier, especially in younger patients.[15] A similar time course of valve failure occurred when aortic homografts were stent mounted. The average time for homograft valve failure exceeds 12 years when freehand sewn, but was approximately 9 years during the short era of stent mounting.[16] The average time for structural failure of a stent-mounted xenograft in the aortic position (depending on the age of the patient) is also 8–9 years.[17] For the last few years of its lifespan the stented xenograft is deformed, calcified and poorly compliant, mimicking native valve pathology (Figure 15.1).

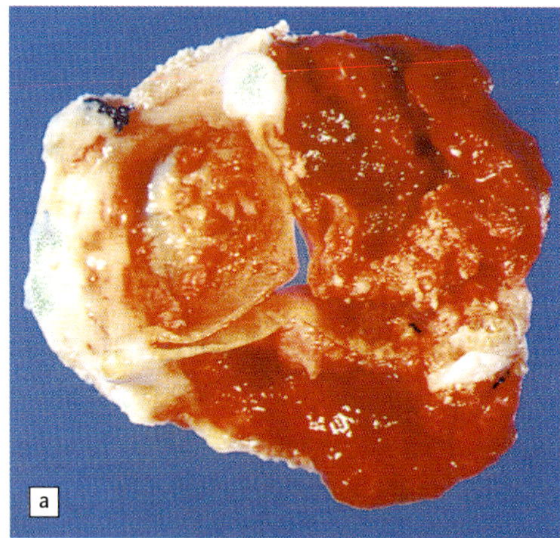

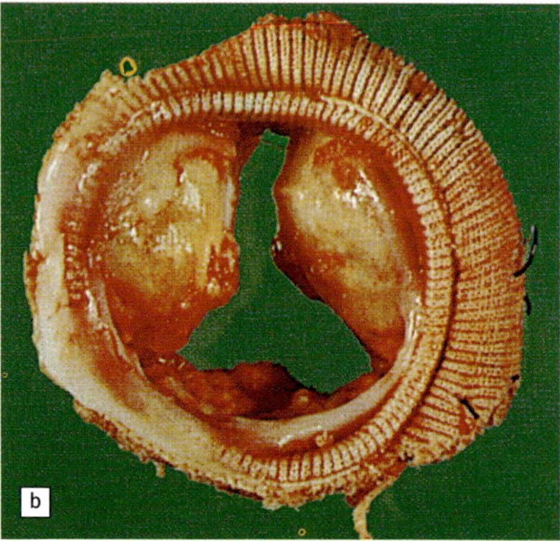

Figure 15.1 Deformed, calcified and clearly pathological stented xenografts (a) in a 14-year-old patient 3 years after implantation and (b) in a 68-year-old patient after 8 years.

Since the native aortic wall provides the best environment for a valve cusp, it is logical to expect that elimination of the stent will reduce stress on the tissue and improve durability. The ideal stentless aortic valve is the patient's own pulmonary valve.[11] When this is used for aortic root replacement, the flow characteristics are perfect and the durability indefinite. However, the Ross procedure exchanges a single valve operation for a double root replacement with an inherent increase in the risk. Aortic homografts convey excellent haemodynamic function, but durability is limited and restricted availability ensures that aortic homografts are not used routinely. By contrast, stentless xenografts are now freely available in all sizes and are user friendly. Reproducible and reliable operative techniques allow widespread application for degenerative aortic valve disease in the elderly.[18] With modern myocardial preservation techniques, the extended ischaemic time required for a more complex procedure has little effect on clinical outcome.[19] On the contrary, the complete relief of increased ejection resistance has an early benefit on left ventricular function which is not seen with stented bioprostheses.[20] The maximum shortening velocity of the myocardium increases to a significantly greater extent after the use of a stentless xenograft than with its stented equivalent. This is explained in part by the alteration in forced velocity relation. The greater the decrease in contracting force (peak wall stress), the greater the increase in contraction velocity. Early changes in ventricular relaxation and end-diastolic pressure are better with stentless valves, indicating that left ventricular diastolic performance also improves within 24 hours of surgery. Stentless valves provide a significant increase in left ventricular stroke volume and stroke work index compared to stented valves. These changes are firmly based on the underlying improvements in left ventricular systolic and diastolic function.[21] These haemodynamic advantages are particularly important in patients with a small aortic root.[22]

David has case matched Toronto SPV valve (St Jude Medical, MN, USA) patients with those receiving the Hancock 2 valve (Medtronic, MN, USA).[13] When the duration of follow-up exceeds 5 years, the actuarial survival of patients with the stentless valve is 93% versus 86% for those with the stented bioprosthesis. Proportional hazard analysis shows valve-related complications to be three times more frequent in stented-valve patients. This suggests that improved valve function and left ventricular mechanics translate directly into improved event-free survival. Another characteristic of the Toronto SPV valves and Freestyle (Medtronic, MN) valves has been the progressive and reproducible improvement in valve function with time. Detailed echocardiographic follow-up shows a consistent fall in mean systolic valve gradients and an increase in effective orifice area progressively from the time of implantation to 18 months postoperatively.[23] At this time, valve gradients are reproducibly less than 10 mmHg, even for sizes between 19 and 23 mm. On exercise or during dobutamine stress echocardiography these gradients remain below 20 mmHg.[24] When the Freestyle valve (Figure 15.2) is implanted by aortic root replacement, the postoperative valve gradients are even lower since a larger valve can be employed in the supra-annular position.[25]

Given these unequivocal and compelling findings for stentless valves in the aortic position, why are they not used for every patient? The answer appears to lie in the modest degree of technical difficulty in patients with calcified aortic sinuses or post-stenotic dilatation in whom additional effort is required to secure a fail-safe implant. In order to test potential surgical problems, we elected to implant the Freestyle valve in all patients (without selection) in whom a tissue valve was appropriate. Candidates for a tissue valve were those over 70 years of age and others who had contraindications for anticoagulant therapy or who elected for a bioprosthesis. After assessing Freestyle valve performance for 2 years, the age limit was reduced to 65 years.

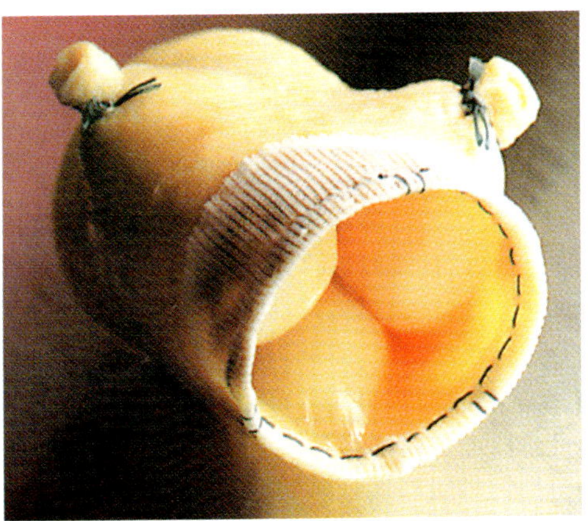

Figure 15.2 The Freestyle valve (Medtronic, MN, USA).

Patients and methods

The group includes 159 consecutive patients aged between 42 and 89 years (mean age 75). Only 13 patients were aged less than 65 years. Ninety-two (58%) were male and 67 (42%) were female. One hundred and forty-five patients (91%) had aortic stenosis with a bicuspid valve or senile degeneration of a tricuspid valve. One had a quadricusp valve and five a failed bioprosthesis. Two patients had extensive calcification of the valve and aortic root from previous radiotherapy for breast cancer. Fourteen patients had pure aortic regurgitation. Two patients with aortic regurgitation had active bacterial endocarditis. Another had acute type A dissection with pre-existing degenerative disease which required valve replacement. Sixty-five (41%) of the patients had concomitant coronary artery disease requiring revascularization (mean 2 ± 1 grafts). For aortic stenosis patients, mean left ventricular mass index (g/m^2) was 162.4 ± 63.7. The upper limit of normal is 125 g/m^2. One hundred and twenty-nine patients (81%) were in sinus rhythm, 28 (18%) were in atrial fibrillation and two were paced. One hundred and forty were in NYHA functional class III or IV.

Surgical methods

The Freestyle stentless porcine xenograft (Figure 15.2) consists of an intact aortic root (equivalent to an aortic homograft) with the coronary arteries ligated and the inflow covered with Dacron cloth to facilitate suture placement. The Dacron cloth is elevated beneath the right coronary to cover the septal muscle aspect of the annulus. The valve cusps are glutaraldehyde fixed at net zero pressure to preserve the collagen architecture. Without loading, the cusps are in a semi-open position.

As for the aortic homograft, either subcoronary implantation or full root replacement can be used. Our preferred technique is the modified subcoronary method

(Westaby), in which the porcine left and right coronary sinuses are scalloped to accommodate the human coronary ostia (Figure 15.3).[23] The porcine non-coronary sinus is left intact in order to facilitate accurate spatial orientation of the commissural pillars since two remain in continuity with the porcine non-coronary sinus. Glutaraldehyde fixation provides the porcine root with a stiffness but flexibility which greatly facilitates implantation. The aim of the modified subcoronary method is to fill the human root with a slightly smaller porcine equivalent. The human valve annulus is sized accurately to select the Freestyle valve. The human aorta is tailored to fit the outflow of the porcine cylinder so that dilatation of the sinotubular junction is not a contraindication for use.

The site of the transverse aortotomy is carefully judged with the aorta distended by blood or cardioplegia. The incision is at least 1 cm above the right coronary ostium and about 0.5 cm above the sinotubular junction. Two-thirds horizontal transection at this level provides excellent access to annulus and coronary arteries. The root is held open with stay sutures so that no retractors are required in the operative field. After

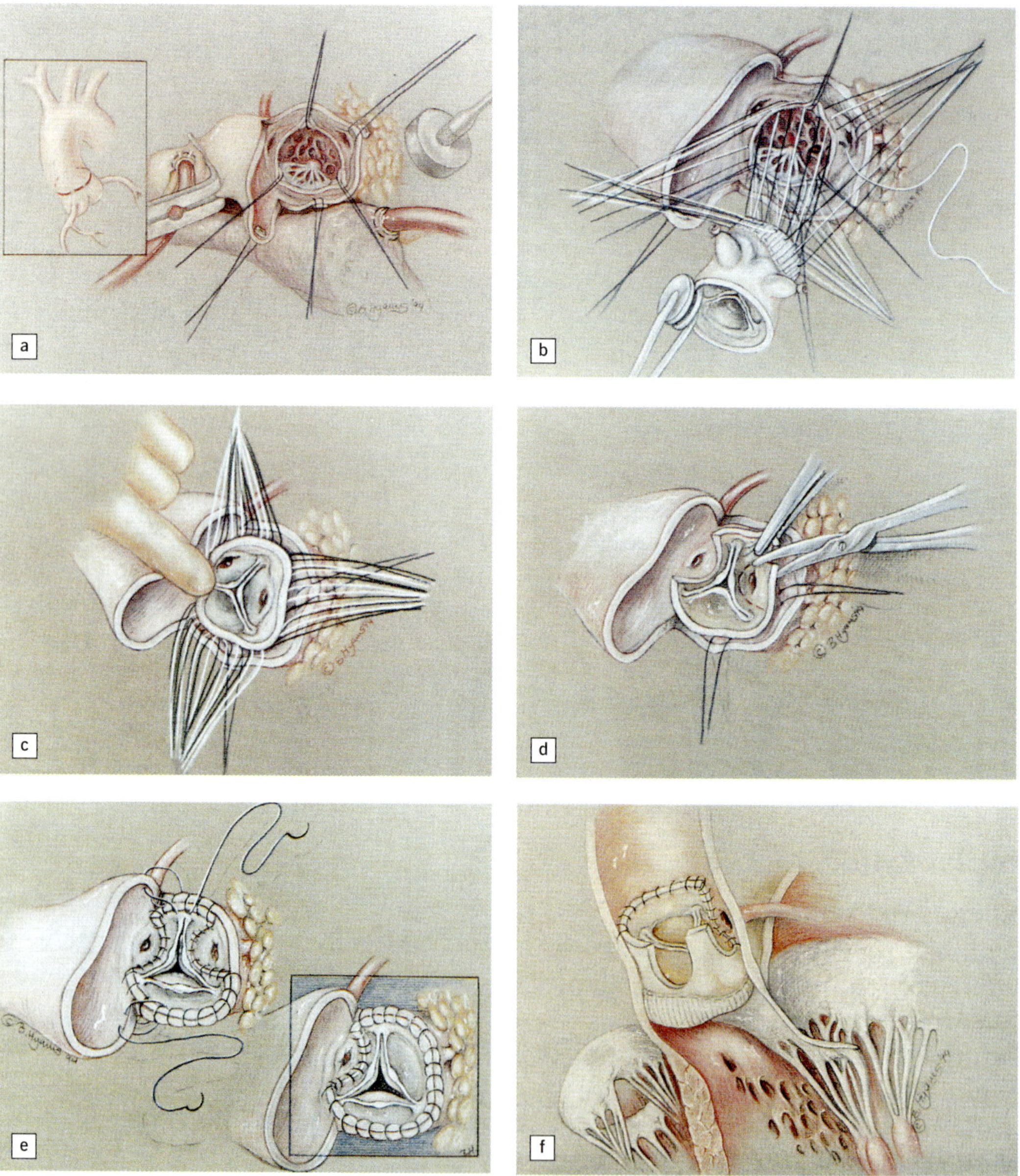

Figure 15.3 (a–f) Surgical technique for Freestyle valve implantation.

excising the native valve, the simple interrupted valve sutures begin at the base of each commissural triangle. The sutures are placed in the same horizontal plane in order to accommodate the inflow of the Freestyle valve. In the middle of the excised cusp, the suture is placed directly through the annulus itself. The Freestyle valve inflow is consequently drawn down well below the apex of the commissural pillars. About five sutures are placed per cusp. This is less than required for a homograft, since the porcine inflow is Dacron covered.

Care must be taken to align the porcine coronaries close to the human coronary ostia. The porcine coronaries are closer together and this must be taken into account. With the correct alignment, the sutures are placed through the Dacron inflow and the valve seated into the annulus. Only then are the two coronary sinuses excised to achieve subcoronary implantation. The outflow of the porcine cylinder is then cut back so that the height corresponds directly to the height of the transverse aortotomy above the annulus. A single running outflow suture of 4/0 Prolene is then started above the freestanding commissural pillar (Figure 15.3). The porcine outflow is directly sutured to the transected native aorta, thus suspending the porcine root within the human root. The first limb of the suture is taken beneath the right coronary artery and around the non-coronary sinus. The remaining limb is then taken beneath the left coronary artery. Partial thickness bites are used to secure the porcine wall to the human aorta in subcoronary position. Both limbs of the suture are brought outside the aorta and tied, after which one limb of the suture is used again to close the aortotomy. This method, which is simple and reliable, was used in all but two who had root replacement. In the presence of severe calcification of the aortic sinuses, a cutting needle was passed backwards and forwards through the aortic wall in preference to tangential bites. Calcification was only insurmountable in the two patients with severe radiotherapy damage, for whom root replacement was performed in preference.

Two modifications of the modified subcoronary method were employed. If the right coronary artery was occluded at the ostium, then the porcine aortic wall was left intact in the right coronary sinus, thereby simplifying the outflow suture line (Figure 15.3). This approach was adopted in eight patients. In four female patients with small aortic root and less than 6 mm between the annulus (above the conduction tissue) and right coronary ostium, the high part of the inflow cloth in the porcine right coronary sinus was rotated to the human non-coronary sinus. This prevents the pitfall of distorting the cloth in order to accommodate the suture line beneath the coronary ostium (Figure 15.4). The Freestyle valve was also employed in two patients with infective endocarditis and aortic root abscesses. In the presence of excavating infection, we usually prefer to use an aortic homograft and no synthetic material but the Freestyle valve is more readily available and user friendly. In one patient with acute type A dissection, the diseased native valve was not suitable for repair and was replaced with the porcine aortic root by the modified subcoronary method. The dissected native aorta was

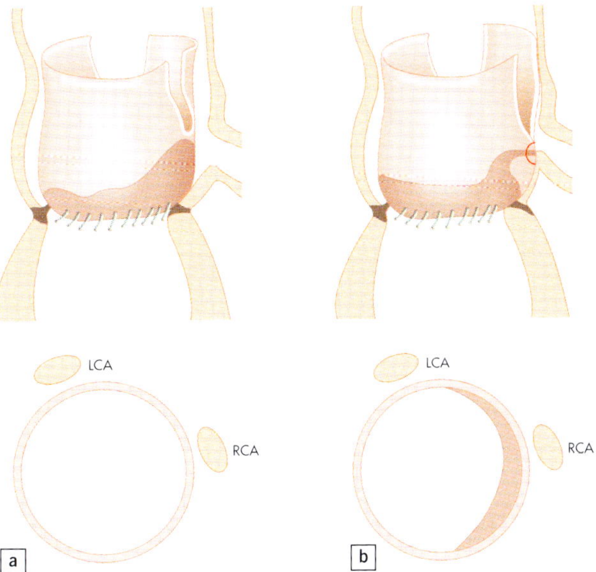

Figure 15.4 The risk of inflow cloth distortion under the right coronary ostium. This leads to unsuspected elevated outflow gradients and the risk of cusp prolapse onto the buckled cloth.

reconstituted with GRF glue and the porcine cylinder reinforced the repair by excluding the dissected tissue (Figure 15.5). The repair was completed by ascending aortic replacement with a Dacron graft using the open distal anastomotic technique. With this combination of surgical methods, the Freestyle valve was suitable in the 159 consecutive patients, and no patient over the age of 70 (first 2 years) then 65 years (subsequently) received a mechanical valve. All operations were performed by the same surgeon (S.W).

Haemodynamic studies

Transthoracic echocardiography was performed at the time of discharge from hospital, then between 3 and 6 months postoperatively, and at 12 and 24 months after operation. Left ventricular cavity size and wall thickness, end-diastolic dimension, septal thickness, posterior wall thickness and end-systolic dimensions were measured from M mode echocardiograms. Dimensional shortening fraction and the ratio of wall thickness to cavity radius at end diastole were determined according to the criteria of the American Society of Echocardiography.[26] Left ventricular muscle mass was calculated and indexed to body surface area.[27] The haemodynamics of the left ventricular outflow tract and stentless valve were determined by measuring Doppler ultrasound flow velocities in the outflow tract and across the stentless valve at recording speeds of 100 mm/s for off-line analysis. Peak flow velocities and the time integral of systolic flow velocity in the left ventricular outflow tract and aortic valve derived from the Doppler recordings.[28] The acceleration (onset to peak flow velocity) and deceleration (peak flow to termination) times, deceleration rate and the total ejection time of the flow velocity across the aortic valve were also determined from the Doppler recordings. Left ventricular stroke volume was calculated as the product of the cross-sectional area and flow velocity time integral in the outflow tract. The effective orifice area of the Freestyle valve was calculated by the continuity equation (stroke volume divided by valve flow velocity time integral), and a conventional calculation of mean pressure drop across the aortic valve was made from the simplified Bernoulli equation. Blood pressure was recorded non-invasively and body surface area was calculated from height and weight. Global stroke volume index and cardiac index were then calculated from stroke volume, heart rate and body surface area. Global stroke work was then determined from the mean arterial pressure and mean net aortic valve pressure drop and indexed to body surface area. Myocardial stroke work was defined as global stroke work divided by muscle mass volume.

Echocardiographic and haemodynamic data are presented as mean ± one

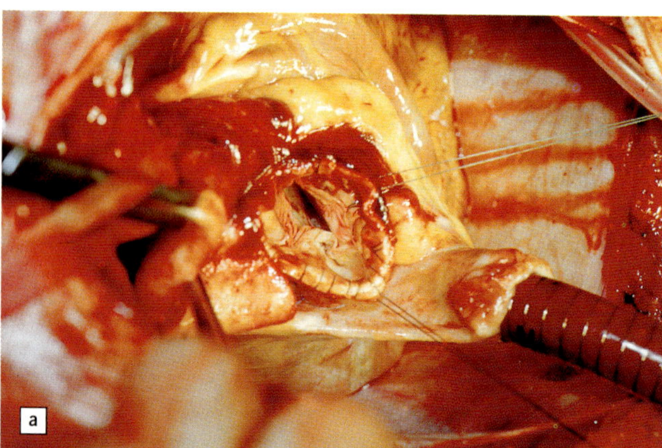

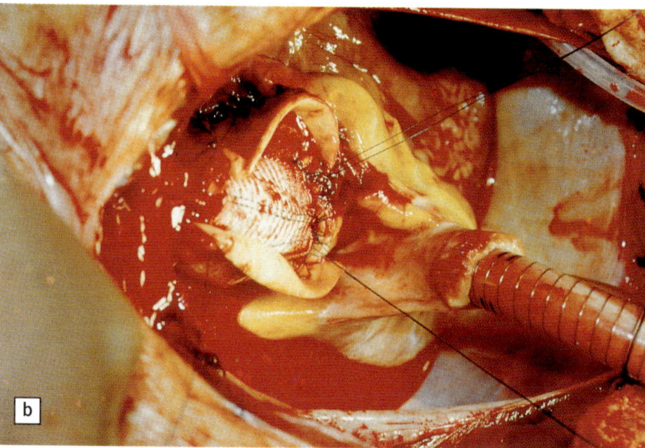

Figure 15.5 (a and b) The Freestyle valve used for valve replacement in acute type A dissection.

standard deviation. One-way analysis of variance was performed to test the significance of changes in each measurement over the follow-up time. When this was significant a further comparison of 95% confidence intervals with respect to the discharge echocardiography was carried out using Dummett's method. Differences were considered statistically significant for a p-value of less than 0.05.

Results

One hundred and thirty procedures were elective (82%) and 29 were emergency operations (18%). One patient (0.6%) required re-entry for bleeding from a vein graft side branch. Mean aortic cross-clamp times with and without coronary bypass were 43 and 61 min, respectively. Three patients with severe diffuse coronary disease required postoperative intra-aortic balloon pumping for up to 4 days. This did not damage the valve implant.

There were eight hospital deaths (5%), all in NYHA IV patients with severe coronary disease. None was valve related. Initially, warfarin was prescribed for 3 months with an INR of between 2.0 and 2.5. Warfarin treatment was discontinued altogether after two elderly patients suffered a cerebral haemorrhage. The patients now receive 75 mg aspirin per day and there have been no thromboembolic events with or without warfarin.

There were no valve-related early or late deaths. One patient underwent reoperation at 3 months for early prosthetic valve endocarditis. After removing the continuous outflow suture, the valve separated easily from the human aortic wall. A second patient underwent urgent repair of acute type A dissection 2 years after Freestyle valve implantation. Whilst the dissection caused valve prolapse and aortic regurgitation, ascending aortic replacement restored competence (Figure 15.6). There were no perceptible degenerative changes in the porcine aortic cusps or wall. There was a fine endothelial covering of the outflow suture line.

Haemodynamic data

A significant fall in heart rate between 3 and 6 months postoperatively was accompanied by a reciprocal increase in global stroke volume index so that cardiac index remained unchanged. By 12 months after surgery, left ventricular mass index had fallen from 162 ± 64 to 109 ± 38 g/m^2. There was also a significant decrease in the thickness of the interventricular septum and posterior wall of the left ventricle to literally normal limits (T/R ratio from 0.61 ± 0.25 to 0.43 ± 0.10). Whilst ventricular cavity size remained unchanged, left ventricular stroke volume index increased from 29.4 ± 10 to 42 ± 17 ml/m^2. Myocardial stroke work progressed from 3.1 ± 1.6 to 5.2 ± 2.2 mJ/cm^3 (all $p < 0.01$ by ANOVA), whilst left ventricular outflow tract diameter remained unchanged. In the meantime, stentless valve effective orifice area increased from 1.84 ± 0.81 to 2.22 ± 0.73. The transvalvular increase in mean flow velocity fell significantly from 82 ± 31 to 49 ± 24 cm/s, whilst mean pressure drop fell from 9.7 ± 5.0 to 5.2 ± 3.7 mmHg (all $p < 0.001$ by ANOVA). Correspondingly, the deceleration time of aortic flow velocity increased from 153.6 ± 64.1 to 202.7 ± 37.6 ms ($p < 0.001$ by ANOVA). These findings show that, as left ventricular hypertrophy regresses, the left ventricular systolic function improves. Left ventricular stroke volume increased as the heart rate fell and cardiac output remained constant. The stroke volume increase was solely due to the changes in flow velocity time integral at outflow tract level. Despite an apparent increase in effective orifice area of the valve and the fall in left ventricular mass and septal thickness, the diameter of the left ventricular outflow tract remained unchanged. By contrast, at aortic valve level, the increased stroke volume was not accompanied by any change in flow velocity time integral so that effective cross-sectional area of the jet at this level must have increased correspondingly. The

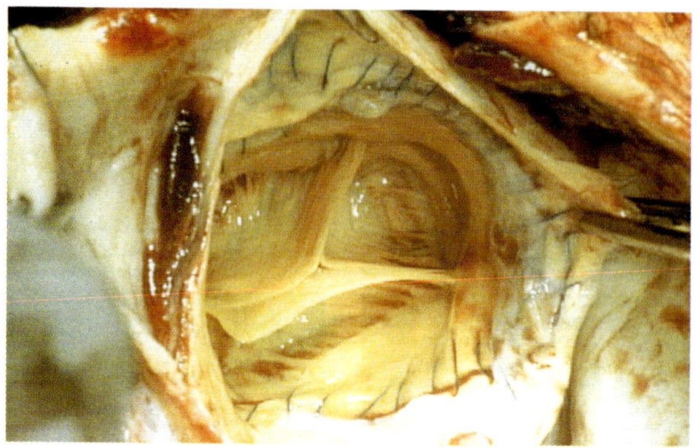

Figure 15.6 Freestyle valve 2 years after implantation in a patient with acute type A dissection. There is no calcification in the aortic wall or cusps.

changes occurred progressively so that by 2 years the effective orifice area had increased by 38% and the mean pressure drop across the Freestyle valve had fallen by 45%. The dramatic improvements in haemo-dynamics were translated into early improvement in exercise tolerance with progression from NYHA III or IV to NYHA I.

Discussion

It was possible to implant the Freestyle valve into all patients irrespective of the condition of the aortic root. In particularly difficult circumstances after extensive radiotherapy damage, the pathological aortic sinuses were excised and the root replaced. This is a more demanding operation with increased hospital mortality when used routinely. For the modified subcoronary method the main aortic cross-clamp time for isolated aortic valve replacement (43.6 ± 6.4 min) does not greatly exceed that for a stented valve, and does not increase hospital mortality. In reoperations we have been able to use a larger (e.g. 25 mm after removing a 23 mm stented prosthesis) Freestyle valve with a substantial increase in orifice area. The degenerate Carpentier–Edwards valves had been implanted in patients in their late 60s, but needed replacement for high gradients and new symptoms at between 3 and 10 years postoperatively. As life expectancy increases, it is necessary to reconsider the use of stented xenografts in patients under 80 years of age.

There is an important relationship between left ventricular ejection dynamics and stentless valve performance. Flow across the normal aortic valve is inertial. Left ventricular pressure is greater than that in the aorta as flow accelerates, but during the latter half of ejection when flow decelerates, the pressure relationship is reversed. Our studies show that this also applies to newly inserted stentless valves. By contrast, for stented bioprostheses, left ventricular pressure is greater than that in the aorta throughout the whole ejection period because of the obstructive nature of stented valve flow.[20,29] This results in a less significant fall in valve pressure gradient with time and a correspondingly less impressive resolution of the left ventricular hypertrophy.[30,31] The progressive fall in transvalvular pressure gradient and an increase in effective orifice area reflect the important benefits of stentless bioprostheses on left ventricular mechanics. The dimensions of the left ventricular outflow tract remain constant after valve replacement, but an increase in blood velocity time integral provides an increase in stroke volume. At valve level, the velocity time integral remains unchanged whilst stroke volume increases. This represents a change in flow pattern, with a wider flow jet and a more rectangular flow profile. The increased stroke volume is also mediated by prolongation of the deceleration period of ejection when left ventricular pressure is below that in the aorta. Improved haemodynamics lead to regression of hypertrophy and relative wall thickness at ventricular level accompanied by a striking (>70%) increase in external ventricular work per cm^3 of myocardium. All of these changes have the effect of lowering energy expenditure during ejection by reducing blood flow velocity and acceleration and thus transvalvular pressure gradients (Table 15.1).[21] By contrast, the stent-mounted xenograft provides a fixed resistance to flow which cannot improve with time, and which provides a dramatic increase in systolic pressure gradients with exercise, even before degeneration of the tissue component.[31,32]

Table 15.1 Three-year follow-up of Freestyle aortic valve haemodynamics and left ventricular (LV) function (mean ± SD)

Item	Follow-up (months)					ANOVA
	0.5 (n=146)	3–6 (n=108)	12 (n=109)	24 (n=85)	36-48 (n=50)	p
Valve size (mm)	23.6 ± 1.8	23.7 ± 2.0	23.6 ± 1.9	23.4 ± 2.0	23.4 ± 2.0	0.732
HR (bpm)	83.9 ± 16.9	73.2 ± 13.1*	73.4 ± 13.3*	68.6 ± 11.5*	67.9 ± 12.7*	<0.0001
EOA (cm^2)	1.84 ± 0.81	1.96 ± 0.69	2.02 ± 0.70	2.21 ± 0.77*	2.22 ± 0.73*	0.002
Mean PG (mmHg)	97 ± 50	5.1 ± 3.0*	5.2 ± 3.7*	5.3 ± 3.8*	5.2 ± 3.9*	<0.0001
Valve resistance (dyne.s/cm^5)	48.6 ± 34.4	30.6 ± 19.0*	30.1 ± 21.7*	26.9 ± 19.6*	27.1 ± 24.5*	<0.0001
LV mass index (g/m^2)	162 ± 64	126 ± 40*	109 ± 38*	108 ± 39*	127 ± 50*	<0.0001
T/R ratio	0.61 ± 0.25	0.51 ± 0.17*	0.43 ± 0.10*	0.45 ± 0.14*	0.52 ± 0.13*	<0.0001
LVEF (%)	55.6 ± 16.8	60.0 ± 14.0	60.9 ± 14.7*	62.2 ± 12.5*	61.2 ± 13.9	0.009

Note: these data included up to 194 patients who had aortic valve replacement with a Freestyle valve, and had one or more echo follow-ups, with a total of 497 echos analysed.

*Significantly different from 0.5 months compared with 95% confidence interval.

HR, heart rate; EOA, effective orifice area; PG, prosthesis pressure gradient;T/R ratio, left ventricular wall thickness to radius ratio; LVEF, left ventricular ejection fraction.

Consequently, the argument for stentless bioprostheses in aortic position is now compelling, particularly for the elderly in whom left ventricular structure and function may normalize within 12 months of operation.

The valve is suitable for endocarditis patients where infection is restricted to the aortic cusps, but we prefer to use a homograft without any foreign material for excavating sepsis and root abscesses. We also found the valve to be particularly effective for repair of the aortic root in acute type A dissection patients who are not amenable to valve resuspension. The porcine root is implanted within the damaged sinuses and reinforces the glue repair (Figure 15.5 a and b). Only a small rim of dissected aortic root around the coronary ostia remains exposed to the circulation.

Whilst life expectancy in elderly patients is limited by other problems, surgically treated aortic stenosis still has an excellent prognosis, with survival of around 75% in 5 years, 60% in 10 years and 40% at 15 years.[33] Hospital mortality for isolated aortic valve replacement under the age of 70 is around 2%. This increases to between 4% and 5% in patients between 70 and 80 years, and up to 10% in those over 80 years.[34,35] Use of a stentless valve has not increased this operative mortality (hospital mortality 6%), despite the fact that 134 patients were NYHA III–V at the time of operation. Midterm results are impressive, with a very low incidence of endocarditis, thromboembolism or sudden death. This is consistent with the improved valve haemodynamics and rapid normalization of left ventricular function found in these patients.

Conclusions

Surgery for aortic stenosis is one of medicine's great success stories, but there is increasing realization that the type of valve prosthesis has an important bearing on outcome. Given the unequivocal differences in rehabilitation of the left ventricle after use of a stentless xenograft, it becomes progressively more difficult to justify the use of first-generation technology.

References

1. Bessone L N, Pupello D F, Hiro S P *et al* 1988 Surgical management of aortic valve disease in the elderly: longitudinal analysis. Ann Thorac Surg 46: 264–269
2. Lindblom D, Lindblom U, Qvist J, Lundstrom H 1990 Long term relative survival rates after heart valve replacement. J Am Coll Cardiol 15: 566–573
3. Jaffe W M, Coverdale H A, Roche A H *et al* 1990 Rest and exercise hemodynamics of 20 to 23 mm allograft Medtronic Intact (porcine) and St Jude medical valves in the aortic position. J Thorac Cardiovasc Surg 100: 167–174
4. Cohn L H, Allred E N, DiSesa V J *et al* 1984 Early and late risk of aortic valve replacement: a 12 year concomitant comparison of the porcine bioprosthetic and tilting disc prosthetic aortic valves. J Thorac Cardiovasc Surg 88: 695–701
5. Barratt-Boyes B G, Christie G W 1994 What is the best bioprosthetic operation for the small aortic root?: allograft, autograft, porcine, pericardial? Stented or unstented? J Card Surg 9: 158–164
6. Dumesnil J G, Yoganathan A P 1992 Valve prosthesis haemodynamics and the problems of high transprosthetic pressure gradients. Eur J Cardiothorac Surg 6(Suppl 1): 34–38
7. Orsinelli D A, Aurigemma F I P, Battista S *et al* 1993 Left ventricular hypertrophy and mortality after aortic valve replacement for aortic stenosis. J Am Coll Cardiol 22: 1678–1683
8. Villari B, Vassali G, Monra E S *et al* 1995 Normalization of diastolic dysfunction in aortic stenosis late after valve replacement. Circulation 91: 2353–2358
9. Jin X Y, Zhang Z M, Gibson D *et al* 1996 Effect of valve substitute on changes in left ventricular function and hypertrophy after aortic valve replacement. Ann Thorac Surg 62: 683–690
10. McGiffen D C, O'Brien M F, Stafford E G *et al* 1988 Long term results of the cryopreserved allograft aortic valve: continuing evidence for superior valve durability. J Card Surg 3(Suppl): 289–296
11. Ross D 1991 Replacement of the aortic valve with a pulmonary autograft: the 'switch' operation. Ann Thorac Surg 52: 1346–1350

12. Binet J P, Duran C G, Carpentier A, Langlois J 1965 Heterologous aortic valve transplantation. Lancet 2: 1275
13. David T E, Feindel C M, Bos J, Sun Z, Scully H E, Rakowski H 1994 Aortic valve replacement with stentless porcine aortic valve. A six year experience. J Thorac Cardiovasc Surg 108: 1030–1036
14. Vesely I, Boughner D, Song T 1988 Tissue buckling as a mechanism of bioprosthetic valve failure. Ann Thorac Surg 46: 302–308
15. Ishihara T, Ferrans V J, Boyce S W *et al* 1981 Structure and classification of cuspal tears and perforation in porcine bioprosthetic cardiac valves implanted in patients. Am J Cardiol 48: 665–677
16. Angell W W, Grehl T M, Buch W, Waerflein R D 1973 Mounted fresh homograft for aortic valve replacement. Med J Aust 21(Suppl): 74–76
17. Pelletier L C, Carrier M, Leclerc Y *et al* 1992 Influence of age on late results of valve replacement with porcine bioprostheses. J Cardiovasc Surg 33: 526–533
18. Westaby S, Huysmans H A, David T E 1998 Stentless aortic bioprostheses: compelling data from the Second International Symposium. Ann Thorac Surg 65: 235–240
19. Menasche P, Tronc F, Nguyen A *et al* 1994 Retrograde warm blood cardioplegia preserves hypotrophied myocardium. A clinical study. Ann Thorac Surg 57: 1429–1435
20. Jin X Y, Gibson D G, Yacoub M H, Pepper J R 1995 Perioperative assessment of aortic homograft, Toronto stentless valve and stented bioprosthesis in the aortic position. Ann Thorac Surg 60: S395–S401
21. Jin X Y, Westaby S, Gibson D *et al* 1997 Left ventricular remodelling and improvement in Freestyle valve haemodynamics. Eur J Cardiothorac Surg 12: 63–69
22. Sintek C F, Fletcher A D, Khonsari S 1995 Stentless porcine aortic root: valve of choice for the elderly patient with small aortic root? J Thorac Cardiovasc Surg 109: 871–876
23. Westaby S, Amarasena N, Long V *et al* 1995 Time-related hemodynamic changes after aortic valve replacement with the Freestyle stentless xenograft. Ann Thorac Surg 60: 1633–1639
24. Walther T, Falk V, Autschbach R *et al* 1994 Hemodynamic assessment of the stentless Toronto SPV bioprosthesis by echocardiography. J Heart Valve Dis 3: 657–665
25. Kon N D, Westaby S A, Amarasena N *et al* 1995 Comparison of implant techniques using the Freestyle stentless porcine aortic valve. Ann Thorac Surg 59: 857–862
26. Sahn D J, DeMaria A, Kisslo J, Weyman A 1978 Recommendations regarding quantitation in M-mode echocardiography: results of a survey of echocardiographic measurements. Circulation 58: 1072–1083
27. Devereux R B, Alonso D R, Lutas E M *et al* 1986 Echocardiographic assessment of left ventricular hypertrophy: comparison to necropsy finding. Am J Cardiol 57: 450–458
28. Chambers J, Shah P M 1995 Recommendations for echocardiographic assessment of replacement heart valves. J Heart Valve Dis 4: 9–13
29. Jin X Y, Pepper J R, Brecker S J *et al* 1994 Non-uniform recovery of left ventricular function after aortic valve replacement for isolated aortic valve stenosis. Am J Cardiol 74: 1142–1146
30. Morris J J, Schaff H V, Mullasny C J *et al* 1993 Determinants of survival and recovery of left ventricular function after aortic valve replacement. Ann Thorac Surg 56: 22–30
31. Hoffmann A, Haefeli R, Weiss P *et al* 1992 Influence of different pressure gradients on later clinical outcome after aortic valve replacement. J Card Surg 7: 9–16
32. Van der Brink B B, Verheul H A, Visser C A *et al* 1992 Value of exercise Doppler echocardiography in patients with prosthetic or bioprosthetic cardiac valves. Am J Cardiol 69: 367–372
33. Lund O 1993 Valve replacement for aortic stenosis: the curative potential of early operation. Scand J Thorac Cardiovasc Surg 40(Suppl): 1–137
34. Elayda M A A , Hull R J, Peul R M *et al* Aortic valve replacement in patients 80 years and older: operative risk and long term results. Circulation 88(Part 2): 11–16
35. He G W, Acuff T E, Ryan W H *et al* 1994 Aortic valve replacement: determinants of operative mortality. Ann Thorac Surg 57: 1140–1146

CHAPTER 16

Root inclusion with stentless bioprostheses

H. A. Huysmans, A. P. Kappetein and L. Baur

The technique of root inclusion was first described by O'Brien for the implantation of homografts.[1] The root inclusion technique for stentless bioprostheses has some important advantages over the most widely used subcoronary implant technique and also over the root replacement technique. In root inclusion a ring of prosthesis aortic wall, including the sinotubular junction, just above the tops of the commissures, is preserved, thereby maintaining distances between the tops of the commissures exactly at their original length. This is essential to obtain normal loading of the valve leaflets with normal stresses and strains, as described by us earlier.[2] Normal loading of the leaflets is probably one of the most important factors for durability of the valve. This also explains the better durability of a stentless valve as compared with a stented valve.[3,4] Especially in a dilated aortic root, root replacement and root inclusion are the only methods to preserve completely the original geometry of the valve, in contrast to the subcoronary implant technique, with which this is very difficult. Root inclusion gives less risk of postoperative bleeding because, in contrast to the root replacement technique, only one suture line is exposed to the pericardium. The aortic wall part of the porcine bioprosthesis will probably calcify in the course of time; this might make a reoperation, if needed, very difficult. With root inclusion the porcine aorta is protected by the patient's aorta, which will probably make reoperation easier. The disadvantage of the root inclusion technique is that it is more difficult than the subcoronary and root replacement techniques and therefore may need somewhat longer cross-clamp times.

In our own experience we found that after a learning curve the root inclusion technique takes little more time than the subcoronary technique. The root inclusion technique can hardly be applied if the aorta is very small or very severely calcified. So far we have not used the technique in aortas smaller than 21 mm.

Technique

In order to be completely successful, the root inclusion technique has to be applied with great attention to detail. As in all implant techniques for stentless bioprostheses and homografts, the proximal suture line should be carefully placed in one plane at the level of the annulus. This means that the suture line runs in the left ventricle below the commissures (Figure 16.1). In the membranous septum below the commissure between the right and the non-coronary sinus, care should be taken to avoid the conduction system. Very exact sizing of the prosthesis is essential.

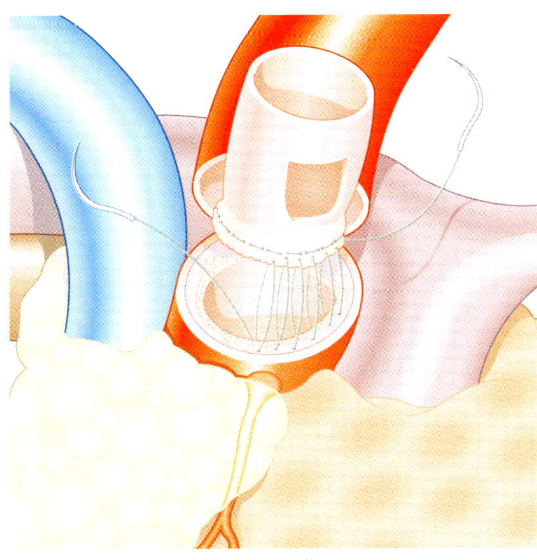

Figure 16.1 Proximal suture line.

It should be measured with the appropriate sizers at the level of the annulus. Too small a prosthesis will lead to dehiscence at the proximal suture line; too large a prosthesis might give good results primarily without regurgitation, but in our experimental work we saw that oversizing causes buckling of the leaflets which will inevitably lead to late damage and regurgitation. Another danger of oversizing is that the porcine sinuses might be compressed in the case of a narrow patient aortic root. The coronary sinuses of the porcine bioprosthesis should be excised as widely as possible. At the distal end the excision should follow the sinotubular junction, just 1 mm below it, whereas the rest of the sinus can be excised keeping at least 2–3 mm from the leaflet attachment. When using a Freestyle stentless bioprosthesis, care should be taken not to damage the Dacron cloth covering the heart muscle on the outside of the right coronary sinus (Figure 16.2). Before suturing the patient's coronary sinuses with the coronary ostia to the edges of the openings in the porcine bioprosthesis, the bioprosthesis should be fixed inside the aorta by three stay sutures above the tops of the commissures of the prosthesis, through the patient's aortic wall. Care should be taken that the prosthesis is thereby fixed in such a way that absolutely no rotation of it is possible and that the length above the annulus is such that the prosthesis is properly suspended in the patient's aorta (Figure 16.3). The patient's sinuses can then be sutured to the prosthesis, avoiding all traction or rotation of the coronary ostia. The suture can be made from inside the prosthesis, but frequently it is easier to make this suture from the space between prosthesis and patient aorta (Figure 16.4). When making the distal suture line, the excess circumference of the patient's aorta can be tailored to fit the prosthesis diameter exactly (Figure 16.5). Rarely, excision of excess aortic tissue is necessary. The whole procedure of implanting a stentless bioprosthesis with the root inclusion technique can be made a lot easier when completely transecting the aorta. One should not hesitate to do this whenever application of this technique seems to be difficult by the usual transverse aortic incision.

Results

Out of 116 patients receiving a Medtronic Freestyle porcine aortic root stentless bioprosthesis for aortic valve replacement between December 1993 and March 1997, 44 patients (38%) were operated upon using the root inclusion technique. There were 27 males and 17 females. The age varied from 34 to 83 years, with a mean of 69.7

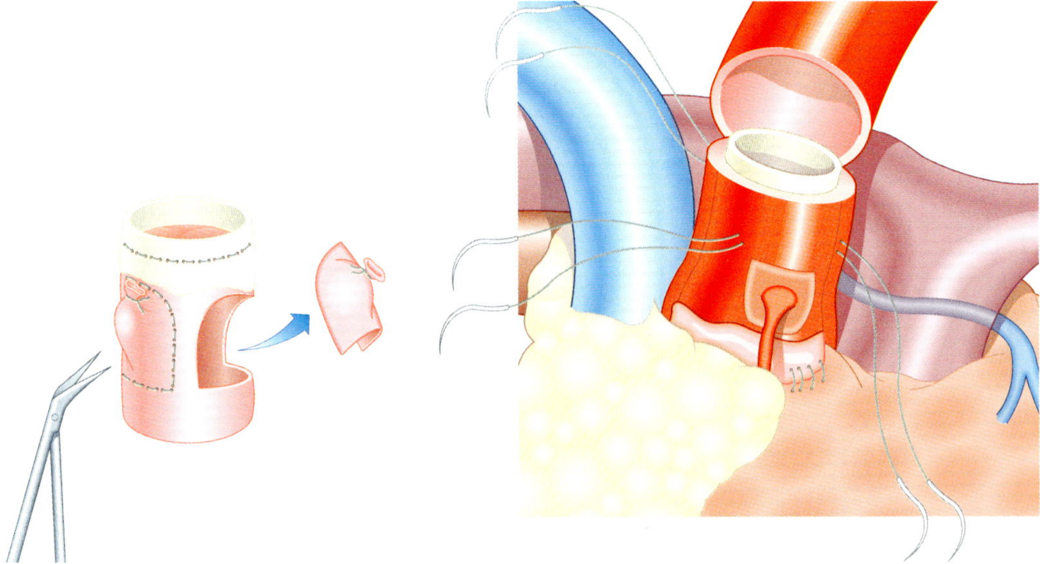

Figure 16.2 Wide excision of both coronary sinuses.

Figure 16.3 Three stay sutures 2 mm above tops of commissure posts.

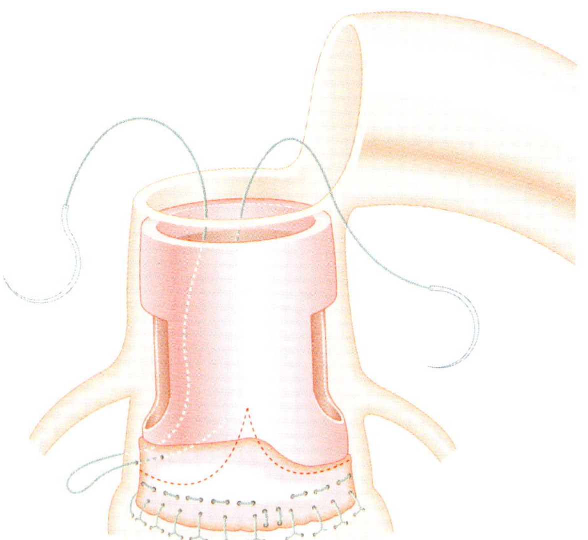

Figure 16.4 Start of suture for fixation of patient's aortic sinuses to prosthesis (lateral view).

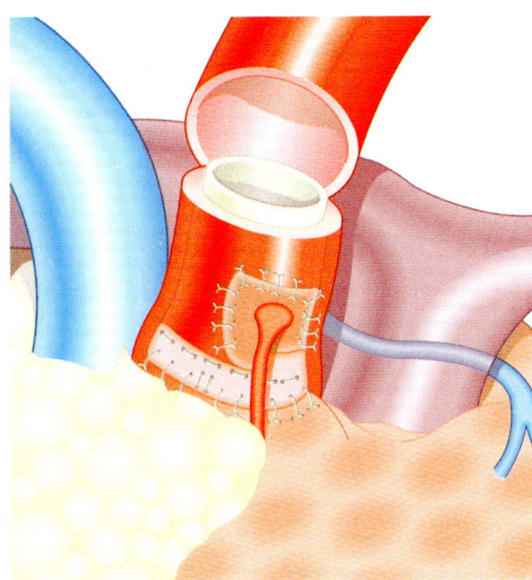

Figure 16.5 Situation before distal suture line; difference in circumference between prosthesis and patient's aorta can easily be corrected.

years. Table 16.1 shows the most important preoperative data of these patients. The previous heart surgery was aortic valve commissurotomy in two patients and aortic valve replacement in three patients. In the two cases of active endocarditis a porcine stentless prosthesis was used because no homograft was available. These two patients were also the youngest ones in the series. Concomitant procedures, prosthesis size and cross-clamp times are listed in Table 16.2. Early postoperative events (within 30 days) are listed in Table 16.3. Two patients died, one of multiorgan failure and the other one after a prolonged state of low cardiac output that occurred after an extremely severe allergic reaction that could never be adequately treated. Other complications were in line with what can be expected in a group of predominantly elderly patients.

There was a complete follow-up in all patients. All patients were seen at 3–6 months, at 1 year and annually thereafter. Extensive echo-Doppler studies were made before discharge, at 3–6 months, 1 year and annually thereafter. Mean follow-up time was 18.6 months. Table 16.4 shows the late postoperative events. Two patients died. One patient developed heart failure postoperatively and was reoperated upon as an emergency after an echo diagnosis of severe regurgitation was made at another hospital. At reoperation no abnormalities of the prosthesis were found and it seems

Table 16.1 Preoperative data

	No. patients
Aortic stenosis (predominantly)	35
Aortic regurgitation	9
Previous heart surgery	5
Active endocarditis	2
Coronary artery disease	8
Mitral regurgitation	2
Heart failure	9
NYHA-class	
I	2
II	22
III	19
IV	1

Table 16.2 Concomitant procedures, prosthesis size, cross-clamp times

	No. patients
Coronary artery bypass surgery	6
Mitral valve repair	2
Prosthesis size (mm)	
21	4
23	20
25	12
27	8
Mean aortic cross-clamp time 96 min (range 58–144 min)	

Table 16.3 Early postoperative data (< 30 days)

	No. patients
Mortality	2 (4.5%)
Low cardiac output	2
Multiorgan failure	1
Arrhythmia (15 atrial fibrillation)	17
Bleeding	3
Respiratory complications	4
Renal complications	4

Table 16.4 Late postoperative events

	No. patients
Mortality	2
Thromboembolism	1
Bleeding	1
Endocarditis	1
Reoperation	2

that the heart failure was mainly myocardial and not valve related. The other patient died at home 6 weeks after surgery from ventricular fibrillation. There was one case of transient ischaemic attack and one case of bleeding in a patient who was on anticoagulants because of atrial fibrillation. One case of late endocarditis could be treated medically. Two patients underwent reoperation. One has already been mentioned above and subsequently died. The other was reoperated for regurgitation due to patient–prosthesis mismatch early in our experience.

Mean postoperative transvalvular gradients, as established by echo-Doppler studies at different times postoperatively, are given in Table 16.5. In all patients a decrease of gradient during the postoperative follow-up was found especially in the period between discharge and the next study at 3–6 months. There were relatively small differences between the different sizes of prostheses. The mean gradients at 1 year were 6.3 mmHg for size 21, 4.3 mmHg for size 23, 4.7 mmHg for size 25 and 3.0 mmHg for size 27. Postoperative regurgitation was more than trivial in only three patients at the time of discharge. Two of those underwent reoperation later on, as decribed earlier; in the third patient the regurgitation went back to trivial during follow-up. In no patient has increase of regurgitation during follow-up been seen so far. The trivial regurgitation could only be recognized by echo-Doppler and was clinically totally irrelevant. The results are shown in Table 16.6.

Table 16.5 Mean and range of postoperative transvalvular gradient

	Mean (mmHg)	Range (mmHg)
At discharge	10.5	2–25
At 3–6 months	4.9	1–12
At 1 year	4.2	2–12
At 2 years	2.0	1–4

Table 16.6 Postoperative regurgitation

	No regurgitation (%)	Trivial (%)	Mild/moderate (%)
At discharge	82	11	7
At 3–6 months	82	18	–
At 1 year	86	14	–
At 2 years	83	17	–

Discussion

The results of the root inclusion technique for implanting the Medtronic Freestyle stentless porcine aortic root bioprosthesis are comparable to those obtained with other stentless valves and homografts with all sorts of techniques. Valve-related events are similar, as are mean transvalvular gradients. Postoperative regurgitation seems to be even less than in other reported series of stentless valves and homografts.[5–7] Reasons for not using the technique could be the need for a short cross-clamp time, when very extensive concomitant procedures have to be performed or when the patient is in a very poor clinical condition. In such cases a subcoronary technique should be preferred or even a stented bioprosthesis be used. In a very small calcified aortic root, it seems difficult to apply the root inclusion technique perfectly and therefore it is probably better avoided. In cases of severely calcified aortic wall around the coronary ostia, the use of any technique for implanting a stentless prosthesis is difficult and dangerous because of the risk of dissection of the coronary arteries.

Conclusion

The root inclusion technique seems to be a good alternative for implanting a stentless bioprosthesis, equivalent to other techniques in the short term and with hopes for better durability results than the subcoronary technique for the long term. This, in combination with the excellent haemodynamic results, might make the use of a stentless bioprosthesis acceptable for aortic valve replacement in patients younger than the elderly group for whom the use of bioprostheses is reserved at present.

References

1. O'Brien M F, McGiffin D C, Stafford E G 1989 Allograft aortic valve implantation: technique for all types of aortic valve and root pathology. Ann Thorac Surg 48: 600–609
2. Rousseau E P M, Van Steenhoven A A, Janssen J D, Huysmans H A 1988 A mechanical analysis of the closed Hancock heart valve prosthesis. J Biomech 7: 545–562
3. Angell W W, Pupello D F, Bessone C U, Hiro S P, Brock J C 1991 Effect of stent mounting on tissue valves for aortic replacement. J Card Surg 6 (Suppl 4): 595–599
4. Hazekamp M G, Goffin Y A, Huysmans H A 1993 The value of the stentless biovalve prosthesis. An experimental study. Eur J Cardiothorac Surg 7: 514–519
5. Del Rizzo D F, Goldman B S, Christakis G T, David T E 1996 Hemodynamic benefits of the Toronto stentless valve. J Thorac Cardiovasc Surg 112: 1431–1446
6. Jin X Y, Gibson D G, Yacoub M H, Pepper J R 1995 Stentless and stented valves in the aortic position: an early postoperative assessment. In: Piwnica A, Westaby S (eds) Stentless bioprostheses. Isis Medical, Oxford, 149–151
7. Kirklin J K, Smith D, Hovick W *et al* 1993 Long-term function of cryopreserved aortic homografts: a ten year study. J Thorac Cardiovasc Surg 106: 154–166

CHAPTER 17

Comparison of results using the Freestyle stentless porcine aortic root bioprosthesis with the cryopreserved aortic allograft

N. D. Kon, S. M. Adair, D. W. Kitzman, A.-M. Nomeir, J. G. Warner, J. E. Dobbins and A. R. Cordell

Aortic stenosis and aortic insufficiency (AI) are correctable mechanical problems of the heart that result in left ventricular dysfunction unless corrected surgically. Among patients with severe symptoms treated medically, only 20% are alive after 8 years.[1–3] In contrast, with surgical treatment the expected 8-year survival with either a mechanical heart valve or a stented porcine bioprosthetic heart valve is 80%.[4,5] However, these improved survival curves do not approach normal life expectancy. The reduced life expectancy is multifactorial, but probably involves factors that relate to the presence of a prosthetic valve. All inserted prosthetic heart valves based on a semi-rigid ring structure are obstructive when compared to a natural aortic heart valve. Mechanical valves have the additional disadvantage of requiring anticoagulation with coumadin. Stented tissue valves have the additional disadvantage of a tendency towards calcific degeneration requiring reoperation after 10 years. In addition, all prosthetic valves are also more prone to endocarditis than are native valves.

In a search for a better bioprosthesis, one that would result in a more normal life expectancy, we began inserting the aortic allograft which has been used for many years[6,7] and has been inserted by a variety of techniques. Another natural valve, the Freestyle stentless porcine valve, was first inserted in 1992.[8,9] This valve is analogous to an allograft in design and therefore has no stent and includes the entire porcine root. The leaflets are fixed with glutaraldehyde at zero pressure and are treated with the antimineralization agent, alpha-amino oleic acid. This report describes our experience with the total root replacement technique, using these two types of stentless aortic valves, the Freestyle stentless porcine aortic root bioprosthesis and the cryopreserved aortic allograft.

Methods

With approval of the Institutional Review Board, prospective clinical trials with both the cryopreserved aortic allograft and the Freestyle stentless porcine bioprosthesis were initiated in 1992. Informed consent was obtained from each of 65 Freestyle patients. One year after initiation of the study, allograft heart valves were no longer considered experimental by the FDA, so informed consent was not required for all of the allograft patients. Of the Freestyle patients, 47.7% were female; 52.3% were male. Of the allograft group, 30.4% were female; 69.6% were male. The age range in both groups is listed in Table 17.1, the preoperative NYHA functional class in Table 17.2, and the predominant valve lesions requiring replacement in Table 17.3. Table 17.4 shows all surgical concomitant procedures performed in each group.

Table 17.1 Preoperative age

Age at implant (years)	Freestyle n (%)	Allograft n (%)
≤ 35	0 (0.0)	26 (20.8)
36–50	1 (1.5)	43 (34.4)
51–64	8 (12.3)	44 (35.2)
65–69	18 (27.7)	6 (4.8)
≥ 70	38 (58.5)	6 (4.8)

Table 17.2 Preoperative clinical data (NYHA functional class)

NYHA classification	Freestyle n (%)	Allograft n (%)
I	2 (3.1)	4 (3.2)
II	13 (20.0)	17 (13.6)
III	42 (64.6)	54 (43.2)
IV	8 (12.3)	50 (40.0)

Table 17.3 Valve lesions requiring replacement

Valvular lesion	Freestyle (*n*)	Allograft (*n*)
Calcification	42	5
Rheumatic	7	9
Congenital	19	45
Myxomatous	5	1
Failed prosthesis	1	34

Table 17.4 Surgical concomitant procedures

Concomitant procedure	Freestyle (*n*)	Allograft (*n*)
Coronary artery bypass	24	24
Ascending aorta repair	10	1
Aortic root enlargement	1	0
Myomectomy	2	0
Ventricular aneurysm repair	0	1
Permanent pacemaker implant	0	3

All 190 patients, whether receiving a cryopreserved aortic allograft or a Freestyle stentless porcine bioprosthesis, underwent a freestanding total aortic root replacement. In performing this technique, the aorta is transected just above the sinotubular ridge (Figure 17.1), and both coronary ostia are mobilized on generous buttons of aortic wall (Figure 17.2). The remaining tissue of the sinus of Valsalva is excised and the diseased aortic valve is removed. The proximal, or inflow, anastomosis is accomplished using from 28 to 35 simple interrupted sutures of 3/0 braided Dacron tied around a 1 mm strip of Teflon felt (Figures 17.3, 17.4). The coronary arteries on their buttons of aortic wall are sewn end-to-side to the prosthetic aorta and a continuous 4/0 polypropylene suture joining graft to native aorta completes the root replacement (Figures 17.5, 17.6).

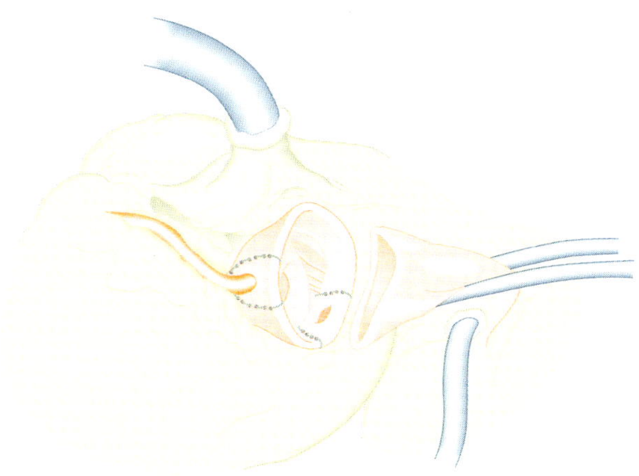

Figure 17.1 The aorta is transected just above the sinus rim.

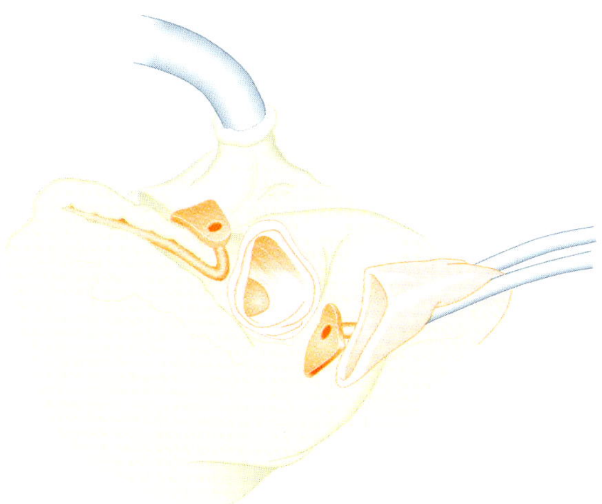

Figure 17.2 Both coronary arteries are immobilized on generous buttons of aortic wall.

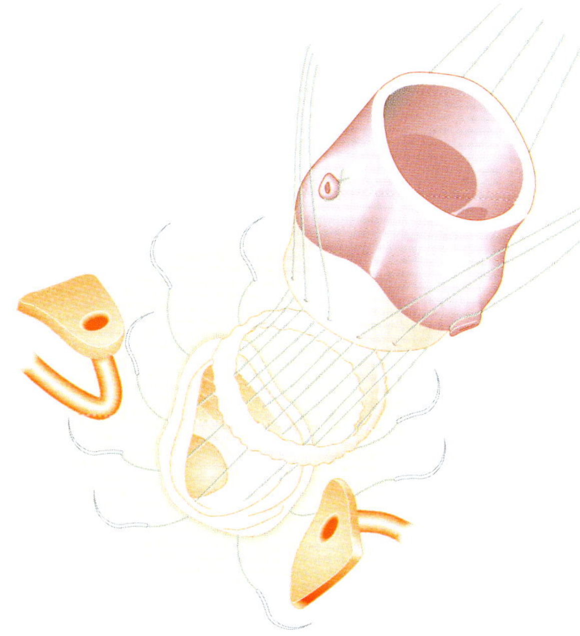

Figure 17.3 The proximal or inflow suture line is accomplished with 28–35 simple interrupted sutures.

All available patients were evaluated by clinical examination at discharge, at 3–6 months, and again at yearly intervals. The valve was assessed using colour-flow Doppler echocardiography at each interval.

Results

Operative mortality (< 30 days in hospital) was 4.6% in the Freestyle group, 3.2% in the allograft group.

No patients in the Freestyle group had haemodynamically significant aortic regurgitation after valve implantation, and there was no increase in the incidence of non-haemodynamically significant AI with time (Figure 17.7).

The incidence of aortic regurgitation in the allograft group is shown in Figure 17.8. One patient developed severe AI at 1 year and another patient developed severe AI at 2 years; both patients required valve replacement. Both had also had initial valve replacement for endocarditis and subsequent valve failure from recurrent leaflet destruction. Figure 17.8 also reveals a higher incidence of non-haemodynamically significant AI in the allograft group, which is increasing over time.

The mean systolic gradients were low and similar in both the allograft and the Freestyle groups, regardless of valve size and regardless of time after implantation (Figure 17.9). The typical laminar flow pattern on echocardiography for the Freestyle valve is shown in Figure 17.10(a), and a similar non-turbulent flow pattern for the allograft valve is depicted in Figure 17.10(b).

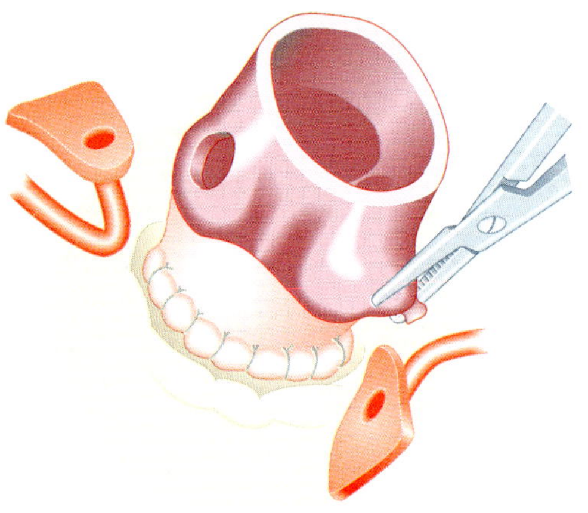

Figure 17.4 Each of the sutures is tied around a ring of Teflon felt.

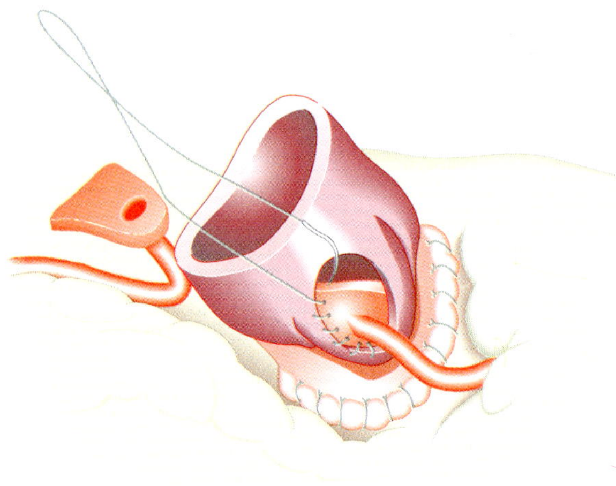

Figure 17.5 The coronary ostia are sewn end-to-side to the respective sinus of Valsalva.

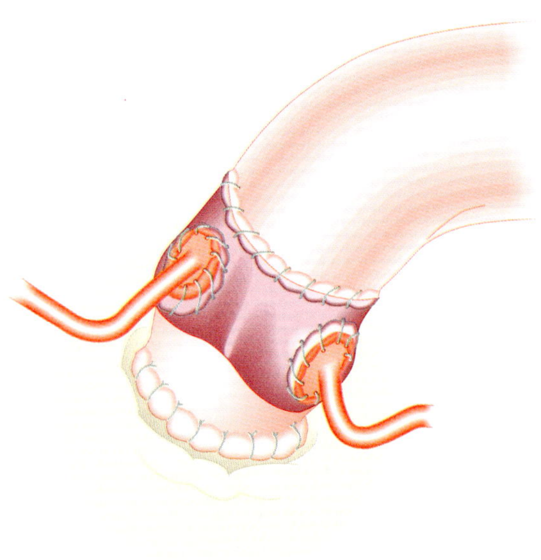

Figure 17.6 The completed total root replacement.

Discussion

Obstructive haemodynamics, calcific degeneration (and therefore limited durability), and the development of prosthetic valve endocarditis are all drawbacks to the conventional stented tissue valves commonly used for aortic valve replacement. The haemodynamic benefits of a stentless tissue valve have been shown repeatedly.[8–14] The main advantage of a stent is that it allows potentially perfect valve mounting, and therefore removes the technical errors associated with freehand (non-stented) valve insertion.

The disadvantages of a stent include the increase in stress forces associated with leaflet opening and closing when leaflets are sewn to a non-flexible structure, the possibility of abrasion of the leaflets against the cloth covering, the potential of paravalvular leaks and, most importantly, the obstructive mass that the stent imposes within the aortic root. Studies have shown that the presence of a stent compared with no stent results in increased valvular gradients and poorer durability.[15,16]

In an effort to eliminate the incidence of technical errors associated with freehand (non-stented) valve insertion, many surgeons are using root replacement techniques in which the entire donor valve mechanism remains intact. These technical demands have been addressed in favour of total root replacement for the aortic allograft,[17,18] pulmonary autograft,[19,20] and stentless porcine aortic valves.[8] Therefore, in this study, the same root replacement technique was used for valve insertion for both the Freestyle stentless porcine valve and the cryopreserved aortic allograft.

	Discharge	3–6 months	1 year	2 years	3 years
No. patients	62	53	36	26	14
Regurgitation (%)					
None/trivial	96.8	98.1	97.2	100	100
Mild	3.2	1.9	2.8	0	0
Moderate	0	0	0	0	0
Moderate/severe	0	0	0	0	0
Severe	0	0	0	0	0

Figure 17.7 Incidence of aortic regurgitation over time in the Freestyle group.

	Discharge	3–6 months	1 year	2 years	3 years
No. patients	114	100	77	40	17
Regurgitation (%)					
None/trivial	91.2	57	35.1	37.5	29.4
Mild	8.8	39	57.1	57.5	64.7
Moderate	0	4	6.5	2.5	5.9
Moderate/severe	0	0	0	2.5	0
Severe	0	0	1.3	0	0

Figure 17.8 Incidence of aortic regurgitation over time in the allograft group.

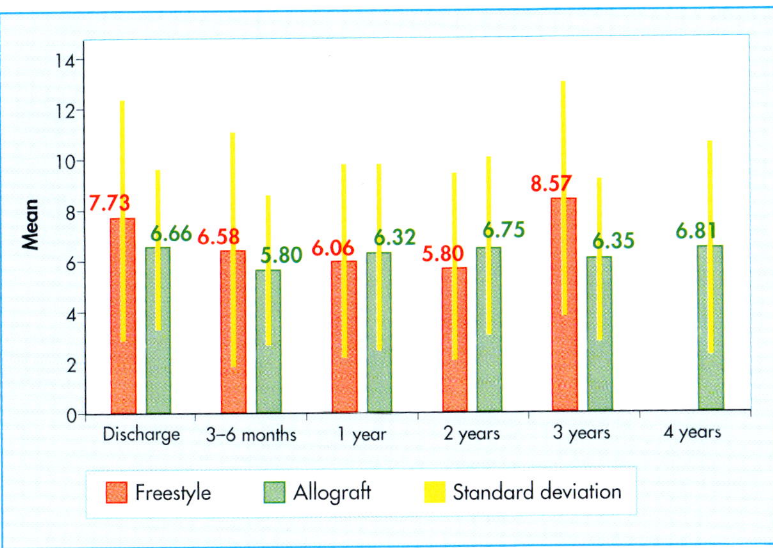

Figure 17.9 Comparison of postoperative gradients in Freestyle and allograft groups over time.

As we had anticipated, patients who received either a stentless porcine biograft or a cryopreserved aortic allograft had equally very low transvalvular gradients. The low gradients would be expected because a freestanding total aortic root replacement procedure had been used in both groups.

An unexpected finding in this study was the increased incidence of AI in the allograft group. The patients who had replacement of their valves for severe AI had had initial surgery for active endocarditis. At reoperation, both these patients were found to have regurgitation secondary to leaflet perforation. It is assumed that recurrent infection caused eventual leaflet perforation, and thus aortic insufficiency, in these two patients.

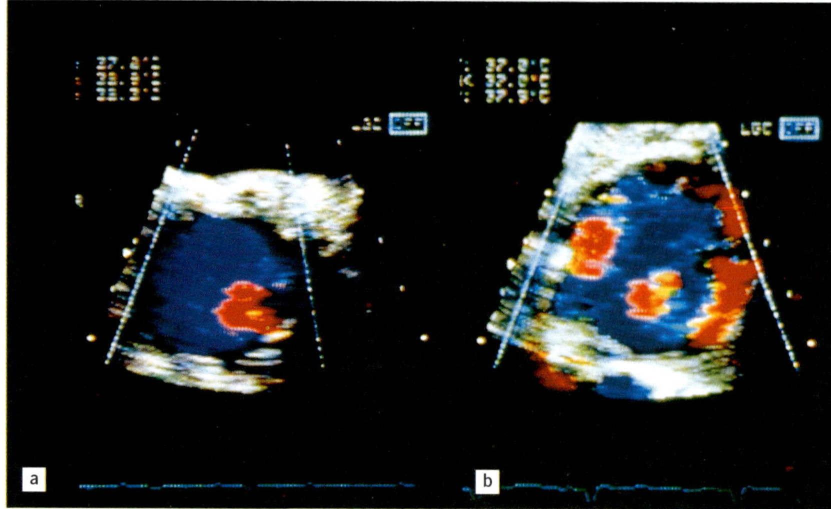

Figure 17.10 Transoesophageal echocardiograms of (a) Freestyle and (b) allograft heart valves demonstrating the laminar flow patterns characteristic of these natural valves.

The increased incidence of non-haemodynamically significant AI is more difficult to explain. Since the annulus size was presumably fixed in both groups with a ring of Teflon felt, one would think that progressive annular dilatation over time would not result in progressive increase in non-haemodynamically significant AI. However, the porcine aorta is thicker and less pliable than the cryopreserved aorta and therefore aortic but not annular dilatation may explain an increase in non-haemodynamically significant AI over time.

The porcine biografts are glutaraldehyde fixed and therefore pose no immunogenic potential. Cryopreserved leaflets, although not strongly immunogenic, might undergo subtle changes in structure secondary to an immune response, thereby producing non-haemodynamically significant AI. A final consideration to explain the increase in non-haemodynamically significant AI may relate to the difference in availability of the two biografts. Porcine biografts may undergo a more scrutinized examination and selection process than do allograft valves, which are a more limited resource.

Conclusions

Excellent short-term results with operative risks no greater than those for a standard valve replacement were obtained with both the Freestyle stentless porcine bioprosthesis and the cryopreserved aortic allograft. In addition, superior haemodynamic performance was demonstrated by both these valves compared with mechanical and stented tissue valves. Neither valve had early haemodynamically significant AI, but the Freestyle stentless porcine valve had a lower incidence of non-haemodynamically significant AI. This difference became more apparent over time. Long-term follow-up will be needed not only to determine valve durability, but also to determine whether age-matched survival curves in these patients will be closer to those of the normal population than the survival curves in patients having a mechanical or stented tissue bioprosthesis inserted.

References

1. Wood P 1958 Aortic stenosis. Am J Cardiol 1: 553–571
2. Frank S, Ross J Jr 1967 The natural history of severe, acquired valvular aortic stenosis [abstract]. Am J Cardiol 19: 128–129
3. Grant R T 1933 After histories for ten years of a thousand men sufferering from heart disease: a study in prognosis. Heart 16: 275
4. Arom K V, Nicoloff D M, Kersten T E, Northrup III W F, Lindsay W G, Emery R W 1989 Ten years experience with the St Jude Medical valve prosthesis. Ann Thorac Surg 47: 831–837

5. Jamieson W R E, Munro A I, Miyagishima R T, Allen P, Burr L H, Tyers G F O 1995 Carpentier–Edwards standard porcine bioprosthesis: clinical performance to seventeen years. Ann Thorac Surg 60: 999–1007
6. Ross D N 1962 Homograft replacement of the aortic valve. Lancet 2: 487–488
7. Barratt-Boyes B G 1964 Homograft aortic valve replacement in aortic incompetence and stenosis. Thorax 19: 131–150
8. Kon N D, Westaby S, Amarasena N, Pillai R, Cordell A R 1995 Comparison of implant techniques using Freestyle stentless porcine aortic valve. Ann Thorac Surg 59: 857–862
9. Sintek C F, Fletcher A D, Khonsari S 1995 Stentless porcine aortic root: valve of choice for the elderly patient with small aortic root? J Thorac Cardiovasc Surg 109: 871–876
10. Westaby S, Amarasena N, Ormerod O, Amarasena G A C, Pillai R 1995 Aortic valve replacement with the Freestyle stentless xenograft. Ann Thorac Surg 60: S422–S427
11. Westaby S, Amarasena N, Long V *et al* 1995 Time-related hemodynamic changes after aortic replacement with the Freestyle stentless xenograft. Ann Thorac Surg 60: 1633–1639
12. Del Rizzo D F, Goldman B S, David T E 1995 Canadian investigators of Toronto SPV™ valve trial. Aortic valve replacement with a stentless porcine bioprosthesis: multicentre trial. Can J Cardiol 11: 597–603
13. David T E, Pollick C, Bos J 1990 Aortic valve replacement with stentless porcine aortic bioprosthesis. J Thorac Cardiovasc Surg 99: 113–118
14. Del Rizzo D F, Goldman B S, Christakis G T, David T E 1996 Hemodynamic benefits of the Toronto stentless valve. J Thorac Cardiovasc Surg 112: 1431–1446
15. Angell W W, Oury J H, Lamberti J J, Koziol J 1989 Durability of the viable aortic allograft. J Thorac Cardiovasc Surg 98: 48–56
16. Angell W W, Pupello D F, Bessone L N, Hiro S P, Brock J C 1991 Effect of stent mounting on tissue valves for aortic valve replacement. J Card Surg (Suppl 4): 595–599
17. Daicoff G R, Botero L M, Quintessenza J A 1993 Allograft replacement of the aortic valve versus the miniroot and valve. Ann Thorac Surg 55: 855–859
18. Jones E L, Shah V B, Shanewise J S *et al* 1995 Should the freehand allograft be abandoned as a reliable alternative for aortic valve replacement? Ann Thorac Surg 59: 1397–1404
19. Kouchoukos N T, Dávila-Román V G, Spray T L, Murphy S F, Perrillo J B 1994 Replacement of the aortic root with a pulmonary autograft in children and young adults with aortic-valve disease. N Engl J Med 330: 1–6
20. Elkins R C, Santangelo K, Stelzer P, Randolph J D, Knott-Craig C J 1992 Pulmonary autograft replacement of the aortic valve: an evolution of technique. J Card Surg 7: 108–116

V Haemodynamics and Left Ventricular Function

CHAPTER 18

Haemodynamic performance of the Toronto SPV valve in stress conditions

C. Zerio, C. Zussa, E. Polesel, P. Pascotto and C. Valfrè

The haemodynamic characteristics of prosthetic heart valves constitute an important part of their functional assessment. The satisfactory haemodynamic performances at rest of aortic stentless bioprostheses have been demonstrated and they compare well with those of matched mechanical ones. However, it has been suggested that *in vivo* resting assessment is inadequate to characterize valve performance fully.[1] In particular, the characteristics of stentless bioprostheses under stress conditions *in vivo* are not well documented and represent the aim of our research.

Cardiac catheterization and Doppler echocardiography are the two established methods for the evaluation of prosthetic valve function at rest.[2] Current methods for *in vivo* assessment of prosthetic heart valves under high flow conditions are dependent on exercise, and are not entirely suitable for wider clinical use. In this study we successfully applied dobutamine stress echocardiography in the *in vivo* evaluation of the haemodynamic performance of the Toronto SPV valve (St Jude Medical, St Paul, MN, USA).

Patients and methods

In the period between 1993 and 1996, 81 patients were operated upon for aortic valve disease with a Toronto SPV valve at our institution. Of the 59 patients operated on for aortic stenosis, 20 were submitted to stress echocardiography. The admission criteria were: age less than 80 years, operation at least 1 year before the beginning of the study, and prosthesis size between 21 and 25 mm. The mean age of our study population was 63 ± 7 years (range 40–71); there were 13 males and seven females. Surgical intervention was isolated aortic valve replacement in all the patients and the valve size was 21 mm in one patient, 23 mm in six and 25 mm in 13.

In three patients there was also a mitral regurgitation, of mild degree in two and mild to moderate in one patient. Mean time since intervention was 26 ± 9 months (range 14–45); sinus rhythm was present in 19 patients (95%), atrial fibrillation in one (5%), mild degree hypertension was present in eight patients (40%) and 19 patients were in NYHA functional class between I and II. Therapy was: beta-blockers in two patients (10%) (the drug was withdrawn 5 days before the echo stress), enalapril in four patients (20%), digoxin in 10 (50%), diuretic in 10 (50%) and oral anticoagulation in one patient (5%).

Dobutamine-stress protocol

Written informed consent was obtained for all patients before every procedure. After a detailed history and physical examination to exclude the presence of any contraindication to stress testing, a complete basal echocardiogram was performed. Stress echocardiographic protocol was performed by a graded i.v. infusion of dobutamine at increments of 5, 10 and 20 μg/kg per min each at intervals of 15 min.

Echo-Doppler measurements were obtained before each increase in the infusion rate. The patients underwent continuous electrocardiographic monitoring and blood pressure was recorded at 5-min intervals. After discontinuation of dobutamine infusion the patient was monitored for a minimum of 20 min.

The criteria for stopping the test were: onset of hypotension (systolic blood pressure < 100 mmHg), onset or worsening of dyspnoea, onset of significant ventricular or supraventricular arrhythmias.

Doppler measurements and calculations

Echocardiography was carried out using a Hewlett Packard Sonos 1000 or Sonos 2500 ultrasound system with a 2.5 MHz transducer with facilities for continuous-wave and pulsed-wave Doppler. The early systolic diameter (D) of the left ventricular outflow tract (LVOT) was measured by the parasternal long axis view, using the inner edge-to-edge methodology. Left ventricular posterior wall thickness (LVPWTh) was measured by the parasternal short axis view. End-systolic (ESV) and end-diastolic volume (EDV) and ejection fraction (EF) were measured by the apical four chambers view. Doppler measurements were taken using the apical four chambers view. We measured peak velocity (pV_{cw}) and mean velocity (mV_{cw}) across the prosthetic aortic valve by means of continuous-wave Doppler; and peak velocity (pV_{pw}) and mean velocity (mV_{pw}) in LVOT by means of pulsed-wave Doppler.

The results shown are the mean of three measurements (six for the patient in atrial fibrillation).

The cross-sectional area (CSA) of the LVOT was calculated as:

$$\text{CSA} = 3.14 \times D^2/4.$$

Cardiac output (CO) was calculated as:

$$\text{CO} = \text{VTI} \times \text{CSA} \times \text{HR},$$

where VTI is the velocity time integral in the LVOT and HR is the heart rate. Cardiac index (CI) was calculated as:

$$\text{CI} = \text{CO} / \text{BSA},$$

where BSA is body surface area. The modified Bernoulli equation was used to calculate peak and mean pressure drop (gradient) across the prosthesis as:

$$\Delta P = 4 \times (V_{cw}^2 - V_{pw}^2),$$

where ΔP is pressure drop, V_{cw} and V_{pw} are the velocities (peak and mean) across the prosthetic valve. The prosthetic effective orifice area (EOA) was calculated with the modified continuity equation as:

$$\text{EOA} = \text{CSA} \times \text{VR},$$

where VR is the ratio of mean subaortic to mean transaortic velocity and gives an approximate behaviour of the orifice, independent of measurements of LVOT diameter.[2] The effective orifice area index (EOAI, which is a measure of how well the flow area matched the body size) was calculated by the ratio:

$$\text{EOAI} = \text{EOA} / \text{BSA}.$$

Results

The dobutamine infusion protocol was well tolerated and no complications or impairments in regional myocardial contractility could be detected in any patient. All the patients had a significant increase in heart rate (85% from rest to stress) (Table 18.1), in the product heart × systolic blood pressure (which is an index of oxygen

Table 18.1 Clinical measurements of patients at rest and at maximum stress

	Rest	Maximum stress	*P*
HR (bpm)	65 ± 10	120 ± 7*	<0.001
BP (mmHg)	137 ± 19	150 ± 8	0.04
HR × BP	9326 ± 1977	17 689 ± 2945	<0.001
CO (l/min)	5.6 ± 1.4	12.2 ± 2.2	<0.001
CI (l/min/m^2)	3.15 ± 1.4	6.8 ± 1.3	<0.001
EF (%)	64 ± 6	78 ± 5	<0.001
EDV (ml)	102 ± 41	102 ± 42	ns
ESV (ml)	36 ± 17	23 ± 13	0.01
LVPWTh (mm)	11.3	12	0.02
LVOT mean vel (m/s)	0.8 ± 0.1	1.2 ± 0.2	<0.001
Peak grad (mmHg)	16 ± 5.6	39 ± 9.4	<0.001
Mean grad (mmHg)	8.9 ± 3.1	18.3 ± 3.5	<0.001
EOA (cm^2)	1.95 ± 0.2	2 ± 0.2	ns
EOAI (cm^2/m^2)	1.11 ± 0.17	1.15 ± 0.2	ns

*Each patient reached the suboptimal HR consistent with their age, with a mean of 80% of the maximal expected HR.

HR, heart rate; BP, systolic blood pressure; CO, cardiac output; CI, cardiac index; EF, ejection fraction; EDV, left ventricular end-diastolic volume; ESV, left ventricular end-systolic volume; LVPWTh, left ventricular posterior wall thickness; LVOT mean vel, left ventricular outflow tract mean velocity; Peak grad, cross-aortic prosthesis peak gradient; Mean grad, cross-aortic prosthesis mean gradient; EOA, effective orifice area; EOAI, effective orifice area index; ns, not significant.

consumption) and in CO which showed a significant increase (110% from rest to maximum stress) and the same for CI (110% from rest to stress). EF also showed a significant increase while systolic blood pressure showed only a slight increase.

EDV did not change, whereas ESV decreased significantly (36% from rest to stress), and LVPWTh showed a slight increase.

Mean velocity in LVOT increased from a mean value of 0.8 m/s to 1.2 m/s, according to the constrictor effect in LVOT, in response to the beta effect of dobutamine. Peak transaortic prosthetic valve gradient showed a significant increase from rest to maximum stress and similarly the mean gradient significantly increased from rest to stress.

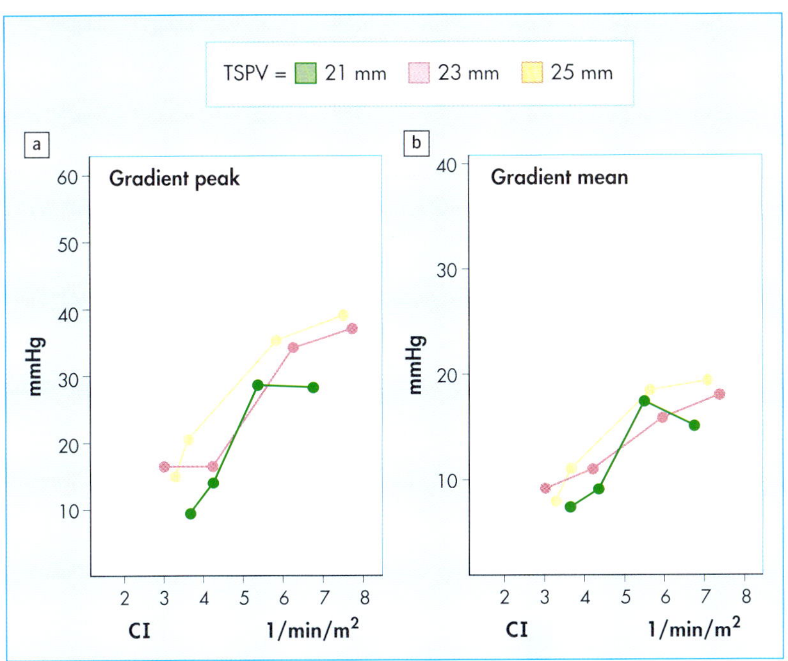

Figure 18.1 The cross-prostheses gradients – peak (a) and mean (b) – for each prosthesis size, related to cardiac index.

EOA remained the same at rest and under maximum stress, and the same for the EOAI. The cross-prosthesis peak and mean gradient are shown in Figure 18.1. It seems evident that the gradient is similar for 21 mm, 23 mm and 25 mm size prostheses and is related to the significant increase in cardiac index.

Discussion

High residual gradients in patients with aortic valve replacement may effectively produce LVOT obstruction, and could account for the unexplained occasional late deterioration of cardiac function reported in the literature.[3,4] Furthermore, the well-documented increase in cross-prosthetic gradients at high flow conditions, such as during exercise, has highlighted the importance of the evaluation of prosthetic valves in such conditions.[1,4] Current methods for *in vivo* assessment of prosthetic heart valves under high flow conditions are dependent on exercise, and are not entirely suitable for wider clinical use. Recently, dobutamine stress echocardiography has been introduced in the evaluation of haemodynamic performance of aortic valve prostheses.[5,6] In fact, dobutamine stress is relatively safe and easy to perform and has proved to be a valid alternative to treadmill exercise testing, with a higher diagnostic yield.[7] Furthermore, the patient is in a recumbent position during the examination, allowing the optimization of the echocardiographic images and precision of the Doppler measurements.

The data reported in the literature regarding the haemodynamics of prosthetic heart valves in the aortic position at rest or under stress are not homogeneous, for a variety of reasons such as small numbers of the series, different type and size of the prosthetic valve, and different methodology (Table 18.2). Furthermore, we did not find papers concerning the haemodynamic performance of the Toronto SPV valve under stress. In our study, peak and mean gradients at rest and under maximum stress are similar to those reported by Tatineni *et al.*[1] in which the authors studied rest and exercise performance of bileaflet aortic prostheses (Table 18.2). The lower gradients reported in other papers are probably related to the lower CO at rest and at maximum stress obtained in those series.[5,6,8] Furthermore, in our study, the EOA is near 2 cm^2 and is similar to the data of Tatineni *et al.*[1] but greater than the EOA reported in other

Table 18.2 Study measurements compared with other studies

	Izzat[5]	Izzat[6]	Tatineni[1]	Laske[8]	Sintek[9]	Present series
Method	Echo-Dob	Echo-Dob	Exercise	Dob Cath	Echo	Echo-Dob
No. patients	10	8	–	13	13	20
Valve size (mm)	CMV 21	CMV 19	StJM 24 ± 3	StJM 25	Freestyle 21	TSPV 24 ± 1
CO rest (l/min)	2.8 ± 0.7	4.1 ± 1.9l	–	12.8 ± 3.6	–	5.6 ± 1.4
CO stress (l/min)	6.8 ± 2.7	6.5 ± 2.0	–	14.6 ± 2.9	–	12.2 ± 2.2
PG rest (mmHg)	–	–	24 ± 7	15.8 ± 9	–	16 ± 5.6
PG stress (mmHg)	–	–	41 ± 12	17.6 ± 9.7	–	39 ± 9.4
MG rest (mmHg)	4.8 ± 3.8	8.1 ± 8.4	11 ± 4	4.9 ± 3.1	8 (2.2–19.3)	8.9 ± 3.1
MG stress (mmHg)	8.8 ± 5.8	15.1 ± 14.2	18 ± 7	5.8 ± 3.9	–	18.3 ± 5
EOA rest (cm^2)	1.2 ± 0.62	1.37 ± 0.56	2.2 ± 1.1	–	1.56 (1.15–2.17)	1.95 ± 0.2
EOA stress (cm^2)	1.23 ± 0.47	1.33 ± 0.59	–	–	–	2 ± 0.2

Echo, echocardiography; Echo-Dob, dobutamine–stress echocardiography (5, 10, 20 μg/kg/min); Exercise, exercise test; Dob Cath, invasive measurements at rest and at stress obtained by dobutamine inotropic support (500 μg/min); CMV, CarboMedics valve; StJM, St Jude Medical valve; TSPV, Toronto SPV valve; CO, cardiac output; PG, cross-prosthesis peak gradient; MG, cross-prosthesis mean gradient, EOA, effective orifice area.

papers (Table 18.2), although in those series[5,6,8,9] the cross-prosthesis gradients were lower than ours. All this evidence demonstrates that the Toronto SPV valve confirmed its optimal haemodynamic characteristics in stress conditions and also for small sizes of valve. The increase of peak and mean gradient under stress conditions is thus only related to a significant increase in CO, while EOA and EOAI are adequate in any conditions.

References

1. Tatineni S, Barner H B, Pearson A C *et al* 1989 Rest and exercise evaluation of St. Jude Medical and Medtronic Hall prostheses. Circulation 80(Suppl 1): 16–23
2. Reisner S A, Meltzer R S 1988 Normal values of prosthetic valve Doppler echocardiographic parameters: a review. J Am Soc Echocardiogr 1: 201–210
3. Arom K V, Nicoloff D M, Kersten T E *et al* 1989 Ten years' experience with the medical valve prosthesis. Ann Thorac Surg 47: 831–837
4. De Paulis R, Sommariva L, Russo F *et al* 1994 Doppler echocardiography evaluation of the CarboMedics valve in patients with small aortic annulus and valve prosthesis–body surface area mismatch. J Thorac Cardiovasc Surg 108: 57–62
5. Izzat M B, Birdi I, Wilde P *et al* 1996 Comparison of haemodynamic performances of St Jude Medical and CarboMedics 21 mm prostheses by means of dobutamine stress echocardiography. J Thorac Cardiovasc Surg 111(2): 408–415
6. Izzat M B, Birdi I, Wilde P *et al* 1995 Evaluation of the haemodynamic performances of small CarboMedics aortic prostheses using dobutamine–stress Doppler echocardiography. Ann Thorac Surg 60: 1048–1052
7. Mertes H, Sawada S G, Ryan T *et al* 1993 Symptoms, adverse effects and complications associated with dobutamine stress echocardiography. Circulation 88: 15–19
8. Laske A, Jenni R, Maloigne M *et al* 1996 Pressure gradients across bileaflet aortic valves by direct measurement and echocardiography. Ann Thorac Surg 61: 48–57
9. Sintek C F, Fletcher A D, Khonsari S 1996 Small aortic root in the elderly: use of stentless bioprostheses. J Heart Valve Dis 5(Suppl III): 308–313

CHAPTER 19

Left ventricular remodelling following aortic valve replacement with the Toronto SPV valve

D. F. Del Rizzo, J. Sever, G. T. Christakis, S. E. Fremes and B. S. Goldman

Although no currently available device is an ideal substitute for the human aortic valve,[1] a bioprosthesis which closely resembles the native valve offers certain theoretical advantages. While homograft aortic valves[2–4] and stentless heterografts[5–7] were successfully used to replace the human aortic valve more than 30 years ago, due to technical difficulties in implantation, and the development of commercially available stent-mounted porcine valves, interest in stentless valves declined while clinical experience with homografts remained limited to a few centres. However, the significant failure rates associated with stented xenografts,[8] especially in younger patients,[9] stimulated the development of an alternative to the conventional stented valve.

In 1988, David reported on a non-stented heterograft,[10] the Toronto SPV valve. Subsequent studies demonstrated that when compared with a conventional stented bioprosthesis, the Toronto SPV valve had superior haemodynamics.[11,12] Further reports have confirmed the haemodynamic benefits of stentless valves[13–21] and in a recent study the haemodynamic performance of the Toronto SPV valve was identical to that of aortic homografts.[22]

Serial echographic studies have demonstrated that transvalvular gradients decrease while effective orifice area (EOA) increases as a function of time following aortic valve replacement (AVR) with the Toronto SPV valve.[12–17] Identical results have also been reported with both the Medtronic Freestyle stentless valve,[18] and with aortic homografts.[22] Ventricular remodelling with regression of left ventricular (LV) mass has also been observed following AVR with the Toronto SPV valve.[14,22] The purpose of the current work is to investigate a possible relationship between changes in transvalvular gradient (Δg) and EOA (ΔEOA) with a reduction in LV mass over time, and to identify the major determinants of these changes in a longitudinal study.

Materials and methods

Patient population

After informed consent, 116 patients underwent aortic valve replacement with a Toronto SPV valve between March 1992 and November 1996 at Sunnybrook Health Sciences Centre. The group consisted of 77 male and 39 female patients with a mean age of 62.7 ± 11.7 years (range 33–82 years). Patient characteristics are described briefly in Table 19.1 and a detailed account can be found in Chapter 11. The primary lesion was stenosis in 71 patients, insufficiency in 19 patients, and 26 patients had a mixed lesion (stenosis with central regurgitation).

Table 19.1 Patient characteristics (n = 116)

Characteristic	*n*	Mean or %	SD	Min	Max
Gender					
Female	39	33.6%			
Male	77	66.4%			
Age group					
<40	11	9.5%			
40–49	6	5.2%			
50–59	18	15.5%			
60–69	49	42.2%			
70–79	29	25.0%			
> 80	3	2.6%			
Age (years)	116	62.6	11.7	33	82
Body surface area (m^2)	116	1.9	0.2	1.4	2.5
Dominant pathology					
Aortic stenosis	71	61.2%			
Aortic insufficiency	19	16.4%			
Mixed	26	22.4%			

Data are presented as absolute percentage or as mean ± 1 standard deviation.

Echocardiography

All patients who undergo AVR with a Toronto SPV valve are followed with serial echocardiograms. The first examination is performed in the immediate postoperative period, prior to discharge. Subsequent follow-up examinations are done at 3 months, 1 year, and annually thereafter. Echocardiographic analyses of the leaflets with continuous-wave and colour Doppler studies are performed at each examination, and are used to assess valve function. Formulas for calculating mean systolic gradient, EOA, and LV mass are provided in the Appendix.

Data analysis

All analyses were performed with the Statistical Analysis System (SAS Institute Inc., Cary, NC, USA) or with BMDP 5V statistical software packages. Regression analysis was performed on Microsoft Excel 4.0. Discrete variables are presented as counts and percentages. Continuous variables are presented as mean ± standard deviation.

All left ventricular mass and gradient data were analysed with the advice of the Department of Research Design and Biostatistics, Sunnybrook Health Science Centre, University of Toronto, Toronto, Canada. The initial change from postoperative to the 3–6 month interval for the continuous variables (peak and mean gradient, EOA, thickness of the intraventricular septum, posterior LV wall thickness, LV mass, and LV mass index) was tested by matched pairs *t*-test. Further analyses of LV mass and the determinants of Δg over time were performed in two steps using statistical models we have recently described.[14] Initially, a multivariate analysis of variance (MANOVA) of both LV mass and gradient was applied to establish the statistical significance of the overall effect of time on both of the primary dependent variables (gradient and LV mass) considered together. Following this, univariate analysis of variance (ANOVA) was used to establish the directional change for each of the dependent variables over time. Finally, linear regression analysis was performed to investigate any possible relationship between Δg and changes in left ventricular outflow tract (ΔLVOT), in the velocity in the LVOT (ΔV_1), in the velocity across the aortic valve (ΔV_2), and in ΔEOA as a function of time. In all instances statistical significance was assumed at the nominal level of $\alpha = 0.05$.

Results

Clinical outcome

The clinical results on the patient population are reported in detail in Chapter 11. At the time of this report, 95 patients have reached the 1-year, 59 patients have reached the 2-year, and 26 patients have reached the 3-year follow-up intervals. Valves implanted by size are shown in Figure 19.1. There were six deaths (two early and four late) in this study, three of which were valve related.

Echocardiographic studies

Transthoracic echocardiography was used to assess both the clinical performance of the valve (leaflet function, insufficiency, thrombosis) and the haemodynamics (transvalvular gradient and EOA). In previous studies we and others have observed a significant decrease in mean systolic gradient with a corresponding increase in EOA over time following AVR with the Toronto SPV valve.[12–17,23] Our current study (Table 11.2, Chapter 11) confirms these observations.

Table 19.2 examines the haemodynamic and LV mass changes from postoperative to the 3–6 months follow-up. In all cases statistical significance was determined by matched pairs *t*-test such that each patient served as his/her own control. Peak gradient decreased by 4.3 ± 7.0 mmHg ($p < 0.0001$) while mean gradient decreased by 1.8 ± 4.0 mmHg ($p < 0.0001$). These changes were associated with an increase in EOA of 0.13 ± 0.43 cm^2 ($p = 0.007$). To determine if these effects were associated with evidence of LV remodelling we examined changes in the thickness of both the intraventricular septum (IVS) as well as the posterior wall of the LV (LVP). We found that IVS decreased by 1.0 ± 1.8 mm ($p < 0.0001$) while LVP decreased by 1.3 ± 1.8 mm ($p < 0.0001$) during the study period. Furthermore, there was a significant decrease in both LV mass (–34.4 ± 56.1 g, $p < 0.0001$) and LV mass index (–18.8 ± 29.6 g/m^2, $p < 0.0001$) from postoperative to the 3–6 months follow-up interval. These results are consistent with the hypothesis that LV remodelling occurs following AVR with the Toronto SPV valve.

The data were then subjected to a MANOVA which demonstrated a statistically discernible relationship between changes in transvalvular gradient and LV mass regression over time ($p < 0.01$ at 1 year; $p = 0.028$ at 3 years). These results are consistent with our previous findings,[14] and indicate that LV mass regression is linked to a change in transvalvular gradient. To determine directional change for LV mass as

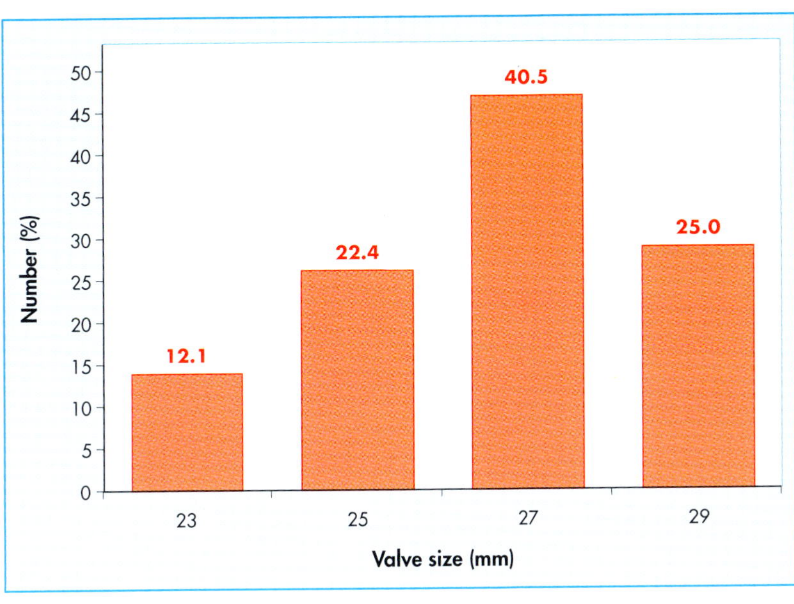

Figure 19.1
Valve sizes implanted were: 23 mm – 14; 25 mm – 26; 27 mm – 47; 29 mm – 29. Number over each bar equals the percentage for each valve size.

Table 19.2 Haemodynamic and left ventricular mass changes

	Peak gradient (mmHg)	**Mean gradient (mmHg)**	**EOA (cm^2)**	**IVS (mm)**	**LV post (mm)**	**LV mass (m)**	**LV mass index (g/m^2)**
Postoperative	19.2 ± 7.6 (86)	8.11 ± 3.2 (86)	1.80 ± 0.57 (81)	13.2 ± 2.5 (76)	12.8 ± 2.3 (76)	262.3 ± 95.5 (75)	138.1 ± 49.9 (75)
3–6 months	14.9 ± 6.5 (84)	6.2 ± 2.8 (84)	1.96 ± 0.67 (81)	12.3 ± 2.3 (74)	11.6 ± 1.9 (74)	226.2 ± 74.1 (73)	119.4 ± 33.8 (73)
Delta (change from postop)	–4.7 ± 7.0 (80)	–1.8 ± 3.0 (80)	0.13 ± 0.43 (74)	–1.0 ± 1.8 (65)	–1.3 ± 1. (65)	–34.4 ± 56.1 (63)	–18.8 ± 29.6 (63)
p	< 0.0001	< 0.0001	0.007	< 0.0001	< 0.0001	< 0.0001	< 0.0001

All data are presented as mean ± 1 standard deviation. The number of patients examined is shown in parentheses. EOA, effective orifice area; IVS, thickness of the intraventricular septum; LV post, thickness of the posterior wall of the left ventricle. Delta is defined as the change in parameter from immediately postoperation to the first follow-up visit (3–6 months). Statistical significance was determined by matched pairs *t*-test such that each patient served as his/her own control.

a function of time, ANOVA was performed. We found there was a significant decrease in LV mass from postoperative to the 3–6 months follow-up interval (262.3 ± 95.5 to 226.2 ± 74.1 g, $p < 0.0001$). A further significant reduction in LV mass was seen from the 3–6 months to the 1-year follow-up interval (226.2 ± 74.1 to 210.4 ± 64.6 g, $p < 0.0001$). The results are shown in Figure 19.2.

Since changes in gradient may be theoretically influenced by ΔV_1, ΔV_2, ΔLVOT, or by ΔEOA, linear regression analysis was carried out to determine the relative importance of each of these variables on Δg. The change in gradient from postoperative to 3–6 months follow-up (Δg) was plotted against ΔV_1, ΔV_2, ΔLVOT, and ΔEOA. These results are shown in Figures 19.3–19.6 and indicate that Δg varied significantly with ΔV_2 ($R = 0.89$, $p_{slope} < 0.0001$) and ΔEOA ($R = 0.49$, $p_{slope} = 0.001$) but occurred independent of ΔV_1 ($R = 0.03$, $p_{slope} = 0.8$) or ΔLVOT ($R = 0.03$, $p_{slope} = 0.16$).

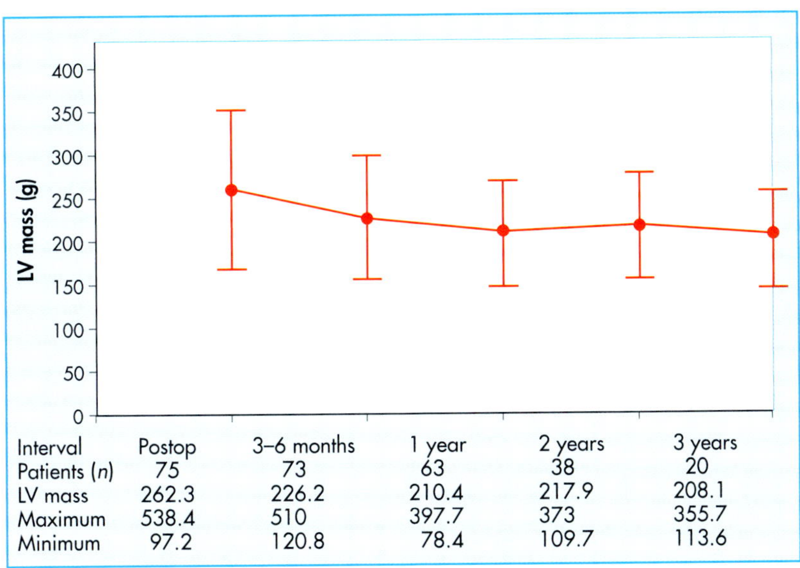

Interval	Postop	3–6 months	1 year	2 years	3 years
Patients (*n*)	75	73	63	38	20
LV mass	262.3	226.2	210.4	217.9	208.1
Maximum	538.4	510	397.7	373	355.7
Minimum	97.2	120.8	78.4	109.7	113.6

Figure 19.2 Data show the change in left ventricular mass as a function of time. LV mass was determined immediately post-AVR, at 3–6 months after surgery, and yearly thereafter. Data are presented as mean ± 1 standard deviation. Statistical significance was determined by ANOVA. There was a significant reduction in LV mass from postoperative to the 3–6 month follow-up interval ($p < 0.0001$) and from the 3–6 month to the 1-year follow-up interval ($p < 0.0001$). The formula used to calculate LV mass is given in the Appendix.

Discussion

The haemodynamic benefits of stentless valves have been repeatedly demonstrated by a number of investigators,[11–21] and in one study the haemodynamic performance of the Toronto SPV valve was identical to that of aortic homografts.[22] Comparative cohort studies have shown the Toronto SPV valve has significantly lower gradients and larger EOAs than conventional stented xenografts;[11,12] it is also superior to mechanical bileaflet prostheses.[22]

The current study corroborates previous reports[12–17] that transvalvular gradients decrease while EOA increases as a function of time following AVR with the Toronto SPV valve. By elimination of a rigid sewing ring, it is believed that the dynamic nature of the aortic root[23] is maintained following AVR with this device. Maintaining normal aortic root function may be responsible, at least in part, for the changes in EOA seen over time.[12,16,17] Identical results have also been reported with both the Medtronic Freestyle stentless valve[18] and with aortic homografts.[22] Ventricular remodelling with regression of LV mass, which has been observed following AVR with the Toronto SPV valve, is also thought to contribute to the changes in EOA and gradient as a function of time.[14,22]

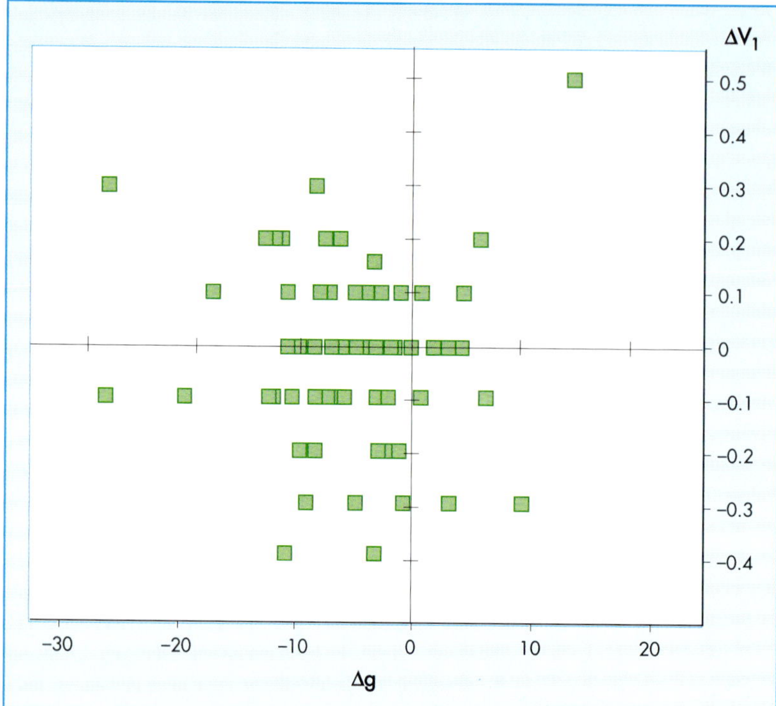

Figure 19.3 Linear regression analysis examining a change in mean transvalvular gradient against a change in V_1 from postoperation to the 3–6 months follow-up interval. The regression equation is $y = -0.001 \times -0.03$; $R = 0.03$; $p_{slope} = 0.8$. V_1 is the maximum velocity in LVOT (m/s).

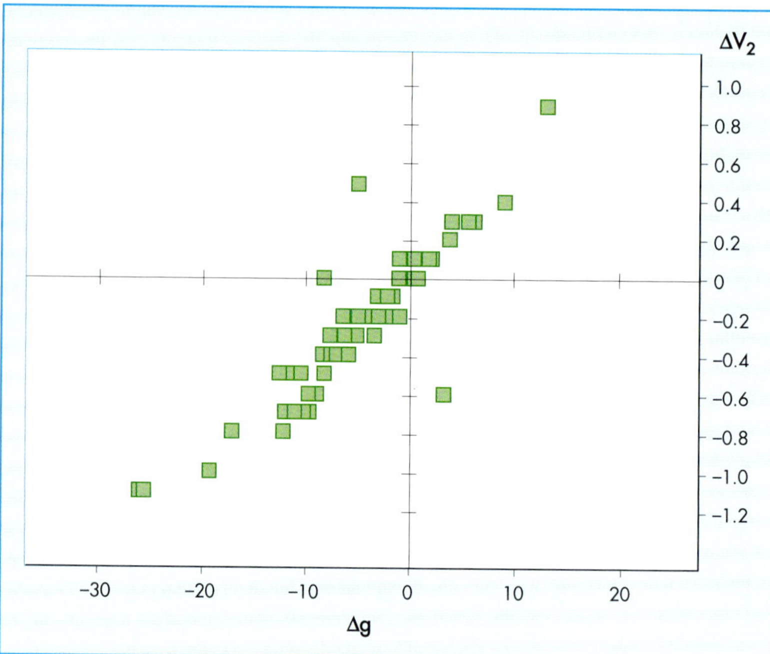

Figure 19.4 Linear regression analysis examining a change in mean transvalvular gradient against a change in V_2 from postoperation to the 3–6 months follow-up interval. The regression equation is $y = 0.047 \times -0.03$; $R = 0.89$; $p_{slope} < 0.0001$. V_2 is the maximum velocity in the aortic valve (m/s).

Mathematical models of ventricular geometry and function have been developed by Dumesnil and his co-workers to study the dynamic geometry of the left ventricle.[24] These investigators demonstrated that ejection fraction is dependent not only on the contraction of the circumferential and longitudinal fibres of the myocardium, but is also related to the specific *R/h* ratio of the ventricle, where *R* is the mid-wall radius, and *h* is the wall thickness. This phenomenon is particularly relevant when studying ventricles with variable *R/h* ratios, as may occur in patients with LVH. In subsequent work, these investigators demonstrated that for two ventricles with identical preload, the ejection fraction will be higher in the ventricle that has undergone LVH when compared to the normal ventricle.[25] Further work from this group demonstrated that EOA and V_2 were the primary determinants of transvalvular

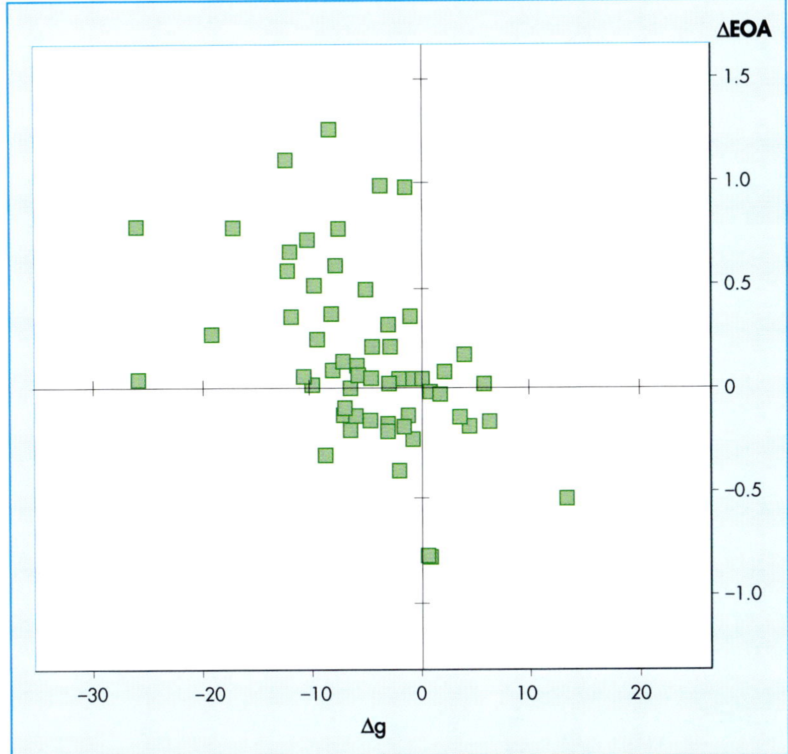

Figure 19.5 Linear regression analysis examining a change in mean transvalvular gradient against a change in effective orifice area (EOA) from postoperation to the 3–6 months follow-up interval. The regression equation is $y = 0.047 \times + 0.03$; $R = 0.49$; $p_{slope} = 0.0001$. The formula to calculate EOA is given in the Appendix.

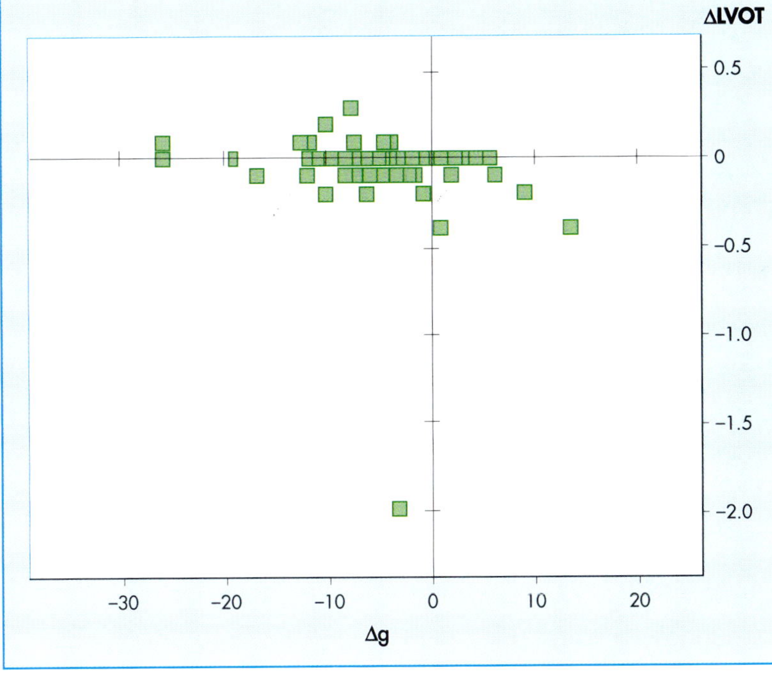

Figure 19.6 Linear regression analysis examining a change in mean transvalvular gradient against a change in left ventricular outflow tract (LVOT) from postoperation to the 3–6 months follow-up interval. The regression equation is $y = -0.007 \times -0.08$; $R = 0.03$; $p_{slope} = 0.16$.

gradient.[26] The current study builds on this conceptual framework. Dumesnil's work predicts that flow velocity across the aortic valve would be higher in patients with LVH than in normal patients. To extend this concept, regression of LVH over time would result in a decreased flow velocity across the valve, which in turn would result in a decrease in transvalvular gradient. Furthermore, if EOA and V_2 are the major determinants of transvalvular gradient at any given time, one could predict that a change in transvalvular gradient as a function of time (Δg) should be dependent on ΔV_2 and ΔEOA. Our results (Figures 19.3, 19.4) are entirely consistent with Dumesnil's findings.

Finally, the haemodynamic performance of the Toronto SPV valve has been excellent to date. The regression of LV mass and ventricular remodelling seen following AVR with this bioprosthesis may have important prognostic implications. Persistence of LVH was shown in the Framingham study to be an important predictor of mortality.[27] We recently reported that actuarial survival data at 3 years exceed 95% in patients who underwent AVR with this valve.[14] These results compare favourably with recently published series on the Carpentier–Edwards pericardial,[28] the Hancock and Carpentier–Edwards porcine,[29] and the St Jude and Medtronic Hall mechanical[30] valves. We believe the unique stentless design of the Toronto SPV valve removes the stimulus which maintains LVH in aortic valve disease-induced hypertrophy, thereby permitting remodelling to occur.[14]

References

1. Yacoub M, Rasmi N R H, Sundt T M 1995 Fourteen-year experience with homovital homografts for aortic valve replacement. J Thor Cardiovasc Surg 110: 186–194
2. Ross D N 1962 Homograft replacement of the aortic valve. Lancet 2: 487–488
3. Barratt-Boyes B, Lowe J B, Cole D S, Kelly D T 1969 Homograft replacement for aortic valve disease. Thorax 20: 489
4. Ross D, Yacoub M 1969 Homograft replacement of the aortic valve: a critical review. Prog Cardiovasc Dis 11: 275–293
5. Binet J P, Duran C G, Carpentier A, Langlois J 1965 Heterologous aortic valve transplantation. Lancet 2: 1275
6. O'Brien M F, Clarebrough J K 1966 Heterograft aortic valve transplantation for human valve disease. Med J Aust 2: 228–230
7. O'Brien M F, Clarebrough J K, McDonald J G, Hale G S, Bray H S, Cade J F 1967 Heterograft aortic valve replacement: initial follow up studies. Thorax 22: 387–396
8. Bloomfield P, Wheatley D J, Prescott R J, Miller H C 1991 Twelve year comparison of a Bjork-Shiley mechanical heart valve with porcine bioprosthesis. N Engl J Med 324: 573–579
9. Jamieson W R E, Rosado L J, Munro A I *et al* 1988 Carpentier–Edwards standard porcine bioprosthesis: primary tissue failure (structural valve deterioration) by age groups. Ann Thorac Surg 46: 155–162
10. David T E, Ropchan G C, Butany J W 1988 Aortic valve replacement with stentless porcine bioprosthesis. J Card Surg 3: 501–505
11. David T E, Pollick C, Bos J 1990 Aortic valve replacement with stentless porcine aortic bioprosthesis. J Thorac Cardiovasc Surg 99: 113–118
12. Del Rizzo D F, Goldman B S, Joyner C P, Sever J, Fremes S E, Christakis G T 1994 Initial clinical experience with the Toronto stentless porcine valve. J Cardiac Surg 9: 379–385
13. Del Rizzo D F, Goldman B S, David T E and the Canadian investigators of the Toronto SPV valve trial 1995 Aortic valve replacement with a stentless porcine bioprosthesis: multicentre trial. Can J Cardiol 11: 597–603
14. Del Rizzo D F, Goldman B S, Christakis G T, David T E 1996 Hemodynamic benefits of the Toronto SPV valve. J Thorac Cardiovasc Surg 112: 1431–1446
15. Goldman B S, David T E, Del Rizzo D F, Sever J, Bos J 1994 Stentless porcine bioprosthesis for aortic valve replacement. J Cardiovas Surg 35(Suppl 1–6): 105–110
16. Mohr F W, Walther T, Baryalei M *et al* 1995 The Toronto SPV bioprosthesis: one year results in 100 patients. Ann Thorac Surg 60: 171–175
17. Walther T, Falk V, Autschbach R *et al* 1994 Hemodynamic assessment of the stentless Toronto SPV bioprosthesis by echocardiography. J Heart Valve Dis 3: 657–665
18. Kon N D, Westaby S, Amarasena N, Pillai R, Cordell A R 1995 Comparison of implantation techniques using Freestyle stentless porcine aortic valve. Ann Thorac Surg 59: 857–862
19. Pillai R, Spriggings D, Amarasena N, O'Regan D J, Parry A J, Westaby S 1993 Stentless aortic bioprosthesis? The way forward: early experience with the Edwards valve. Ann Thorac Surg 56: 88–91
20. Konertz W, Weyand M, Sidiropoulos A, Schwammenthal E, Breithardt G, Scheld H H 1992 Technique of aortic valve replacement with the Edwards stentless aortic bioprosthesis 2500. Eur J Cardiothorac Surg 6: 274–277

21. Hvass U, Chatel D, Ouroudji M *et al* 1994 The O'Brien–Angell stentless valve. Early results of 100 implants. Eur J Cardiothorac Surg 42: 36–39
22. Jin X Y, Zhang Z, Gibson D G, Yacoub M H, Pepper J R 1996 Changes in left ventricular function and hypertrophy following aortic valve replacement using aortic homograft, stentless, or stented valve. Ann Thorac Surg 62: 683–690
23. Vesely I, Menkis A H, Rutt B, Campbell G 1991 Aortic valve/root interactions in porcine hearts: implications for bioprosthetic valve sizing. J Card Surg 6: 482–489
24. Dumesnil J G, Shoucri R M, Laurenceau J L, Turcot J 1979 A mathematical model of the dynamic geometry of the intact left ventricle and its application to clinical data. Circulation 59: 1024–1034
25. Dumesnil J G, Shoucri R M 1991 Quantitative relationships between left ventricular ejection and wall thickening and geometry. J Appl Physiol 70: 48–54
26. Dumesnil J G, Yoganathan A 1992 Valve prosthesis hemodynamics and the problem of high transprosthetic gradients. Eur J Cardiothorac Surg 6(Suppl 1): S34–S38
27. Levy D, Garrison R J, Savage D D, Kannel W B, Castelli W P 1990 Prognostic implications of echocardiographically determined left ventricular mass in the Framingham heart study. N Engl J Med 322: 1561–1566
28. Cosgrove D M, Lytle B W, Taylor P C *et al* 1995 The Carpentier–Edwards pericardial aortic valve: ten-year results. J Thorac Cardiovasc Surg 110: 651–662
29. Jones E L, Weintraub W S, Craver J M *et al* 1990 Ten-year experience with the porcine bioprosthetic valve: interrelationship of valve survival and patient survival in 1,050 valve replacements. Ann Thorac Surg 49: 370–384
30. Masters R G, Pipe A L, Walley V M, Keon W J 1995 Comparative results with the St. Jude Medical and Medtronic Hall mechanical valves. J Thorac Cardiovasc Surg 110: 663–671

Appendix

The mean systolic gradient and effective orifice area are calculated by:

$$\text{Mean systolic gradient} = 4[(0.65V_2)^2 - (0.65V_1)^2]$$

$$\text{Effective orifice area} = \frac{0.8 \times (0.65V_1) \times A_{\text{LVOT}} \times 100}{100 \times \sqrt{[(0.65V_2)^2 - (0.65V_1)^2]}}$$

where: V_1 is the maximum velocity in LVOT (m/s);
V_2 is the maximum velocity in the aortic valve (m/s);
A_{LVOT} is the area of the LVOT (cm^2).

The LV mass (g) is calculated by:

$$\text{LV mass} = 0.000\,83\,[(\text{LV}_{\text{post}} + \text{IVS} + \text{LV}_{\text{end}})^3 - (\text{LV}_{\text{end}})^3] + 0.6$$

where: LV_{post} is the LV posterior wall thickness at end-diastole (mm);
IVS is the thickness of the intraventricular septus at end-diastole (mm);
LV_{end} is the LV end-diastolic size (mm).

The LV mass index (g/m^2) is calculated by:

$$\text{LV mass/BSA}$$

where: BSA is the body surface area (m^2).

CHAPTER 20

Clinical and haemodynamic performance of the Freestyle aortic root bioprosthesis

P. C. Cartier, J. Métras, J. G. Dumesnil, D. Doyle, D. Desaulniers, M. Lemieux and G. Raymond

The Medtronic Freestyle aortic root bioprosthesis was released by the FDA in July 1992 for human investigational use. Since then, over 800 prostheses have been implanted around the world.

The advantages of the porcine bioprostheses are well known: central flow, low embolic rate and no anticoagulation therapy. Its disadvantages are limited durability, calcification, especially in children and young adults, and significant residual gradient in small sizes.[1]

Stent modification and use of antimineralization processes have improved valve performance and durability, but high gradients are still encountered in small sizes. To alleviate this, stentless porcine devices have been proposed. In the absence of a stent, improved haemodynamic results are obtained because of improved effective orifice area.[2]

The Medtronic Freestyle aortic root bioprosthesis is a full aortic root with porcine coronary ostia intact. The porcine aortic root is preserved in a buffered 0.2% glutaraldehyde solution, and fixed with zero pressure across the leaflets and a pressure of 40 mmHg across the aortic wall. This method of fixation preserves the natural collagen structure of the leaflets and maintains the native valve anatomy. The Freestyle is treated with an antimineralization process, alpha-aminooleic acid (AOA), synthesized from oleic acid, a naturally occurring fatty acid.

A thin polyester cloth covering has been added to strengthen the proximal suture line and cover any exposed porcine myocardium.

Patients and methods

Clinical investigation of the Freestyle aortic root bioprosthesis began in January 1993 in our institution. Since May 1, 1997, there have been 270 implants at Laval Hospital in Quebec City. Included in the study were patients 20 years of age or older requiring aortic valve or aortic root replacement. Patients undergoing concomitant procedures such as coronary artery bypass or valve reconstruction were eligible to participate. However, those requiring concomitant valve replacement or having a pre-existing prosthetic valve in another position were excluded from the study. Data from 242 patients were available for this study.

There are three techniques commonly used for homograft, autograft or stentless bioprostheses: aortic root replacement, intra-aortic cylinder and valve replacement. At Laval Hospital 217 (89.6%) were valve replacements with or without scalloping the non-coronary sinus and 24 (9.9%) were aortic root replacements; there was one root inclusion.

The total patient group consisted of 134 males (55.4%) and 108 females (44.6%). Patient age averaged 68 years (SD = 7). A majority of patients were in NYHA functional class III or IV (85.6%). Risk factors or concomitant diseases consisted of left ventricular dysfunction which included left ventricular hypertrophy, wall motion abnormality or dilatation, coronary artery disease present in 42.6%, ejection fraction less than 50% present in 15.3% of the patients. Hypertension and angina disease were also frequently encountered. Additional patient characteristics are summarized in Tables 20.1 and 20.2.

Table 20.1 Patient demographics and preoperative data

Gender	
Male	134 (55.4%)
Female	108 (44.6%)
Age (years)	
Mean (SD)	68 (7)
Range	38–85
Cardiac rhythm	
Normal sinus	212 (87.6%)
Atrial fibrillation	12 (4.9%)
Paced	4 (1.7%)
Heart block	14 (5.8%)
NYHA classification	
I	2 (0.8%)
II	33 (13.6%)
III	180 (74.4%)
IV	27 (11.2%)

Table 20.2 Risk factors/coexisting diseases

Left ventricular dysfunction	214 (88.4%)
Hypertension	144 (59.5%)
Angina	142 (58.7%)
Cigarette smoker	133 (55.0%)
Coronary artery disease	103 (42.6%)
Hyperlipidaemia	78 (32.2%)
Ejection fraction < 50%	37 (15.3%)
History of TIA/CVA	17 (7.0%)

CVA, cerebrovascular accident; TIA, transient ischaemic attack.

Surgical information is presented in Tables 20.3–20.5. Distribution of implant sizes for all patients was 19 mm for 8 implants (3.3%); 21 mm for 36 implants (14.9%); 23 mm for 58 implants (24%); 25 mm for 76 implants (31.4%); and 27 mm for 64 implants (26.4%). Total cross-clamp time averaged 103 min without concomitant surgery, and 134 min with a concomitant procedure. The most common concomitant surgical procedure was coronary artery bypass in 84 (34.7%). Over 75% of the patients needed either a moderate or extensive annular debridement.

Management of operation was done according to the preferences of the implanting surgeon. Mild hypothermia with double stage single venous cannula was the rule but myocardial protection varied according to the preferences of the surgeon from cold intermittent antegrade to warm continuous retrograde.

Definitions of morbid prosthesis-related complication follow the guidelines of the American Association for Thoracic Surgery and the Society of Thoracic Surgeons. Morbidity included structural deterioration, non-structural dysfunction, thromboembolism, antithromboembolic-related haemorrhage and endocarditis. Consequences of morbid events included reoperation, explant and prosthesis-related mortality.[3]

Haemodynamic performance of the Freestyle bioprosthesis was assessed by echocardiography. Echo-Doppler assessments were made on all operative survivors prior to discharge. Additional assessments were made during the late postoperative period (3–6 months after implant) and annually beginning with the first anniversary of the implant date. Measurements were made of cardiac output, mean pressure gradient, effective orifice area, and regurgitation.

Statistical methods

Continuous data were expressed as mean ± standard deviation. Percentages were determined for categorical variables. Comparisons of mean gradient, effective orifice area and cardiac output at discharge, 3–6 months, 1 year and 2 years were analysed

Table 20.3 Surgical information: size of bioprosthesis

Size (mm)	No.	%
19	8	3.3
21	36	14.9
23	58	24.0
25	76	31.4
27	64	26.4

Table 20.4 Surgical information: cross-clamp time; cardioplegia

Cross-clamp time (min)	
Without concomitant surgery (n = 99)	
Mean (SD)	103 (20)
Range	43–168
With concomitant surgery (n = 89)	
Mean (SD)	134 (30)
Range	80–244
Cardioplegia	
Cold	36 (14.8%)
Warm	145 (60.0%)
Both	61 (25.2%)

Table 20.5 Surgical information: concomitant procedures; annular debridement

Concomitant procedures	
CABG	84 (34.7%)
Ascending aortic repair	28 (11.6%)
Annuloplasty	4 (1.7%)
Aortic root enlargement	3 (1.2%)
IABP	8 (3.3%)
VSD repair	1 (0.4%)
Perm. pacemaker	1 (0.4%)
Others	9 (3.7%)
Annular debridement	
None	2 (1.0%)
Minimal	32 (13.2%)
Moderate	142 (58.6%)
Extensive	66 (27.2%)

using a repeated ANOVA design with a sphericity test on orthogonal components. This test determines whether or not the F statistics from the univariate procedure are valid. As p-values of F test were significant at the 0.05 level, only repeated measures designs were performed. Categorical data were analysed using Fisher's exact test. Product-limit analyses (also called Kaplan–Meier analyses) were used to report the time-dependent cumulative probabilities of the outcome for complications. Plots of negative log of the survival function versus time revealed that parametric models were not appropriate for survival data. All reported p-values are two-tailed and were declared significant at $\alpha = 0.05$. The statistical package program SAS (SAS Institute Inc., Cary, NC, USA) was used to perform the analyses.

Results

Patient follow-up

Follow-up data were available for 227 patients, with 163 followed for more than 1 year, 92 for more than 2 years and 35 for more than 3 years. This is a short follow-up; however, the NYHA class remained stable, with 95% of the group being in either class I or II (Table 20.6). Sinus rhythm was present at follow-up in almost 90% of the patients. The antithrombo-embolic therapy of choice was aspirin. Warfarin was reserved for patients in atrial fibrillation or with higher risks of thromboembolism (Table 20.7).

Prosthesis-related complications

There were four cases of endocarditis; two were reoperated almost a year after the original operation and two were treated medically. One patient was reoperated 33 days postoperatively for a paravalvular leak.

Mortality

There were ten early deaths and nine late deaths. The one early valve-related death was a reoperated patient with significant risk factors who failed to come off bypass despite the fact that the valve had been replaced. Seven of the early deaths were cardiac but not related to the valve. The one late valve-related death was secondary to ileofemoral

Table 20.6 Follow-up data: NYHA class

NYHA classification	3–6 months	1 year	2 years	3 years
Population	202	163	92	35
Class I	161 (79.7%)	133 (81.6%)	78 (83.8%)	27 (77.2%)
Class II	35 (17.3%)	25 (15.3%)	11 (11.8%)	7 (20%)
Class III	5 (2.5%)	3 (1.8%)	2 (2.2%)	1 (2.8%)
Class IV	0	2 (1.3%)	0	0
Unable to assess	1 (0.5%)	0	1 (1.1%)	0

Table 20.7 Follow-up data

	Discharge	3–6 months	1 year	2 years	3 years
Numbers of implants	227	202	163	92	35
Cardiac rhythm					
Normal sinus	204 (89.9%)	180 (89%)	143 (87.7%)	80 (87%)	31 (88.6%)
Atrial fibrillation	14 (6.2%)	9 (4.5%)	8 (4.9%)	6 (6.5%)	3 (8.6%)
Paced	9 (4.0%)	8 (4.0%)	9 (5.5%)	4 (4.4%)	1 (2.8%)
Heart block	0	4 (2.0%)	3 (1.8%)	2 (2.1%)	0
Junctional	0	1 (0.5%)	0	0	
Antithromboembolic therapy					
None	15	38	30	17	1
Warfarin	31	23	18	9	4
Aspirin	180	143	116	67	30
Warfarin and aspirin	1	0	1	0	0
Unknown	0	0	0	0	0

Table 20.8 Mortality and valve-related morbidity

Event	Number of early events	Number of late events	Percentage actuarial freedom at 3 years (SE)
Endocarditis	0	4	
Reoperation	0	3	98.7 (0.7)
Death	10	9	91.3 (1.9)
Valve-related	1	1	99.2 (0.6)
Sudden/unexplained	0	1	99.6 (0.4)
Cardiac	7	0	97.1 (1.1)
Non-cardiac	2	7	95.4 (1.5)

embolism and renal insufficiency. Seven of the late deaths were non-cardiac, the one sudden death was suspected to be myocardial infarction (Table 20.8).

The overall mortality was 4.1%, with a mortality of 2.4% for valve replacement and 16.6% for root replacement (Table 20.9). Although some might think this mortality for root replacement is high, if you compare it to the data from Summit Medical, the STS database, the mortality for aortic root reconstruction was 14.9% for people under 70 years old and 21.7% for those over 70. In our own series of Ross procedures where root replacement is done almost routinely, the mortality is 3.5%. It is not the technique used that causes mortality but the underlying disease.

Table 20.9 Mortality and valve-related morbidity: early mortality

Valve replacement	2.4%
Root replacement	16.6% (p = 0.011)
Root inclusion	0

Neurological events

Neurological events are always tragic. In our series, there were 10 valve-related events and 14 non-valve-related events. Of those, 17 were early and seven late. Fifteen were permanent with seven who recuperated completely and six partially. The freedom from valve-related neurological events at 3 years was 97.5% for permanent and 98.4% for transient events (Table 20.10).

Table 20.10 Mortality and valve-related morbidity: neurological events

	Early	Late	Percentage freedom at 3 years, (SE)
Valve related			
Permanent	3 (2, 1)	3 (2, 1)	97.5 (0.9)
Transient	2	2	98.4 (0.9)
Non-valve related			
Permanent	9 (3, 4, 2)	0	
Transient	3	2	

Haemodynamic performance

Haemodynamic performance was assessed by echocardiography. Echo-Doppler assessments were made of all operative survivors prior to discharge, at 3–6 months and annually thereafter. Measurements were made of cardiac output, mean pressure gradient, effective orifice area and regurgitation.

The most interesting data encountered concerned the mean gradient and the effective orifice area. Although there is no statistical difference between cardiac output at discharge, at 3–6 months and at 1 year, there was a statistically significant decrease in average mean gradient from discharge to 3–6 months for all sizes and this trend seems to persist for sizes 19, 25 and 27 mm at 1- and 2-year follow-up, but it was not statistically significant (Figures 20.1, 20.2). Similarly, there was a statistically significant increase in the average effective orifice area from discharge to 3–6 months for all sizes and this trend seems to persist at 1- and 2-year follow-up (Figures 20.3, 20.4). This trend was seen in all valve sizes. These findings were confirmed with other

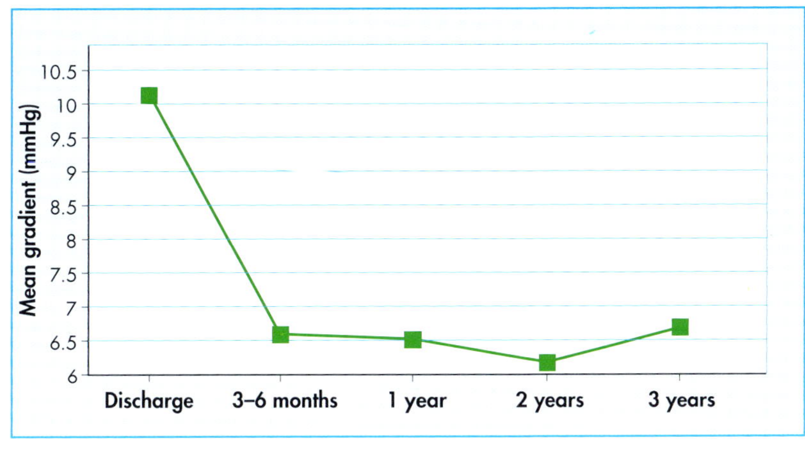

Figure 20.1 Mean gradient.

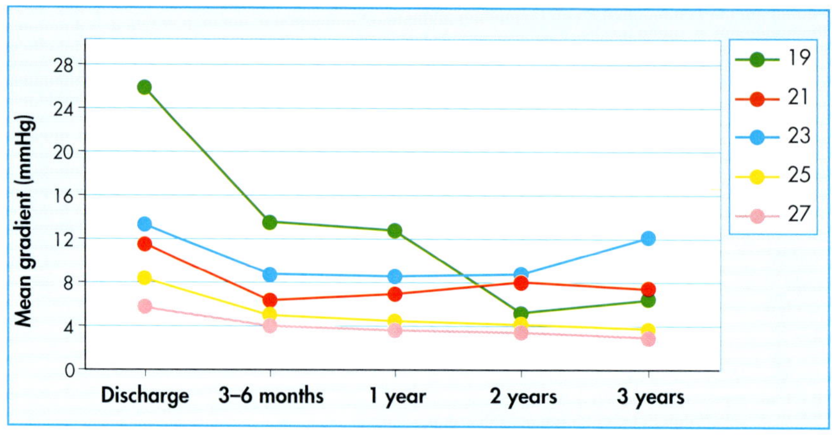

Figure 20.2 Mean gradient for various valve sizes used.

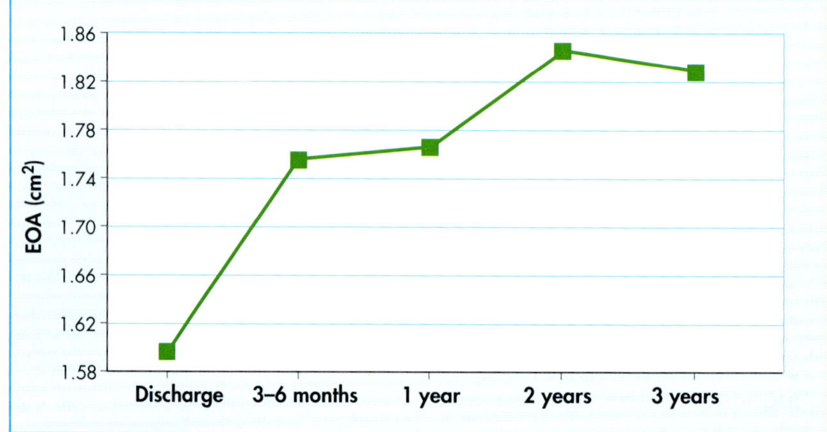

Figure 20.3 Freestyle effective orifice area.

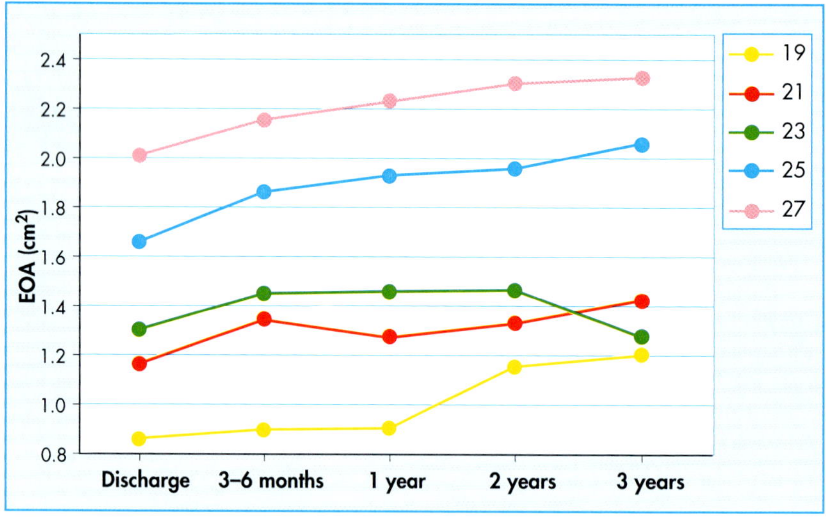

Figure 20.4 Freestyle effective orifice area for various valve sizes used.

stentless bioprostheses. One of the reasons could be a remodelling of the left ventricular outflow tract which usually does not occur with a rigid ring.

Regurgitation was trivial or mild in the majority of the patients and was not haemodynamically significant. There was no evidence that the regurgitation progresses; on the contrary, it actually seems to get better with time (Figure 20.5).

Discussion

The Freestyle aortic root bioprosthesis is part of a new generation of stentless bioprostheses. The haemodynamics are remarkable, with low gradient and higher effective orifice area that are without comparison with previous bioprostheses. Their

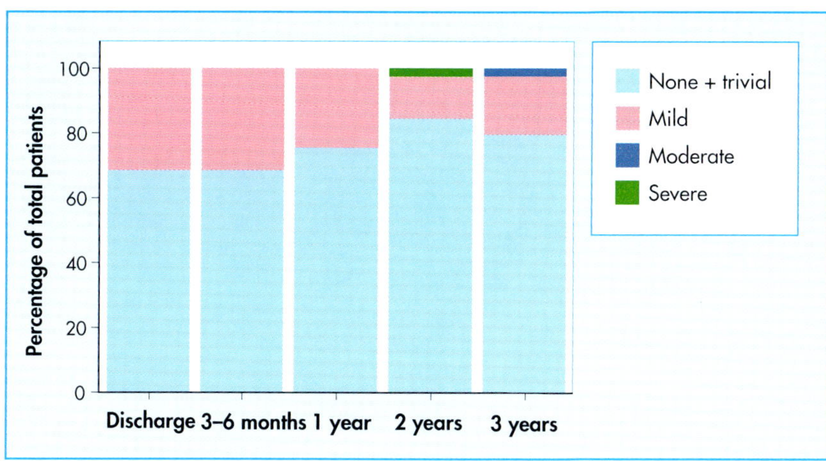

Figure 20.5
Aortic regurgitation.

introduction has changed the thinking on aortic valves, when considering replacement, from just an annulus to a complex entity including a flexible annulus, sinuses and a sinotubular junction. The implantation technique is also different and has raised a lot of controversy — continuous or interrupted, scalloped or not, root or subcoronary implantation. Despite strong advocates for each technique, it is still too early to conclude who will be right.

The early results are very encouraging. The actuarial survival at 3 years is 91.3% (SE = 1.9%). The freedom from valve-related complications at 3 years is: for valve-related death 99.1% (SE = 0.6%), for permanent neurological events 97.5% (SE = 0.9%), for endocarditis 98.3% (SE = 0.9%) and for reoperation 98.7% (SE = 0.7%).

The increased effective orifice area and the lower mean gradient are the main advantages of this valve compared with the stented bioprosthesis. Will it affect long-term survival? There is much concern about regurgitation. It is important to remember that in the majority of the cases it is not haemodynamically significant and that there is no progression at follow-up; on the contrary, there seems to be an improvement. There was no reoperation for prosthesis regurgitation in our series except for one patient who was reoperated at 1 month for a paravalvular leak at the beginning of our experience.

Acknowledgements

We thank Louise Côté and Jacinthe Aubé for their technical assistance, Martine Fleury for the secretarial support and Serge Simard for all the statistical analysis.

References

1. Dumesnil J G, Yoganathan A P 1992 Valve prosthesis hemodynamics and the problem of high transprosthetic pressure gradients. Eur J Cardiothorac Surg 6(Suppl I): 34–38
2. Yoganathan A P, Eberhardt C E, Walker P G 1994 Hydrodynamic performance of the Medtronic Freestyle aortic root bioprosthesis. J Heart Valve Dis 3(5): 571–580
3. Edmunds L H, Clark R E, Cohn L H, Miller D C, Weisel R D 1988 Guidelines for reporting morbidity and mortality after cardiac valvular operations. Ann Thorac Surg 46: 257–259

CHAPTER 21

Left ventricular remodelling after stentless aortic valve replacement

T. Walther, V. Falk, C. Weigl, A. Diegeler, L. Schilling, R. Autschbach and F. W. Mohr

Left ventricular hypertophy (LVH) is an an important and independent cardiac risk factor in patients with aortic valve disease.[1–7] Aortic stenosis is the most common underlying pathology in patients requiring aortic valve replacement (AVR). With aortic valve replacement, physiological haemodynamics and regression of LVH, namely left ventricular remodelling, can be achieved. Therefore valve replacement therapy improves the prognosis for the patient.[1,8]

Nevertheless, the ideal aortic valve prosthesis does not yet exist.[9–11] In addition to mechanical or biological stented valves, stentless bioprostheses have been used more frequently in the past 10 years with good results.[12–15] Morphologically, stentless bioprostheses resemble the native aortic valve.

Left ventricular remodelling is present to some degree in all patients after AVR, irrespective of the valve type implanted. But little is known about the exact time course and the influence of different valves upon left ventricular remodelling. This study was performed to compare prospectively mechanical, conventional and stentless bioprostheses with regard to postoperative haemodynamics and left ventricular remodelling.

Methods

Two hundred and ninety-four consecutive patients who had aortic valve replacement were entered in a prospective clinical trial from March 1996 onwards. Informed consent was obtained after outlining the study in detail. Patients younger than 70 years received a bileaflet mechanical prosthesis (group 1: ATS, Carbomedics, SJM) whereas patients older than 70 years were randomized to receive a conventional bioprosthesis (group 2: Carpentier–Edwards) or a stentless bioprosthesis (group 3: Freestyle, Toronto SPV valve). Follow-up at the hospitals' outpatient clinic was performed at 6 months and annually thereafter, 6 months follow-up was complete in 114 patients. Demographics are shown in Table 21.1.

Intraoperatively the aortic valve annulus was measured using one exact standard sizer. With this technique a comparable measure for the annulus could be achieved in all patients. The operation was performed using a standard technique with cold crystalloid cardioplegia (Bretschneider) and moderate hypothermia. All stented valves were implanted using a standard technique with interrupted pledgetted sutures in a supra-annular position. The stentless valves were implanted in a subcoronary position with interrupted sutures and a running suture line at the top using the freehand technique.

Echocardiography was performed pre- and postoperatively using standard views with the patient at haemodynamically stable conditions (heart rate 60–100/min, mean

Table 21.1 Demographics of the 294 patients according to the three different study groups

Group	Mechanical	Conventional	Stentless
No. patients	201	30	63
Age (years)	60.3	74.7	72.5
AS (%)	85	92	91
Annulus (mm)	25	22.2	24.3
AVR (mm)	23.9	22.2	25.5
Bypass no.(%)	24 (1.7)	30 (1.5)	29 (1.9)
Cross-clamp (min)	57.5	58.4	71.9
Mortality	1	1	2

AS, aortic stenosis; AVR, aortic valve replacement.

arterial blood pressure 60–90 mmHg). All parameters were averaged from five cardiac cycles in sinus rhythm and from 10 cardiac cycles when atrial fibrillation was present. Pressure gradients were calculated according to the Bernoulli formula with correction for left ventricular outflow tract (LVOT) velocities. Valve orifice areas were calculated according to the continuity equation and calculated per body surface area.

Postoperative valve-related morbidity and mortality are reported according to standard guidelines.[16] Left ventricular posterior wall (LVPW) hypertrophy was defined as tissue thickness >12 mm at the suprapapillary level on M-mode recordings or as left ventricular mass >220 g as calculated from M-mode recordings using the Devereux formula.

Results are given as mean ± standard deviation. Statistical analysis was performed using the SPSS statistical package (SPSS Inc., Chicago, IL, USA); the Student's *t*-test was applied.

Results

No major valve-related problems, e.g. endocarditis, stuctural or non-structural dysfunction, have been encountered during follow-up thus far. One patient had to be reoperated for paravalvular leakage after mechanical AVR. Overall mortality (n = 4, 1.3%) was not valve related. Postoperative echocardiographic results were compared to 6-month follow-up data. Ventricular dimensions, haemodynamic data and left ventricular hypertrophy were analysed (Tables 21.2–21.4).

Assessment of the left ventricle was performed using two-dimensional echocardiography applying the Simpson method. Left ventricular end-diastolic volumes were in the normal range in all patients preoperatively and there was a slight decrease at follow-up in all three groups. Left ventricular ejection fraction was in the range of 48–54% preoperatively and there was a slight increase at follow-up. The exact data are given in Table 21.2.

Table 21.2 Left ventricular (LV) dimensions from two-dimensional echocardiographic measurements according to Simpson

LV dimensions	Mechanical	Conventional	Stentless
ED (ml)			
Postop	112	85	87
6 Months	99	73	83
EF (%)			
Postop	51	48	54
6 Months	52	56	56

ED, end-diastolic volume; EF, ejection fraction.

Transvalvular flow velocities were in the normal range for all patients in the three different groups. After stentless AVR, maximum flow velocity and transvalvular pressure gradients were lower. There was an increase in valve orifice areas at follow-up in all patients; however, this was most pronounced after stentless AVR. Haemodynamic data are given in Table 21.3.

Left ventricular hypertrophy was analysed from parasternal M-mode echocardiographic recordings. Preoperatively all patients had marked LVH, with no statistically significant difference between groups. At follow-up there was a significant decrease of LVH in all three groups compared with preoperative measurements. After stentless AVR the decrease of LVH was significantly larger compared with patients having mechanical AVR ($p<0.05$). Left ventricular posterior wall diameter was within the normal range as early as at the 6-month follow-up and left ventricular mass was close to normal in the patients with stentless AVR. All data concerning left ventricular hypertrophy are shown in Table 21.4.

Discussion

The beneficial impact of left ventricular remodelling on the prognosis for patients after aortic valve replacement is well known. In several studies it was shown that there is some postoperative left ventricular remodelling no matter what type of prosthesis was implanted. Nevertheless, little is known about the exact time course of left ventricular remodelling.

Since the introduction of stentless bioprostheses about 10 years ago, a physiological aortic valve prosthesis has become available. With its increasing use, the possible advantages of stentless bioprostheses in terms of early left ventricular remodelling became evident.[15] Thus far, most clinical studies consisted of a linear analysis of one valve only. No prospectively randomized trials comparing conventional and stentless

Table 21.3 Haemodynamic measurements from Doppler echocardiography

Haemodynamics	Mechanical	Conventional	Stentless
V_{max} (m/s)			
Postop	2.6 ± 0.5	2.7 ± 0.4	2.2 ± 0.4
6 Months	2.5 ± 0.3	2.5 ± 0.4	2.1 ± 0.3
AOA (cm^2)			
Postop	1.14 ± 0.3	1.07 ± 0.4	1.21 ±0.2
6 Months	1.16 ± 0.2	1.15 ± 0.2	1.55 ± 0.6

Maximum flow velocity (V_{max}) is derived from continuous-wave Doppler measurements; valve orifice area is calculated using the continuity equation.The maximum flow velocity is used to calculate transvalvular pressure gradients (Bernoulli equation: pressure gradient = $4 \times V_{max}^2$). AOA, aortic valve orifice area.

Table 21.4 Left ventricular hypertrophy (LVH), given as left ventricular posterior wall diameter (LVPWd) and left ventricular mass (LV mass)

LVH	Mechanical	Conventional	Stentless
LVPWd (mm)			
Postop	14.6	14.3	15.3
6 Months	12.6*	11.1*	10.8*
LV mass (g)			
Postop	397	280	359
6 Months	333*	242	244*

* Indicates $p< 0.05$ versus postop.

valves have yet been performed. The results of this trial comparing several prostheses in a prospectively randomized fashion are therefore of clinical importance.

Surgically the implantation of stentless valves is more difficult and time consuming than conventional AVR. In our study this resulted in slightly longer cross-clamp times without any additional morbidity or mortality.

Exact sizing of the patient's annulus is of utmost importance in a study in which the haemodynamic and morphological data of different patient groups are compared.[17] Therefore, one exact standard sizer, as applied in this study, should be used in each patient. In this study it was shown that in patients having the same annular diameter a 2 mm larger stentless bioprosthesis could be implanted. This can be partially attributed to the oversizing technique. Thus, in a given patient, better valve performance can be anticipated.

With regard to the left ventricle, end-diastolic volumes slightly decreased in all three groups and there was an increase in ejection fraction. This result underlines that there is some recovery for the left ventricle in all patients postoperatively.

After stentless AVR, laminar transvalvular blood flow can be demonstrated by colour Doppler examinations. This is in contrast to the turbulence that can be seen with stented aortic valves. The laminar flow profile of stentless bioprostheses can be explained by the flexible structure of the aortic root in these patients.

On average, all patients included in this study had preoperative left ventricular hypertrophy. Left ventricular remodelling was present in all three groups at follow-up ($p<0.05$). Nevertheless, left ventricular remodelling was pronounced in patients having stentless in comparison to mechanical AVR ($p<0.05$). As early as 6 months after the implantation of stentless bioprostheses, normal parameters for left ventricular posterior wall thickness and an almost normal left ventricular mass were found.

The earlier and more extensive left ventricular remodelling after stentless AVR can be explained by several factors. First, the implantation of larger valves in a given patient leads to a lower transvalvular pressure gradient. Secondly, with the flexible design of stentless bioprostheses the elasticity on the aortic root can be preserved. Both factors lead to a laminar transvalvular flow profile which might have an additional impact upon early left ventricular remodelling.

Conclusion

In conclusion, left ventricular remodelling was present after conventional and after stentless AVR at 6-month follow-up. This was in conjunction with early haemodynamic improvements. After stentless AVR, left ventricular remodelling was much more pronounced ($p<0.05$). Thus, the stentless design by early decrease of LVH leads to a decrease of the cardiac risk for the patient. This might be advantageous to enhance further the postoperative quality of life for the patient.

In this clinical trial the advantages of stentless bioprostheses have been proven using a prospectively randomized study design. Although long-term follow-up is warranted, stentless valves are the bioprostheses of choice.

References

1. Acar J, Elias J, Luxereau P 1995 Aortic stenosis and mixed aortic valve disease. In: Acar J, Bodnar E (eds) Textbook of acquired heart valve disease. ICR Publishers, London. Vol 1, pp 454–486
2. Diez J 1994 Current work in the cell biology of left ventricular hypertrophy. Curr Opin Cardiol 9: 512–519
3. Liao Y, Cooper R S, Mensah G A, McGee D L 1995 Left ventricular hypertrophy has a greater impact on survival in women than in men. Circulation 92: 805–810
4. Aronow W S 1994/95 Diagnostic and prognostic value of left ventricular hypertrophy in elderly patients. Editorial. J Cardiovasc Diagn Proc 12: 151–157

5. Messerli F H, Ketelhut R 1993 Left ventricular hypertrophy: a pressure-independent cardiovascular risk factor. J Cardiovasc Pharmacol 22(Suppl I): S7–S13
6. Gordon T, Kannel W B 1971 Premature mortality from coronary heart disease. The Framingham study. JAMA 215: 1617
7. Anderson K P 1984 Sudden death, hypertension, and hypertrophy. J Cardiovasc Pharmacol 6 (Suppl 3): S498
8. Kirklin J W, Barratt-Boyes B G 1993 Aortic valve disease. In: Kirklin, J W, Barratt-Boyes B G, (eds) Cardiac surgery, 2nd edn. Churchill Livingstone, New York, 554–555
9. Collins J J 1991 The evolution of artificial heart valves. Editorial. N Engl J Med 324: 624–626
10. Wernly J A, Crawford M H 1991 Choosing a prosthetic heart valve. Cardiol Clin 9: 329–338
11. Davila J C 1989 Where is the ideal heart valve substitute? What has frustrated its realization? Ann Thorac Surg 48: S20–S23
12. David T, Feindel C M, Bros J, Sun Z, Scully H E, Rakowski H 1994 Aortic valve replacement with a stentless porcine aortic valve. A six year experience. J Thorac Cardiovasc Surg 108: 1030–1036
13. Westaby S, Amarasena N, Ormerod O, Amarasena C, Pillai R 1995 Aortic valve replacement with the Freestyle stentless xenograft. Ann Thorac Surg 60: S422–S427
14. Mohr F W, Walther T, Baryalei M *et al* 1995 The Toronto SPV bioprosthesis: one-year results in 100 patients. Ann Thorac Surg 60: 171–175
15. Walther T, Falk V, Autschbach R *et al* 1994 Hemodynamic assessment of the stentless Toronto SPV™ bioprosthesis by echocardiography. J Heart Valve Dis 3: 657–665
16. Edmunds L H, Clark R E, Cohn L H, Miller D C, Weisel R D 1988 Guidelines for reporting morbidity and mortality after cardiac valvular operations. Ann Thorac Surg 46: 257–259
17. Walther T, Falk V, Weigl C *et al* 1997 Discrepancy of sizers for conventional and stentless aortic valve implants. J Heart Valve Dis 6(2): 145–148

CHAPTER 22

Functional haemodynamic performance of the Toronto SPV valve versus the annular Carpentier–Edwards aortic valve per patient annulus size

P. C. Strike, T. Edwards, I. A. Simpson, S. A. Livesey and V. T. Tsang

Bioprosthetic valve replacements are now widely used in the aortic position, but there are several disadvantages to the conventional stented bioprostheses. Conventional stented porcine bioprostheses have an effective orifice area less than that of the left ventricular outflow tract[1] and this may leave unacceptable outflow tract obstruction, especially in the small aortic root or if there is mismatch between the valve and the patient.[1–3] The physical presence of the stent itself also leads to a degree of outflow obstruction and consequently to a less favourable haemodynamic profile.

Other disadvantages of the presence of the stent are that it leads to increased stresses on the valve cusps themselves because of the inability of the stent to change shape during the various stages of the cardiac cycle.[4] The stent itself cushions impact of the cusps less well than the native aortic root[2,5] and the leaflets may abrade against the cloth covering.[6] In effect, in a stentless valve, the host aortic root itself acts as a stent for the valve. The fact that the aortic root is effectively used as a stent is also beneficial haemodynamically in that in systole the leaflets are more fully opened as the commissural areas are pulled apart, allowing decreased resistance to flow.[7,8]

Stented xenografts have unfortunately compared badly with homograft valve replacements as a result of valve calcification and degeneration, and stentless xenografts may be a possible solution to this problem.[9] It has been shown that stent mounting adversely affects tissue valve durability with aortic valve replacements in homografts.[10]

The stentless design of the Toronto SPV valve (St Jude Medical Inc., St Paul, MN, USA) allows a larger valve size (usually 2–3 mm larger) to be implanted for a given patient annulus size than the conventional stented annular valves.[1,4,11] This is especially useful in the small aortic root.[12,13] There have been previous favourable comparisons with the Hancock II valve[1,14] and with other stented porcine and pericardial bioprostheses.[13] The purpose of this study was to ascertain if the benefits outlined above translate to a superior haemodynamic profile as measured by Doppler echocardiography compared with the commonly used annular Carpentier–Edwards aortic bioprosthesis.

Patients and methods

Between 1993 and 1996, 34 Toronto SPV valves were implanted in the aortic position. Over the same time period, 44 annular Carpentier–Edwards valves were similarly implanted.

In general, upon sizing the aortic annulus at the time of surgery it was found that a Toronto SPV valve of at least one size larger than the annulus could be implanted; for example in an annulus sized to take a conventional size 23 mm prosthesis, a size 25 mm Toronto SPV valve was able to be inserted.

The surgical technique used in implanting the Toronto SPV valve was as follows. Initially the inflow suture line was secured with multiple interrupted runs of continuous 3/0 Prolene sutures. Next, the commissures were suspended with 4/0 Prolene and then the outflow scalloped suture line was performed with continuous 4/0 Prolene sutures to the aortic sinuses without compromising the coronary artery ostia. The Carpentier–Edwards bioprostheses were implanted conventionally using multiple interrupted runs of continuous 2/0 Prolene sutures.

Of the 34 Toronto SPV valves implanted, 21 patients consented to undergo repeat echocardiography and examination. Of the 44 annular Carpentier–Edwards valves, 23 patients consented to undergo repeat echocardiography and examination. The distribution of annulus size into which they were implanted is shown in Table 22.1.

Table 22.1 The distribution of aortic annulus size into which the Toronto SPV valve and the Carpentier–Edwards valves were implanted

Patient annulus size (mm)	**Toronto SPV valve** n **= 21**	**Carpentier–Edwards** n **= 23**
21	4	7
23	4	10
25	8	4
27	5	2

The demographics, resting pulse, blood pressure, height, weight, and body surface area of the study populations are shown in Table 22.2.

Table 22.2 Patient demographics of the study groups

	Toronto SPV valve	**Carpentier–Edwards**
Number	21	23
Age at operation (years)	71.2 ± 7.4	74.9 ± 5.44
Age range (years)	51–86	61–83
Concurrent CABG	7	10
Male / female	15 / 6	11 / 13
Mean resting systolic BP (mmHg)	137.7 ± 19.1	145.1 ± 23.7
Pulse (bpm)	73.2 ± 10.5	70.8 ± 9.1
Height (cm)	169.1 ± 8.1	166.3 ± 12.7
Weight (kg)	76.4 ± 11.0	74.1 ± 17.9
Body surface area (m^2)	1.87 ± 0.16	1.87 ± 0.29
Time to follow-up (months)	11.1 ± 5.5	26.86 ± 16.4

CABG, coronary artery bypass grafting.

There was no significant difference in age at operation, resting pulse and blood pressure or in height, weight or body surface area, giving two well-matched groups.

It was not possible to obtain accurate estimates of left ventricular systolic function in all patients due to the difficulties in two-dimensional imaging in this elderly group of patients post-cardiac surgery. However, a semiqualitative estimate of left ventricular function was possible in all cases based on the presence of left ventricular dilatation and global and segmental left ventricular performance. The systolic function was independently assessed as being normal, moderate or poor in function. The results of this were comparable and are shown in Table 22.3.

Table 22.3 Semiqualitative analysis of left ventricular function for the two groups

	Toronto SPV valve (*n* = 21)	**Carpentier–Edwards (*n* = 23)**
Normal	12	14
Moderate	7	7
Poor	2	2

Doppler echocardiography

Detailed two-dimensional and full Doppler echocardiographic studies were performed on all patients. All studies were undertaken using a Hewlett Packard Sonos 1500 machine and a 2.5 MHz transducer by the same experienced operator. The diameter of the left ventricular outflow tract (LVOT) was measured via the parasternal long axis view in early systole from inner edge to inner edge and the left ventricular outflow tract area was calculated from this. Great care was taken to locate the Doppler window yielding the maximal transvalvular velocities from the apical views with well-defined envelopes and peaks. If these were suboptimal then right parasternal or suprasternal positions were used. Between three and five consecutive cardiac cycles were examined to ensure accuracy.

Colour-flow mapping was used in both long axis parasternal views and apical views to look for any evidence of valvular regurgitation.

Aortic valve gradient (AVG)

Both peak (AV_{max}) and mean (AV_{mean}) aortic valve gradients were calculated from the modified Bernoulli equation using the velocities recorded as above, i.e. AVG = 4 V^2.

Effective orifice area (EOA)

EOA was calculated from the continuity equation:

$$EOA = (LVOT\ CSA \times LVOT\ VTI) / AV\ VTI$$

where CSA is the cross-sectional area and VTI is the velocity time integral.

Effective orifice area index (EOAI)

EOAI is a measure of how well the valve orifice area matches the body surface area (BSA):

$$EOAI = EOA / BSA.$$

Results

The operative and 30-day mortality of the Toronto SPV valve group was zero out of 34 patients. The 30-day mortality for the Carpentier–Edwards group was four deaths out of 44 cases, all of whom had undergone concurrent coronary artery bypass grafting (CABG).

Tables 22.4–22.8 show the mean values ± standard deviation for the parameters assessed comparing the Toronto SPV valve and the Carpentier–Edwards valve for all annulus sizes and then per patient annulus size. Statistical significance was assessed by means of Student's *t*-test.

It can be seen that there is a highly significant difference ($p < 0.001$) between the Toronto SPV valve and the Carpentier–Edwards valve when considering peak aortic velocity, peak aortic gradient, mean aortic velocity, mean aortic gradient, aortic valve

Table 22.4 Comparative haemodynamic data for all patient annulus sizes

	Toronto SPV valve	Carpentier–Edwards
Peak AV (m/s)	1.78 ± 0.46*	2.4 ± 0.44*
Mean AV (m/s)	1.17 ± 0.31*	1.62 ± 0.30*
Peak AVG (mmHg)	13.53 ± 6.7*	23.8 ± 8.5*
Mean AVG (mmHg)	5.46 ± 3.16*	10.9 ± 3.89*
AVA (cm^2)	2.01 ± 0.78*	1.17 ± 0.41*
EOAI (cm^2/m^2)	1.06 ± 0.37*	0.62 ± 0.21*

AV, aortic velocity; AVA, aortic valve area; AVG, aortic valve gradient; EOAI, effective orifice area index.
* $p < 0.001$ Toronto SPV valve versus Carpentier–Edwards valve.

Table 22.5 Comparative haemodynamic data for 21 mm patient annuli

	Toronto SPV valve	Carpentier–Edwards
Peak AV (m/s)	1.98 ± 0.42	2.39 ± 0.50
Mean AV (m/s)	1.27 ± 0.17*	1.70 ± 0.28*
Peak AVG (mmHg)	16.2 ± 7.1	23.7 ± 9.80
Mean AVG (mmHg)	6.43 ± 1.75*	11.72 ± 4.0*
AVA (cm^2)	1.57 ± 0.60*	0.94 ± 0.22*
EOAI (cm^2/m^2)	0.86 ± 0.23	0.58 ± 0.20

AV, aortic velocity; AVA, aortic valve area; AVG, aortic valve gradient; EOAI, effective orifice area index.
* $p < 0.05$ Toronto SPV valve versus Carpentier–Edwards valve.

Table 22.6 Comparative haemodynamic data for 23 mm patient annuli

	Toronto SPV valve	Carpentier–Edwards
Peak AV (m/s)	2.23 ± 0.30	2.38 ± 0.37
Mean AV (m/s)	1.43 ± 0.32	1.58 ± 0.30
Peak AVG (mmHg)	20.1 ± 5.70	23.3 ± 7.20
Mean AVG (mmHg)	8.21 ± 4.0	10.3 ± 3.60
AVA (cm^2)	1.47 ± 0.37	1.26 ± 0.40
EOAI (cm^2/m^2)	0.81 ± 0.19*	0.66 ± 0.21*

AV, aortic velocity; AVA, aortic valve area; AVG, aortic valve gradient; EOAI, effective orifice area index.
* $p < 0.05$ Toronto SPV valve versus Carpentier–Edwards valve.

Table 22.7 Comparative haemodynamic data for 25 mm patient annuli

	Toronto SPV valve (n = 8)	Carpentier–Edwards (n = 4)
Peak AV (m/s)	1.65 ± 0.45	2.31 ± 0.42
Mean AV (m/s)	1.12 ± 0.34	1.48 ± 0.16
Peak AVG (mmHg)	11.7 ± 5.9*	21.9 ± 8.22*
Mean AVG (mmHg)	4.98 ± 2.91	8.72 ± 1.78
AVA (cm^2)	2.01 ± 0.66	1.45 ± 0.59
EOAI (cm^2/m^2)	1.10 ± 0.27*	0.67 ± 0.31*

AV, aortic velocity; AVA, aortic valve area; AVG, aortic valve gradient; EOAI, effective orifice area index.
* $p < 0.05$ Toronto SPV valve versus Carpentier–Edwards valve.

Table 22.8 Comparative haemodynamic data for 27 mm patient annuli

	Toronto SPV valve (n = 5)	Carpentier–Edwards (n = 2)
Peak AV (m/s)	1.48 ± 0.35	1.84 ± 0.13
Mean AV (m/s)	0.96 ± 0.20*	1.37 ± 0.01*
Peak AVG (mmHg)	9.11 ± 4.25	13.5 ± 1.97
Mean AVG (mmHg)	3.70 ± 1.53*	7.50 ± 0.15*
AVA (cm^2)	2.58 ± 0.72	1.75 ± 0.35
EOAI (cm^2/m^2)	1.42 ± 0.52	1.0 ± 0.17

AV, aortic velocity; AVA, aortic valve area; AVG, aortic valve gradient; EOAI, effective orifice area index.
* $p < 0.05$ Toronto SPV valve versus Carpentier–Edwards valve.

area and effective orifice area index as measured by Doppler echocardiography for all sizes of patient annulus, with the Toronto SPV valve producing a superior haemodynamic profile. Looking across the range of annulus sizes there is a noticeable trend in favour of the Toronto SPV valve which, as can be seen from the tables, often reaches statistical significance despite relatively small numbers.

Aortic regurgitation was found to be present in two of the Carpentier–Edwards valves and in five Toronto SPV valves. In all cases in the Toronto SPV valves this was mild, valvular and of no clinical significance. In the Carpentier–Edwards group, one case was mild valvular regurgitation and the other case was mild paravalvular regurgitation; again neither of these was of clinical significance.

The respective aortic cross-clamp times for the operations performed are shown in Table 22.9. There was a trend towards longer aortic cross-clamp times and operative times with the Toronto SPV valve although these were not statistically significant and there was no noticeable trend regarding annulus size. The NYHA status for all patients was ascertained at follow-up and is displayed in Table 22.10. As can be seen, the patients in both groups were symptomatically very similar both pre- and post-operatively, with good operative results as would be expected.

Table 22.9 Operative aortic cross-clamp times (min)

	Toronto SPV valve	Carpentier–Edwards
All annulus sizes (mm)	66.0 ± 11.75	58.92 ± 17.92
21	64.0 ± 16.9	61.0 ± 11.3
23	66.0 ± 8.8	54.1 ± 22.5
25	66.9 ± 12.9	63.3 ± 10.4
27	66.0 ± 10.86	56.0 ± 5.7

Table 22.10 Pre- and postoperative NYHA status for the Toronto SPV valve and the Carpentier–Edwards valve

	Toronto SPV valve (n = 21)		Carpentier–Edwards (n = 23)	
NYHA	Pre	Post	Pre	Post
I	0	11	0	13
II	4	8	3	7
III	12	2	14	3
IV	5	0	6	0

Discussion

This study supports the theory that the Toronto SPV valve bioprosthesis provides superior haemodynamics to the stented annular Carpentier–Edwards bioprosthesis, as assessed by Doppler echocardiography, in the aortic position. This difference is highly statistically significant when considering all annulus sizes ($p < 0.001$) for peak and mean aortic velocity, peak and mean aortic valve gradient and for valve area. There was a marked trend across the range of annulus sizes in favour of the Toronto SPV valve and this again was statistically significant for mean aortic velocity and gradient and for aortic valve area in the smallest, 21 mm, size of annulus.

Doppler ultrasound is extremely sensitive for the detection of even trivial valve regurgitation[15] in normally functioning valves. Its presence is well described with the insertion of the stentless valve and for other stentless bioprostheses and it has been well demonstrated that the incidence of this decreases as more implants are undertaken by individual surgeons. Hvass *et al.* showed that an initial rate of central regurgitation of 6–12% could be expected, decreasing with experience.[16] Also it has been noted that despite an incidence of mild aortic regurgitation seen in the early postoperative period, this becomes undetectable at 1 year in the majority of these patients.[17] The Freestyle insertion technique is a more demanding procedure than the insertion of a stented bioprosthesis. It is felt that an initial incidence of aortic regurgitation may be due to undersizing of the valve and because in diastole the bulging of the sinuses (which are functionally acting as stents for the SPV) causes the valve leaflets to be pulled apart.[8]

Although one would expect a longer cross-clamp time for the Toronto SPV valve, there was only a slightly increased cross-clamp time for the Toronto SPV valve versus the Carpentier–Edwards valve (mean 66.0 ± 11.75 min versus 58.92 ± 17.92 min). This can partly be explained by the fact that all Toronto SPV valve cases were performed by senior consultant staff whereas a number of the Carpentier–Edwards valves were implanted by trainee surgeons under consultant supervision, and by the increased number of other procedures that were undertaken in the Carpentier–Edwards group. (In the Toronto SPV valve group seven out of the 21 patients studied underwent concurrent CABG, and in the Carpentier–Edwards group 10 patients underwent CABG and one patient had aortic root replacement.)

The figures obtained in this study correlate well with the previously published echocardiographic data available for the Carpentier–Edwards annular bioprosthesis[18–21] and for the Toronto SPV valve.[1,4,5,11,22]

It has been shown[22,23] that over the course of time the haemodynamic profile of the Toronto SPV valve improves further, with a decrease in transvalvular gradients, an increase in effective orifice area and a decrease in left ventricular mass seen. These features are thought to be due to ventricular remodelling and, to a lesser extent, to regression of postoperative tissue oedema or haematoma.[7]

It is interesting to note that although the valves were implanted over the same time period, the mean follow-up time of the Toronto SPV valves was less than that for the Carpentier–Edwards valves, due to a large number of Toronto SPV valves being inserted towards the end of the study period. It is possible that the haemodynamic differences observed may be even greater as time progresses.

This effect on regression of left ventricular mass is seen to a lesser degree with stented bioprostheses.[23]

Conclusion

Per patient annulus size, the Toronto SPV valve provides superior haemodynamics over the annular Carpentier–Edwards aortic bioprosthesis as assessed by Doppler echocardiography. The aortic cross-clamp times are slightly longer for the Toronto SPV valve group and there is a greater incidence of mild valvular aortic regurgitation, both of which are due to the increased complexity of the operation as well as to valve design and should decrease with increasing operator experience. The aortic regurgitation described remains clinically insignificant.

References

1. David T E, Polick C, Bos J 1990 Aortic valve replacement with stentless porcine aortic bioprosthesis. J Thorac Cardiovasc Surg 99: 113–118
2. Rahimtoola S H 1978 The problem of valve prosthesis patient mismatch. Circulation 58: 20–24
3. Teoh K H, Fulop J C, Weisel R D *et al* 1987 Aortic valve replacement with a small prosthesis. Circulation 76(Suppl III): 111–123
4. Wong K, Shad S, Waterworth P D, Khaghani A, Pepper J R, Yacoub M H 1995 Early experience with the Toronto stentless porcine valve. Ann Thorac Surg 60: S402–S405
5. Meloni L, Ricchi A, Cirio E *et al* 1995 Echocardiographic assessment of aortic valve replacement with stentless porcine xenografts. Am J Cardiol 76: 294–296
6. Barrett-Boyes B G, Christie G W, Raudkivi P J 1992 The stentless bioprosthesis: surgical challenges and implications for long term durability. Eur J Cardiothorac Surg 6(Suppl 1) S39–S43
7. Del Rizzo D, Goldman B, Christakis G, David T 1996 Hemodynamic benefits of the Toronto stentless valve. J Thorac Cardiovasc Surg 112: 1431–1446
8. Del Rizzo D F, Goldman B S, David T E 1995 Aortic valve replacement with a stentless porcine bioprosthesis: multicentre trial. Can J Cardiol 11(7): 597–603
9. Gross C, Harringer W, Mair R *et al* 1995 Aortic valve replacement: is the stentless xenograft an alternative to the homograft? Early results of a randomized study. Ann Thorac Surg 60: S418–S421
10. Angell W W, Pupello D F, Bessone L N, Hiro S P, Brock J C 1991 Effect of stent mounting on tissue valves for aortic valve replacement. J Card Surg (4): 595–599
11. Mohr F W, Walther T, Baryalei M *et al* 1995 The Toronto SPV bioprosthesis: one year results in 100 patients. Ann Thorac Surg 60: 171–175
12. Vilela Batista R J, Dobrianskij A, Comazzi M *et al* 1987 Clinical experience with stentless pericardial aortic monopatch for aortic valve replacement. J Thorac Cardiovasc Surg 93: 16–26
13. Casabona R, De Paulis R, Zattera G F *et al* 1992 Stentless porcine and pericardial valve in the aortic position. Ann Thorac Surg 54: 681–685
14. Del Rizzo D F, Goldman B S, Joyner C P, Sever J, Fremes S E Christakis G T 1994 Initial experience with the Toronto stentless porcine valve. J Card Surg 9(4): 379–385
15. Edwards T, Livesey S A, Monro J L, Ross Sir J K 1995 Biological valves beyond fifteen years; the Wessex experience. Ann Thorac Surg 60: A211–A215
16. Hvass U, Chatel D, Assayag P *et al* 1995 The O'Brien–Angell stentless porcine valve: early results with 150 implants. Ann Thorac Surg 60: S414–S417
17. Walther T, Falk V, Autschbach R *et al* 1994 Hemodynamic assessment of the stentless Toronto SPV bioprosthesis by echocardiography. J Heart Valve Dis 3: 657–665
18. Cosgrove D M, Lytle B W, Williams G W 1985 Hemodynamic performance of the Carpentier–Edwards pericardial valve in the aortic position in vivo. Circulation 72(3 Pt II), II: 146–152
19. Frater R, Salomon N, Rainer G, Cosgrove D, Wickham E 1992 The Carpentier–Edwards pericardial aortic valve: intermediate results. Ann Thorac Surg 53: 764–771
20. Rothkopf M, Davidson T, Lipscomb K *et al* 1979 Hemodynamic evaluation of the Carpentier–Edwards bioprosthesis in the aortic position. Am J Cardiol 44: 209–213
21. Chaitman B, Bonan R, Lepage G *et al* 1979 Hemodynamic evaluation of the Carpentier–Edwards porcine xenograft. Circulation 60: 1170–1182
22. David T E, Feindel C M, Bos J, Sun Z, Scully H E, Rakowski H 1994 Aortic valve replacement with a stentless porcine aortic valve. A six year experience. J Thorac Cardiovasc Surg 108: 1030–1036
23. Jin X Y, Zhang Z, Gibson D G, Yacoub M H, Pepper J R 1996 Changes in left ventricular function and hypertrophy following aortic valve replacement using aortic homograft, stentless, or stented valve. Ann Thorac Surg 62: 683–690

Echocardiographic assessment of the Freestyle aortic root with particular reference to aortic regurgitation

X. Y. Jin and S. Westaby

The new stentless bioprostheses provide improved haemodynamics, rapid resolution of left ventricular hypertrophy and the promise of improved durability with mitigation from early calcification through biochemical treatments.[1–6] Superlative valve function and avoidance of anticoagulation with warfarin are compelling arguments for the use of stentless bioprostheses in elderly patients with aortic stenosis.[1–3] The only conceivable argument against these valves is the modest degree of operative difficulty and a risk of aortic regurgitation similar to the aortic homograft. Aortic root replacement can be used for patients with severe calcification of the aortic sinuses or an ascending aneurysm. However, the operative mortality for root replacement exceeds that of subcoronary implantation through increased duration of ischaemic time and surgical complexity (Medtronic Freestyle study data). We have now used the Freestyle valve in 200 consecutive patients to receive a tissue valve in the aortic position, irrespective of the morphology of the aortic root or preoperative clinical condition. Having documented excellent valve haemodynamic function with rapid resolution of left ventricular hypertrophy,[4,5] we prospectively studied the structure and function of the aortic root and the propensity for postoperative aortic regurgitation over a 3-year follow-up.

Methods

Patients

This prospective clinical study includes 190 patients (110 men, 80 women) who underwent Freestyle aortic valve replacement for predominant aortic stenosis with follow-up from 0.5 to 36 months. Age at valve replacement ranged from 50 to 91 years (mean 73 ± 6 years). Seventy-three patients underwent concomitant coronary artery bypass. The series was consecutive and unselected irrespective of anatomical difficulties or NYHA functional class. In this series, no patient over 70 years old received a mechanical valve and no patient received a stented bioprosthesis. In all isolated aortic replacements, the aortic cross clamp time was between 30 and 50 min (mean 43 min). The sizes of stentless valves ranged from 19 mm (in two patients only) to 27 mm, with a mean size of 23.4 ± 1.9 mm. At latest follow-up, the NYHA functional class was 1.1 ± 0.4. The study was part of a prospective clinical assessment of efficacy and safety of the Freestyle stentless porcine aortic valve (Medtronic Inc., Minneapolis, MN, USA) approved by the Central Oxford Research Ethics Committee with data submitted to the Food and Drug Administration. All operations were performed by one surgeon (SW).

Surgical technique

This has been described in detail but several key points relate to this study.[3,7] The modified subcoronary technique has been referred to as the 'cylinder within a cylinder' method, because the valve size is chosen to provide a snug fit within the human aortic root. The glutaraldehyde-fixed porcine aortic sinuses retain about 10% of the distensibility of native aorta and this allows a degree of expansion of the Freestyle aortic wall when pressure loaded. The valve may therefore expand to fit the human root. By contrast, the inflow of the valve is supported by Dacron cloth which cannot expand. The height of this cloth beneath the porcine right coronary is difficult to accommodate under the human right coronary when the distance between the annulus and ostium is short. Distortion through bending of the Freestyle inflow may cause obstruction or incompetence. Avoidance of this problem is part of the surgical learning curve. If necessary, the valve is rotated so that the elevated part of the Dacron cloth is positioned in the human non-coronary sinus.

The ligated porcine coronaries are situated closer together than the human coronary ostia, particularly in patients with bicuspid valves (where the human coronaries may be diametrically opposite). Attempts to accommodate substantial discrepancies between the porcine and human coronaries may lead to commissural pillar distortion. Because of this, the inflow of the valve should be secured with the closest approximation between porcine and human coronaries before the porcine coronaries are removed. With this approach, the porcine sinuses are excised to accommodate directly the human coronary ostia.

The aorta is first opened 2–3 mm above the sinotubular junction and about 1 cm above the right coronary ostium. A two-thirds transection is made, leaving only the aorta above the left coronary sinus intact. Stay sutures are then used to hold the aortic root open so that no retractors are required in the operative field. The human aortic root should not be distorted. One stay suture is applied directly above the right coronary ostium, so the position of this is kept in mind. The left coronary ostium is always easily visible. The angle between the coronary ostia is noted in preparation for orientation of the Freestyle valve. The diseased valve is excised and calcium excavated from the annulus. Decalcification may be required for troublesome plaques in the aortic sinuses or around the coronary ostia.

Valve sizing relies entirely on the native valve annulus and only a thin rim of this should be left. The diameter of the sinotubular junction is irrelevant, since this part of the aorta is tailored to fit the outflow of the Freestyle valve. Leaving the porcine non-coronary sinus intact prevents distortion of two commissures and allows accurate alignment of the third. Care is taken not to splay the commissures when suturing under the left and right human coronaries.

Simple inflow sutures (in a single plane) begin in the base of the triangle of each commissure. This ensures undistorted seating of the inflow. The outflow is secured with a single running suture of 4/0 polypropylene, beginning at the commissure between left and right coronary sinuses. The outflow of the Freestyle valve is trimmed to a height just above the porcine commissures with the object of suturing the crest of the valve to the two-thirds transected aorta. This method effectively suspends the Freestyle valve from the transverse aortotomy and ensures competence as long as the commissures are not distorted. The aortic closure then further reinforces the outflow suture line.

Echocardiography

Transthoracic echocardiography was performed at the time of discharge from hospital, then at 3–6 months, 12 months, 24 months, and 36 months after the operation. Echocardiograms were recorded using a Toshiba 380A Echocardiographic System, with a 2.5 MHz phased array transducer. From the parasternal left ventricular long axis view, the internal diameters of outflow tract, aortic sinus, sinotubular junction (commissure level), and the ascending aortic root (3–4 cm above aortic annulus level) were measured from a two-dimensional image at early systole when the valve was fully opened.[8–11] Serial M-mode echocardiograms of the left ventricle, aortic sinus level, and ascending aorta (at 2 years) follow-up were also recorded and stored on video tape at a speed of 50 or 100 mm/s, with simultaneous electrocardiogram and phonocardiogram. From an apical five chamber view (from which the outflow tract and aortic valve can be imaged parallel to the Doppler ultrasound beam), flow velocities in the outflow tract (2.5 MHz pulsed Doppler) and the maximum velocity across the stentless valve (2.5 MHz continuous-wave Doppler) were recorded at a speed of 100 cm/s.[5]

All video recordings were read and analysed off line. Systemic blood pressure was also recorded non-invasively by the Hewlett Packard 66S Haemodynamic Monitoring System. Body surface area was calculated from each patient's height and weight. A preoperative echocardiogram was not feasible in the study protocol because many patients referred from other hospitals needed emergency surgery.

Aortic root diameters and aortic distensibility

The internal diameters of left ventricular outflow tract, aortic sinus, sinotubular junction, and aortic root were measured at early ejection from two-dimensional echocardiographic images. Aortic distensibility was calculated by the formula:[12] [2 × (change in aortic diameters)/(diastolic aortic diameter × change in aortic pressure)]. Aortic pressure was estimated from brachial pressure. Changes in aortic diameters were determined from M-mode aortogram between end diastole (onset of QRS complex of electrocardiogram) and end systole (beginning of A_2, second heart sound).

Stentless aortic valve haemodynamics

The effective orifice area of the aortic valve was calculated by the continuity equation, i.e. stroke volume divided by valve flow velocity time integral.[10] Left ventricular stroke volume was calculated as the product of the cross-sectional area and flow velocity time integral in the outflow tract.[9] Mean pressure drop across the aortic valve was made from the modified Bernoulli equation, i.e. by taking the subvalvular (V_1) and valvular (V_2) mean velocities into account, mean pressure drop = 4 ($V_2^2 - V_1^2$), in mmHg.[10]

Left ventricular mass index

Left ventricular end-diastolic dimension, septum thickness and posterior wall thickness were measured from M-mode echocardiograms, and the wall thickness to cavity ratio (*T*/*R* ratio) was calculated. Left ventricular muscle mass was quantified according to the formula of the American Society of Echocardiography, and indexed to body surface area.[11,13]

Statistical analysis

Echocardiographic and haemodynamic data are presented as mean ± one standard deviation. Data were analysed using Minitab statistic software (Release 11 for Windows, 1996; Minitab Inc., USA).[14] One-way analysis of variance was performed to test the significance of changes in the mean value of each measurement over the follow-up time. When this was significant, a further comparison of 95% confidence intervals with respect to the measurement at discharge was carried out using Dunnett's method, with an overall error rate of 0.05 and an individual error rate of 0.02. The paired *t*-test was used to determine the significant difference of aortic distensibility between sinus and ascending levels at 2-year follow-up. A *p*-value of less than 0.05 was considered statistically significant.

Results

A total of 436 echocardiograms were obtained with adequate imaging quality for off-line reading and data analysis. Mean values for each measurement were derived from three heart beats in patients in sinus rhythm (84%), and from five beats in patients with atrial fibrillation (12%) or having a VVI pacemaker (4%).

Changes in left ventricular hypertrophy and aortic valve haemodynamics are presented in Chapter 15. In summary, there was a progressive fall in relative wall thickness, left ventricular mass index and transvalvular mean systolic pressure drop, together with an increase in valve effective orifice area. By 2 years after surgery, left ventricular mass index had fallen to within normal limits. These remarkable changes were associated with symptomatic relief and return to NYHA I.

Changes in aortic root diameter and distensibility

During the 3-year follow-up, the size of the Freestyle valve inflow remained constant, as did the diameter of the left ventricular outflow tract. Changes in effective orifice area were not caused by anatomical changes but rather through marked improvement in physiological function of the left ventricle. However, at the level of the aortic sinuses, there was a small but measurable decrease in diameter, which became statistically significant at 12 and 24 months after the operation. This process may represent the resolution of post-stenotic dilatation, haematoma and the adhesion of the porcine and human aortic walls. By contrast, the internal diameter of the stentless valve at commissure level (sinotubular junction, i.e. the outflow of the Freestyle valve) and the diameter of the ascending aorta both remained unchanged (Table 23.1). Furthermore, despite the fall in internal diameter, the distensibility at aortic sinus level did not change significantly. In fact, the level of aortic sinuses remained more distensible than that of ascending aorta (1.1 ± 1.0 versus $0.5 \pm 0.6 \cdot 10^{-6} cm^2/dyne$, $p < 0.01$).

Residual aortic regurgitation

The presence and degree of aortic regurgitation from 436 echocardiographic studies are presented in Table 23.2. The grade of aortic regurgitation was measured by colour flow mapping of the regurgitant jet length. Aortic regurgitation was graded as absent (0/4), mild (1/4), moderate (2/4) or moderately severe (3/4). No patient was found to have moderately severe or severe regurgitation (4/4). The use of the term *trivial aortic regurgitation* was avoided, since this is apparently of little haemodynamic significance and often reflects the closing volume of the valve. At discharge from hospital, 92% of the valves were fully competent; this figure remained consistent through the 3-year follow-up. No patient with an initially competent valve developed aortic regurgitation. Six per cent of patients had between mild and moderate aortic regurgitation at hospital discharge; this remained stable and no patient in the series had moderate to severe aortic regurgitation at any stage. Consequently, the slight alterations in aortic root anatomy were not associated with any changes in the incidence of aortic regurgitation.

Discussion

The modified subcoronary implant technique can be applied in virtually all patients who require a tissue valve in the aortic position. The only exceptions in our series were two patients who had undergone radical radiotherapy for breast cancer many years before, and had a small porcelain aortic root.

Mild to moderate aortic regurgitation occurred in approximately 9% of patients, probably through slight inaccuracy of the commissural pillar alignment. Aortic regurgitation was not seen to be progressive in any patient, and in some patients there was an impression that the regurgitation decreased. These medium-term results are reassuring since the aortic root, remains somewhat distensible, the cusps open as in a

Table 23.1 Changes in left ventricle cavity size, wall thickness, aortic root diameters and valve haemodynamics (mean ± SD)

Variable	Time after AVR (months)					ANOVA
	0.5	3–6	12	24	36	*p*-Value
Left ventricular end-diastolic dimension (mm)	48±9.7	48±7.7	49±7.2	48±6.4	48±6.0	0.876
Ratio of wall thickness to cavity radius	0.59±0.22	0.49±0.15	0.43±0.10*	0.45±0.10*	0.50±0.13	<0.001
Left ventricular mass index (g/m^2)	149±59	126±39*	109±39*	109±37*	125±50*	<0.001
Aortic valve effective orifice area (cm^2)	1.6±0.8	1.8±0.6	1.9±0.6*	2.2±0.8*	2.2±0.7*	<0.001
Aortic valve mean pressure gradient (mmHg)	8.7±4.9	5.1±3.0*	5.2±3.6*	5.3±3.5*	5.2±3.8*	<0.001
Implanted valve size (mm)	23.6±1.9	23.7±2.0	23.4±1.9	23.4±2.0	23.4±2.0	0.732
Left ventricular outflow tract diameter (mm)	20.5±3.1	20.4±2.3	20.5±2.4	20.7±2.4	20.4±2.7	0.870
Aortic sinus level diameter (mm)	29.8±6.0	29.4±5.3	27.3±4.8*	26.2±4.8*	26.8±4.0*	<0.001
Aortic sinotubular junction diameter (mm)	24.4±3.4	24.5±4.3	24.7±4.5	23.9±4.8	25.2±4.3	0.493
Ascending aortic root diameter (mm)	36.7±5.2	37.1±7.3	36.6±6.1	37.4±7.5	38.4±6.0	0.648
Aortic distensibility at sinus level (10^{-6} cm^2/dyne)	1.2±0.9	1.0±0.7	1.1±1.2	1.0±1.0	1.2±1.0	0.896
Aortic distensibility at root level (10^{-6} cm^2/dyne)	0.4±0.6	0.6±0.7	0.6±0.6	0.6±0.5	0.5±0.7	0.786

p-Value determined by one-way analysis of variance with respect to follow-up time.
* Significant difference compared with 95% confidence interval with respect to discharge study.

Table 23.2 Incidence of Freestyle aortic valve regurgitation: Oxford data based on 436 echocardiographic studies

Grade of regurgitation*	0.5 month (*n*=119)	3–6 months (*n*=102)	12 months (*n*=100)	24 months (*n*=79)	36 months (*n*=36)	*p*-Value†
None	109 (92%)	92 (90%)	91 (91%)	70 (89%)	31 (86%)	>0.05
Mild (1/4)	3 (2%)	3 (3%)	4 (4%)	5 (6%)	4 (11%)	>0.05
Moderate (2/4)	7 (6%)	8 (7%)	5 (5%)	4 (5%)	1 (3%)	>0.05
Moderate severe (3/4)	0	0	0	0	0	N/A

* Grade of aortic regurgitation was based on colour-flow mapping of the length and width of regurgitant jet with respect to that of left ventricular outflow tract.
† *p*-Value was determined by χ^2, with respect to follow-up time.

nearly normal aortic root, and the stresses of stent mounting are eliminated. With time, valve function improves in tandem with rehabilitation of the left ventricle. Our data show that with an effective orifice area of 1.7 cm^2 at hospital discharge, the calculated flow jet width was 1.47 cm, accounting for 49% of the aortic sinus diameter. However, by 2 years postoperatively, the effective orifice area has increased to 2.2 cm^2 with a flow jet width of 1.66 cm; it thus increases to 66% of sinus diameter. It is possible that the slight fall in sinus diameter within the range of the present study may improve valve haemodynamics by forming a more efficient downstream physical geometry.[15]

The distensibility of the aortic wall at sinus level $1.7 \pm 2.0 \cdot 10^{-6} cm^2/dyne$ falls below the published normal range, and reflects the combination of the physical properties of the fused native aortic sinuses and porcine graft.[12,16] Distensibility at sinus level nevertheless remained 55% greater than that of the ascending aorta (3–4 cm above the sinuses), where distensibility is also affected by age or concomitant coronary disease.[12,16,17] This suggests that the Freestyle valve remains distensible for up to 3 years after implantation. Whether this indicates that the porcine graft is free from calcification remains to be seen, but warrants further prospective investigation to determine whether a fall in distensibility can be used to monitor valve degeneration. However, with advanced age the human root is subject to fibrosis and calcification, which limits distensibility of the porcine graft. With repeated measurements, it was reassuring to find that the diameter of the stentless valve at commissural level remained virtually identical to that of the valve size itself, and that this relationship was unaltered with time. The normal anatomical configuration of the Freestyle valve (and native root) over time confirms the reliability of the implant technique and promotes leaflet coaptation during diastole with a low risk of aortic regurgitation. It has been argued that it is necessary to keep the outflow portion of the Freestyle aortic root intact in order to maintain the normal geometric relationship of the three commissures and prevent aortic regurgitation. This so-called 'root inclusion technique' is technically challenging, requiring circumferential suture lines around the coronary ostia as well as inflow and outflow suture lines. Calcification around the coronary ostia or in the aortic sinuses contraindicates this method, and if coronary bypass grafts are required, the ischaemic time may be prohibitive.

Of the suggested implant methods, the modified subcoronary technique is the simplest and provides excellent haemodynamics with minimal risk of aortic regurgitation. Mild to moderate aortic regurgitation may rarely occur through inaccurate implantation (during the learning curve), but does not progress with time. Full aortic root replacement has little risk of aortic regurgitation, but there is no haemodynamic advantage to this method after 6 months.[18] By contrast, the hospital mortality is virtually the same as the risk of mild to moderate regurgitation with the modified subcoronary method.

Conclusions

After Freestyle valve implantation, the morphology and mechanics of the aortic root are preserved whilst valve gradients fall progressively and effective orifice area increases through improvement in ventricular function. In a consecutive unselected series which includes patients with post-stenotic dilatation and severe calcification of the aortic root, more than 90% had no aortic regurgitation. The remainder had either mild or mild-to-moderate regurgitation, which may be caused by malalignment of the commissure between the scalloped left and right coronary sinuses. Aortic regurgitation was never seen to progress with time. The modified subcoronary technique is expeditious, with the advantage of simplicity, long-term stability and excellent haemodynamic function.

References

1. David T E, Feindel C M, Bos J, Sun Z, Scully H E, Rakowski H 1994 Aortic valve replacement with a stentless porcine aortic valve. A six year experience. J Thorac Cardiovasc Surg 108: 1030–1036
2. Sintek C F, Fletcher A D, Khonsari S 1995 Stentless porcine aortic root: valve of choice for the elderly patient with small aortic root? J Thorac Cardiovasc Surg 109: 871–876
3. Westaby S, Amarasena N, Long V *et al* 1995 Time-related hemodynamic changes after aortic replacement with the Freestyle stentless xenograft. Ann Thorac Surg 60: 1633–1639
4. Jin X Y, Zhang Z M, Gibson D G, Yacoub M H, Pepper J R 1996 Effects of valve substitute on changes in left ventricular function and hypertrophy after aortic valve replacement. Ann Thorac Surg 62: 683–690
5. Jin X Y, Westaby S, Gibson D G, Pillai R, Taggart D 1997 Left ventricular remodelling and improvement in Freestyle stentless valve haemodynamics. Eur J Cardiothorac Surg 12: 63–69
6. Myers D 1997 New tissue-processing techniques. In: Piwnica A, Westaby S (eds) Surgery for acquired aortic valve disease. ISIS Medical Media, Oxford, 448–459
7. Westaby S, Amarasena N, Ormerod O, Amarasena G A C, Pillai R 1995 Aortic valve replacement with the Freestyle stentless xenograft. Ann Thorac Surg 60: S422–S427
8. Dubin J, Wallerson D C, Cody R J, Devereux R B 1990 Comparative accuracy of Doppler echocardiographic methods for clinical stroke volume determination. Am Heart J 120: 116–123
9. Lewis J F, Kuo L C, Nelson J G, Limacher M C, Quiones M A 1984 Pulsed Doppler echocardiographic determination of stroke volume and cardiac output: clinical validation of two new methods using the apical window. Circulation 70: 425–431
10. Chambers J, Shah P 1995 Recommendation for the echocardiographic assessment of replacement heart valves. J Heart Valve Dis 4: 9–13
11. Sahn D J, Demaria A, Kisslo J, Weyman A 1978 The committee on M–mode standardization of American Society of Echocardiography: recommendations regarding quantitation in M-mode echocardiography: results of a survey of echocardiographic measurements. Circulation 58: 1072–1083
12. Stefanadis C, Wooley C F, Bush C A, Kolibash A J, Boudoulas H 1988 Aortic distensibility in post–stenotic aortic dilatation: the effect of co-existing coronary artery disease. J Cardiol 18: 189–195
13. Devereux RB, Alonso DR, Lutas EM *et al* 1986 Echocardiographic assessment of left ventricular hypertrophy: comparison to necropsy finding. Am J Cardiol 57: 450–458
14. Minitab Inc. Minitab reference manual, release 11, Windows version. Minitab Inc., Philadelphia, pp 3.3–3.6
15. Yoganathan A P, Cape E G, Sung H W, Williams F P, Jimoh A 1988 Review of hydrodynamic principles for the cardiologist: applications to the study of blood flow and jets by imaging techniques. J Am Coll Cardiol 12: 1344–1353
16. Stefanadis C, Wooley C F, Bush C A, Kolibash A J, Boudoulas H 1987 Aortic distensibility abnormalities in coronary artery disease. Am J Cardiol 59: 1300–1304
17. Hirata K, Triposkiadis F, Sparks E, Bowen J, Wooley C F, Boudoulas H 1991 The Marfan syndrome: abnormal aortic elastic properties. J Am Coll Cardiol 18: 57–63
18. Kon N D, Westaby S, Amarasena N, Pillai R, Cordell A R 1995 Comparison of implantation techniques using Freestyle stentless porcine aortic valve. Ann Thorac Surg 59: 857–862

VI Implantation Techniques

CHAPTER 24

The Ross operation and aortic annulus reduction

R. C. Elkins, C. J. Knott-Craig, K. Chandrasekaran and M. M. Lane

The Ross operation[1] or pulmonary autograft replacement of the aortic valve was introduced in 1967[2] and was originally accomplished as an intra-aortic implant, either as a scalloped subcoronary implant or as an inclusion cylinder. By 1986 experience with the autograft operation had increased and its use was extended to younger patients and to patients with disease processes of the aortic valve and left ventricular outflow tract that were not amenable to an intra-aortic implant. In these patients the autograft was performed as a root replacement.[3,4] Many of these early root replacements were in young children and patients with complex left ventricular outflow tract obstruction.[3,5,6] Because of concern over using a pulmonary root that was not similar in size to the aortic root, especially the aortic annulus, surgeons avoided the Ross operation in patients with significant mismatch of the aortic and pulmonary annulus.[7,8] Young patients who otherwise would have been good candidates for a Ross operation were often not considered if dilatation of the aortic annulus secondary to long-standing aortic insufficiency was present. Frequently, those who had a Ross operation had a less satisfactory result with early failure from autograft insufficiency.[9]

With the advent of routine postoperative echocardiographic surveillance of patients having a Ross operation, it became apparent that early failure of the autograft was associated with a preoperative diagnosis of aortic insufficiency, usually associated with a non-stenotic bicuspid aortic valve.[10,11] The autograft failure was frequently associated with dilatation of the autograft annulus and inadequate leaflet coaptation, producing progressive central autograft valve insufficiency. In the absence of leaflet coaptation, leaflet prolapse, especially of the non-coronary leaflet, also occurs. At reoperation, the autograft leaflets frequently appeared normal except for a slight increase in thickness, and in most of these patients a reduction annuloplasty of the aortic valve was associated with improved autograft function and avoided autograft replacement.[11]

Recognition of these early failures and a desire to continue to use the autograft aortic valve replacement in patients with aortic annulus dilatation led to modification of the autograft insertion technique. Early efforts involved fixation of the aortic annulus by tying the interrupted sutures of the proximal suture line over an external strip of Dacron or Teflon. It was hoped that if one did this in an arrested heart, the aortic annulus would tend to conform to the pulmonary annulus as this suture line was completed. However, postoperative echocardiographic measurement did not always indicate a significant reduction in the aortic annulus and this led to the use of a modification of the annulus reduction technique proposed by Carpentier.[12]

Methods

The medical records of the 270 Ross operations performed at the University of Oklahoma Health Sciences Center were reviewed. Forty-seven patients who had fixation and attempted reduction of the aortic annulus with the use of external synthetic material, formal aortic annulus reduction or autograft reoperation with aortic annulus reduction were included in the present study. Fifteen patients received the early fixation technique described in the previous section, and are identified as group 1. Twenty-four patients (group 2) received the Carpentier-modified annular reduction technique at the time of their original Ross operation, and eight patients (group 3) underwent this procedure at the time of reoperation. Patient characteristics for the three groups are summarized in Table 24.1. Current follow-up is available on all patients and echocardiographic assessment is available within 1 year on all patients. Assessment of aortic annulus size and autograft valve function at the time of the most recent echocardiogram were compared to the echocardiographic assessment at the time of the Ross operation or at the time of their autograft reoperation. These echocardiographic measurements of aortic annulus size are also compared to the operative measurements in those patients who had an aortic annulus reduction. The patient's autograft valve function and clinical status were also assessed.

Table 24.1 Patient characteristics

Group	Age (years)	Aortic valve pathology	Aortic valve morphology	Aortic root pathology
1 (*n* = 15) (1992–1996)	11–47 (median 29)	AS: 0 AI: 10 AS+AI: 5	BI: 15 TRI: –	DILN: 2 ANEUR: 2
2 (*n* = 24) (1995–1997)	13–47 (median 29)	AS: 1 AI: 16 AS+AI: 7	BI: 21 TRI: 3	DILN: 6 ANEUR: 8
3 (*n* = 8) (1992–1996)	7–47 (median 22)	AS: 2 AI: 6	BI: 4 TRI: 2	DILN: 1 ANEUR: 1

AI, aortic insufficiency; AS, aortic stenosis; BI, bilateral; TRI, trilateral; DILN, ascending aortic dilatation; ANEUR, aortic aneurysm.

Operative technique

The operative technique for the Ross operation has previously been described.[13] In groups 1 and 2, all patients had their Ross operation as a root replacement. In group 3, four patients had a root replacement, three had a scalloped subcoronary implant and one had an inclusion cylinder implant.

In the annulus reduction procedure used in group 2 patients, the proximal aortic root is excised to the level of the aortic annulus following excision of the aortic valve and measurement of the aortic annulus. Two polypropylene sutures (2/0 or 3/0) are placed as purse-string sutures at the aortic annulus in the nadir of the coronary sinuses and below the aortic annulus in the interleaflet triangle between the left coronary sinus and the non-coronary sinus and the triangle between the left coronary sinus and the right coronary sinus. At the interleaflet triangle between the right coronary sinus and the non-coronary sinus and along the membranous septum, the suture line is kept close to the aortic annulus to avoid the bundle of His (Figure 24.1). The sutures are brought external to the aorta at the aortic annulus in the midpoint of the non-coronary sinus and tied over a felt pledget with a Hegar dilator of appropriate size in the aortic annulus (Figure 24.2). The size of the Hegar dilator is selected using a nomogram of aortic annulus size based on the

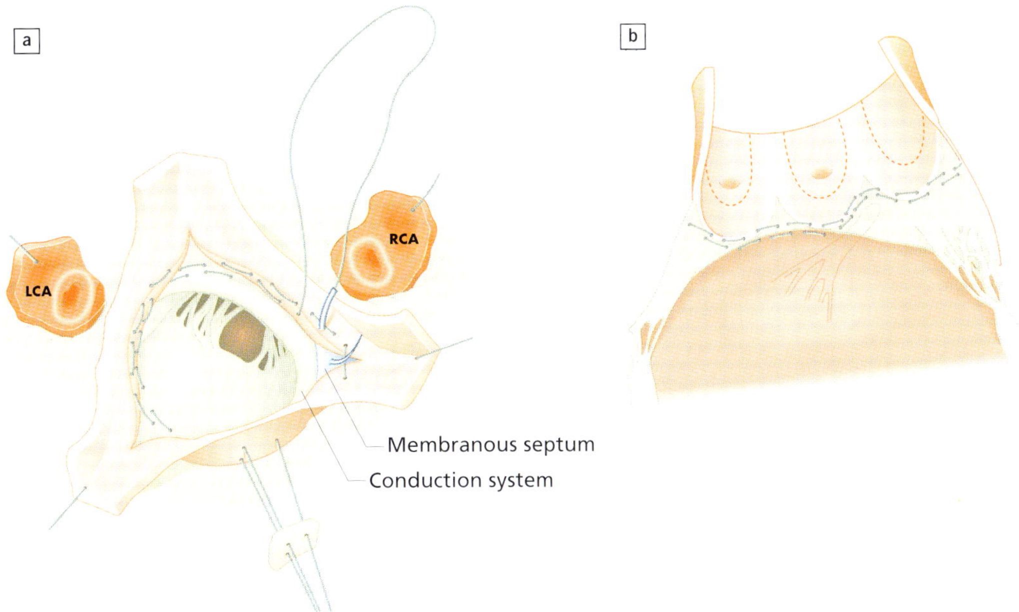

Figure 24.1 (a) Two purse-string sutures of 2/0 polypropylene are placed at the aortic annulus in the nadir of the coronary sinuses, in the lateral fibrous trigone in the interleaflet triangle between the left and non-coronary sinus, in the muscle of the ventricular septum at the commissure between the left and right coronary sinuses and in the membranous septum between the right and non-coronary sinus. The sutures are brought through the aortic annulus external to the aorta in the midpoint of the non-coronary sinus and passed through a felt pledget. (b) An opened view of the aortic annulus showing the exact placement of the sutures. Notice the placement of the sutures in the membranous septum to avoid the conduction system.

patient's body surface area.[14] The proximal suture line between the aortic annulus and the autograft root is composed of interrupted sutures of 4/0 polypropylene, carefully placed so that they include the previously placed purse-string sutures in the aortic annulus (Figure 24.3). These sutures are then tied over a thin strip of woven Dacron to ensure fixation of the aortic annulus and the left ventricular outflow tract (Figure 24.4). After implantation of the left coronary artery to the posterior sinus of the pulmonary autograft, the pulmonary root is trimmed 3–4 mm distal to the sinotubular junction of the pulmonary root and the Ross operation is completed.

Most patients with aortic insufficiency and aortic annulus dilatation will also have dilatation of the ascending aorta. Some will also have an aortic aneurysm of the ascending aorta. In patients with an aneurysm of the ascending aorta, the ascending aorta is replaced with a Dacron graft of appropriate size. This was required in eight patients in group 2 (Figure 24.5), and ascending aortic dilatation requiring a vertical reduction aortoplasty was performed in six patients (Figure 24.6).

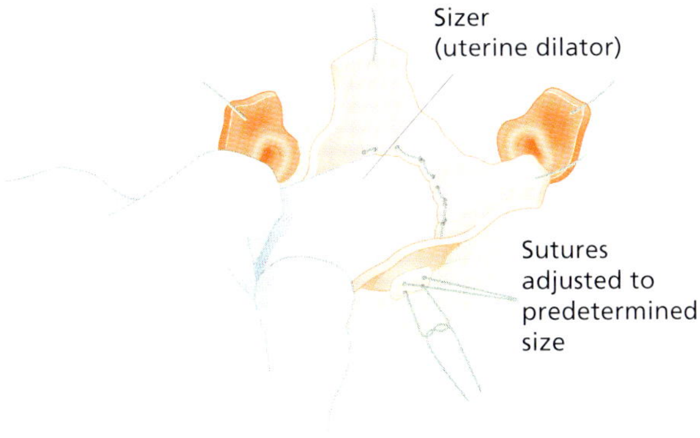

Figure 24.2 The two sutures are tied over the felt pledget with a graduated dilator in the aortic annulus of appropriate size for the patient.

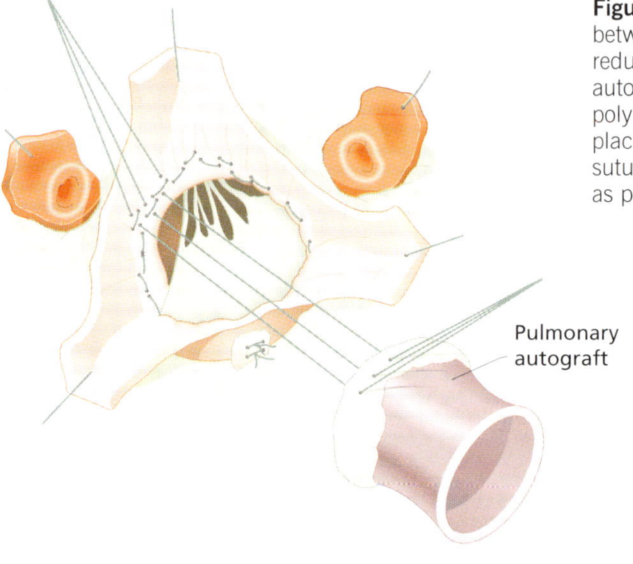

Figure 24.3 The proximal suture line between the aortic annulus that has been reduced in size and the pulmonary autograft is interrupted sutures of 4/0 polypropylene. The sutures are carefully placed beneath the reduction annuloplasty sutures and through the autograft as close as possible to the pulmonary annulus.

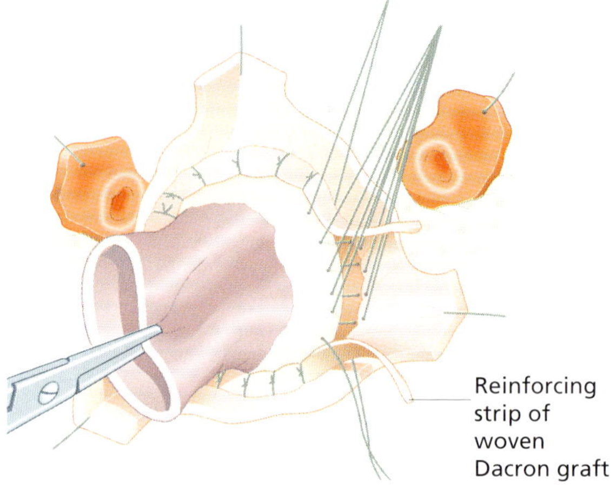

Figure 24.4 The proximal suture line is tied over a thin strip of woven Dacron graft, being careful to keep the Dacron material external to the autograft and not between the apposition line of the aortic annulus and the autograft. The two ends of the Dacron graft are tied together with the last two sutures to complete the 'fixation' of the aortic annulus.

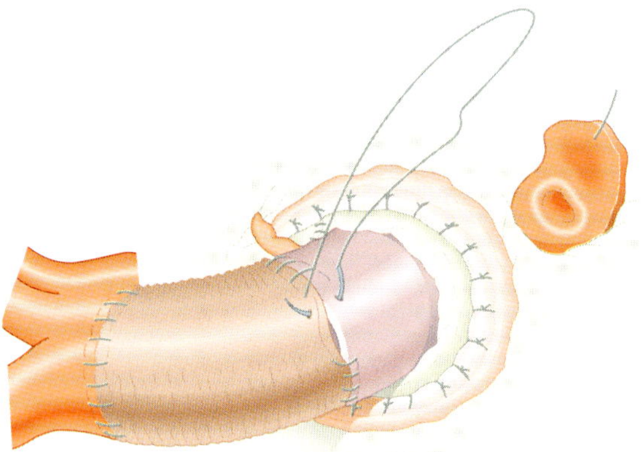

Figure 24.5 Replacement of an ascending aortic aneurysm with a knitted Dacron graft, similar in size to the size of the aortic annulus following annulus reduction. The graft is anastomosed to the pulmonary autograft 4–5 mm distal to the sinotubular junction of the autograft. This anastomosis is completed prior to implantation of the right coronary artery so that the autograft can be distended and the proper site for implantation of the right coronary can be selected.

Results

There were no operative deaths. In the group 1 patients, operative annulus measurement of the aortic annulus following excision of the aortic valve ranged from 24 to 33 mm with a median of 30 mm. Thirteen of the 15 patients had an aortic annulus size of 28 mm or greater. Postoperative echocardiographic measurement of the aortic annulus demonstrated a 1–9 mm decrease in the aortic annulus in 13 patients and no change in the aortic annulus size in the remaining two patients (Figure 24.7). Autograft valve insufficiency by colour-flow Doppler in the most recent

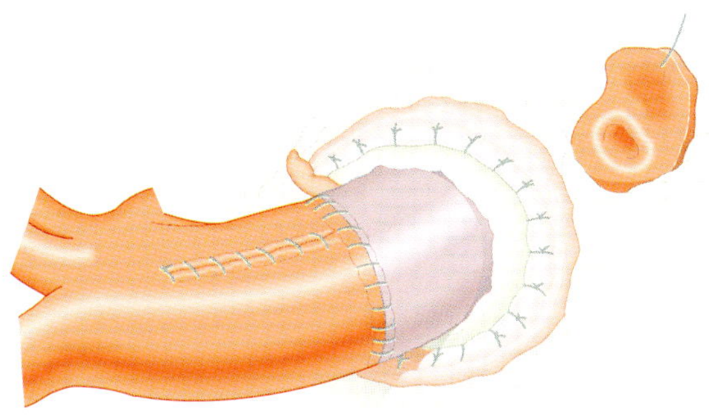

Figure 24.6 In patients with significant dilatation of the ascending aorta, a vertical aortoplasty is performed to reduce the size of the ascending aorta to the size of the sinotubular circumference of the pulmonary autograft.

echocardiogram is 0 or trace in six patients, 1+ in eight, and one patient developed progressive autograft valve insufficiency requiring reoperation at 1.8 years following his Ross operation. The length of follow-up in this group of patients is a total of 32.3 years with a range of 0.6–4.1 years and a mean of 2.2 years.

In the group 2 patients, the aortic annulus measured 26–55 mm (median 31 mm) prior to annulus reduction, with 21 patients having an aortic annulus of 28 mm or more. The largest was a very dysplastic annulus in a patient with a previous aorta-to-left-ventricular tunnel repair that measured 55 mm in its greatest diameter. Annulus reduction was 2–31 mm with a mean of 7.2 mm, and in 18 patients the aortic annulus reduction was 5 mm or more (Figure 24.7). Total follow-up in this group of patients is limited: 12.9 patient-years and a mean of 0.6 patient-years. Postoperative autograft valve insufficiency by colour-flow Doppler is 0 to trace in 13 patients, 1+ in 10 patients and 1–2+ in one patient. No patient has required reoperation of the autograft valve.

Group 3 patients required reoperation for autograft insufficiency 0.2–9 years following their Ross operation. During this period of follow-up, the aortic annulus dilated 3–10 mm, mean 5.8 mm, and leaflet prolapse was identified in one patient. The aortic annulus was reduced at reoperation from 3 to 9 mm with an average of 5.6 mm (Table 24.2). The length of follow-up after reoperation is 0.6–4 years. Six of the eight patients have good results: five patients have trace to 1+ autograft valve insufficiency by colour-flow Doppler and one has 2+ autograft valve insufficiency. Two patients have required autograft valve replacement, one with a prosthetic valve and one with a homograft valve based on patient choice.

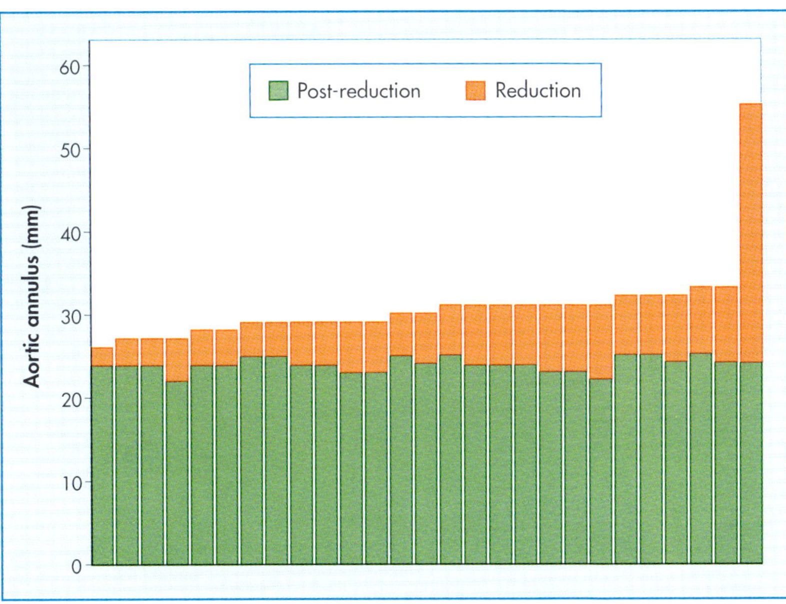

Figure 24.7 The aortic annulus size of the group 1 and group 2 patients prior to aortic annulus reduction, intraoperative measurement by a graduated sizer, and the post-reduction aortic annulus size are displayed graphically. In the group 1 patients the post-reduction annulus size was measured by echocardiography and in the group 2 patients the reduction annulus size was measured with a graduated sizer.

Table 24.2 Autograft valve reoperation (group 3)

Patient	Time to reoperation (years)	Aortic annulus at Ross op (mm)	Aortic annulus at reop (mm)	Aortic annulus reduction (mm)
1	9.0	20	27	23
2	7.6	27	32	24
3	5.4	20	30	23
4	4.0	27	30	27
5	1.8	25	32	25
6	1.4	25	28	23
7	1.0	18	23	16
8	0.2	23	29	23

Discussion

Experience with the Ross operation has increased dramatically during the past 10 years. As an increasing number of surgeons have gained experience with this complex operation, the indications for the operation have been extended and the pathological abnormalities of the aortic valve and of the aortic root that are being treated with this operation are more complex. The operation has been used in neonates and in all ages including some patients in the fifth and sixth decades.[15] It has been proposed as the operation of choice for young patients with aortic valve endocarditis[16–18] and has been identified as the aortic valve replacement of choice for the child and young adult.[9,19] The demonstration that the pulmonary autograft root could be used to replace the aortic valve and root has hastened these developments but has also led to the recognition of an increased risk of autograft valve failure in patients with a bicuspid aortic valve and aortic insufficiency and in patients with significant mismatch between the pulmonary autograft root and the aortic root.[10,11,20]

The advantages of a tissue valve have encouraged surgeons to develop techniques of valve repair and valve replacement that maintain anatomical and structural relationships such that valve competence can be maintained and will be lasting. The advent of good echocardiographic assessment prior to, during and following surgery has increased our understanding and knowledge of valve anatomy and function. This continued expansion of knowledge has demonstrated the important relationships of annulus and sinotubular dimensions as well as previously unrecognized pathology involving these structures and the ascending aorta. This recognition has directed surgeons in altering their approach to the management of patients with a significant array of pathological entities involving the aortic valve and the aortic root.

A previous publication by our group has called attention to the need for an alteration in operative technique if one uses the Ross operation in patients with aortic annular dysplasia,[10] and recently David *et al.* have described the importance of geometric mismatch of the aortic and pulmonary roots in producing aortic insufficiency after the Ross operation.[20] They have described a correction of this mismatch which involves reducion of the aortic annulus by plication of fibrous tissue beneath the commissures of the non-coronary sinus. This is combined with an aortic annuloplasty between the membranous interventricular septum and the lateral fibrous trigone when necessary to reduce the annulus size to a determined size of the pulmonary valve annulus. The pulmonary annulus size was predicted to be 10% greater than the measured size of the sinotubular junction of the pulmonary root. This size of the pulmonary sinotubular junction was measured directly with graduated dilators. These techniques have produced excellent results but follow-up is still limited.

Durham *et al.*[19] have recently reported the use of aortic root tailoring in 11 patients with an aortic annulus measurement of at least 2 mm greater than the pulmonary annulus (range 2–9 mm, mean 4.3 mm). A triangular wedge of tissue was excised from the aortic valve annulus at the level of the commissure between the left and non-coronary cusps extending into the anterior leaflet of the mitral valve. The edges of the mitral leaflet and the aortic annulus were then reapproximated over a calibrated dilator to make the aortic annulus 2 mm smaller than the measured pulmonary annulus. Postoperative colour-flow Doppler demonstrated no more than trace to 1+ autograft valve insufficiency and no aortic stenosis. The size of the reduced aortic annulus was not restrained or fixed. Short-term follow-up in this group of patients has shown no recurrence of aortic insufficiency. These authors felt that this technique allowed the use of the Ross operation in patients with excessive aortic annular dilatation, while maintaining the potential for growth in the paediatric patient.

Our experience with the Ross operation suggests that progressive aortic annulus dilatation can occur in both children and adult patients and that this is associated with premature autograft valve failure due to autograft valve insufficiency. This is a relatively unusual process, but it is more likely to occur in patients with a bicuspid aortic valve and aortic valve insufficiency. It is our impression that in this group of patients reduction of the aortic annulus is indicated when the annulus size is larger than the normal size expected for the patient's body surface area.[14] The presence of aortic stenosis appears to be associated with a lower incidence of autograft valve failure.[9,11] In six of the eight patients in group 3, the patient's first aortic valve operation was for aortic valve insufficiency (five Ross operations, one prosthetic valve) and five had a bicuspid aortic valve.

Associated ascending aortic pathology was frequent in the group 1 and 2 patients. Of the group 1 patients, two required replacement of the ascending aorta with a Dacron graft and two required a vertical reduction aortoplasty. In the group 2 patients, eight required replacement of their ascending aorta with a Dacron graft and six required a vertical aortoplasty to reduce the size of the ascending aorta to the size of the pulmonary root. The need to deal with these significant abnormalities of the patients' ascending aorta did not substantially complicate their operative management and allowed the patients to have the benefit of the Ross operation. Eight of these patients were 21 years of age or younger and the oldest patient was 46. Long-term evaluation of this proposed modification of the Ross operation is limited, but in the patients with an external cuff fixation in whom annular reduction was successful (group 1), follow-up is available for two patients for 4 years each and one patient in group 3 has been followed for 5 years. In these three patients there has been no increase in aortic annulus size and their autograft valve function has remained excellent during this follow-up period. It is anticipated that continued follow-up on the group 2 patients will demonstrate the efficacy of this modification of the Ross operation. Its use in patients with aortic insufficiency and aortic annular dilatation may be expected to produce results similar to those for patients without this constellation of aortic root pathology and the indications for the Ross operation may be safely extended.

References

1. Ross D 1988 Pulmonary valve autotransplantation (the Ross operation). J Card Surg 3: 313–319
2. Ross D N 1967 Replacement of aortic and mitral valves with a pulmonary autograft. Lancet 2: 956–958
3. Stelzer P, Jones D J, Elkins R C 1989 Aortic root replacement with pulmonary autograft. Circulation 80: III209–III213

4. Gerosa G, McKay R, Ross D N 1991 Replacement of the aortic valve or root with a pulmonary autograft in children. Ann Thorac Surg 51: 424–429
5. Elkins R C, Santangelo K, Randolph J D *et al* 1992 Pulmonary autograft replacement in children. The ideal solution? Ann Surg 216: 363–371
6. Reddy V M, Rajasinghe H A, Teitel D F, Haas G S, Hanley F L 1996 Aortoventriculoplasty with the pulmonary autograft: The 'Ross–Konno' procedure. J Thorac Cardiovasc Surg 111: 158–167
7. David T E 1995 An anatomic and physiologic approach to acquired heart disease. Eur J Cardiothorac Surg 9: 175–180
8. Kouchoukos N T, Davila-Roman V G, Spray T L, Murphy S F, Perrillo J B 1994 Replacement of the aortic root with a pulmonary autograft in children and young adults with aortic valve disease. N Engl J Med 330: 1–6
9. Elkins R C, Knott-Craig C J, Ward K E, Lane M M 1997 The Ross operation in children: ten-year experience. Ann Thorac Surg 65: 496–502
10. Elkins R C, Knott-Craig C J, Howell C E 1996 Pulmonary autografts in patients with aortic annulus dysplasia. Ann Thorac Surg 61: 1141–1145
11. Elkins R C, Lane M M, McCue C 1996 Pulmonary autograft reoperation: incidence and management. Ann Thorac Surg 62: 450–455
12. Carpentier A 1983 Cardiac valve surgery – the 'French correction'. J Thorac Cardiovasc Surg 86: 323–337
13. Elkins R C, Santangelo K, Stelzer P, Randolph J D, Knott-Craig C J 1992 Pulmonary autograft replacement of the aortic valve: an evolution of technique. J Card Surg 7: 108–116
14. Kirklin J W, Barratt-Boyes B G 1993 Cardiac surgery, 2nd edn. Churchill Livingstone, New York, pp 40–45
15. Oury J H 1997 The International Registry of the Ross Procedure: 1996 results. J Heart Valve Dis 6(4): 333–334
16. Oswalt J D, Dewan S J 1993 Aortic infective endocarditis managed by the Ross procedure. J Heart Valve Dis 2: 380–384
17. Joyce F, Tingleff J, Aagaard J, Pettersson G 1994 The Ross operation in the treatment of native and prosthetic aortic valve endocarditis. J Heart Valve Dis 3: 371–376
18. Joyce F S, Oswalt J D, Tingleff J, Pettersson G 1997 The Ross operation: treatment of choice for aortic valve endocarditis? (Abstract in Program of 33rd Annual Meeting, The Society of Thoracic Surgeons)
19. Durham L E, des Jardins S E, Mosca R S, Bove E L 1997 Ross procedure with aortic root tailoring for aortic valve replacement in the pediatric population. Ann Thorac Surg 64: 482–486
20. David T E, Omran A, Webb G, Rakowski H, Armstrong S, Sun Z 1996 Geometric mismatch of the aortic and pulmonary roots causes aortic insufficiency after the Ross procedure. J Thorac Cardiovasc Surg 112: 1231–1239

Coronary stenosis following AVR with a stentless bioprosthesis: complication or coincidence?

B. S. Goldman, E. Schampaert, G. T. Christakis, J. Sever and S. E. Fremes

There are numerous possible reasons for the development of angina pectoris following aortic valve replacement (AVR): new, progressive or recurrent coronary disease, direct injury to the coronary artery, coronary embolism, the sequelae of coronary perfusion, malposition of the valve or encroachment by excessive pannus. Ostial stenosis has been recognized as a complication of balloon perfusion catheters and plaque disruption or a jet lesion may result from cardioplegic infusion.[1–3] Subcoronary implantation of a stentless porcine bioprosthesis raises the concern of intimal hyperplasia (tissue creep) obstructing the coronary orifice.

Clinical material

Between March 1992 and November 1996, 265 patients at our institution received stented aortic valve prostheses (mechanical 106, bioprosthetic 159), with concomitant coronary artery bypass in 43%; one patient developed angina pectoris and new ostial left main stenosis at 3 months postoperatively. During that same time interval, 116 patients received stentless aortic valve bioprostheses (Toronto SPV valves), with concomitant bypass in 38%. Subsequently, six patients presented with new (four patients) or recurrent (two patients) angina, 3–7 months postoperatively. We reviewed these latter patients to evaluate possible factors contributing to coronary stenosis after aortic valve replacement with a stentless porcine valve.

Clinical characteristics

The clinical characteristics of the six patients with a stentless porcine valve (SPV) implant are listed in Table 25.1. Review of the operative records for any evidence of direct surgical injury revealed three patients to have had heavily calcified valves with difficult excision, one patient with inadvertent excision of the posterior (left coronary) annulus which required pericardial patch repair below the left coronary ostium, and two patients (early in the series) who had extensive dissection around the base of the aorta and origin of the coronary arteries prior to aortotomy. Two patients had documented coronary artery disease and received bypass grafts at the time of the SPV implant. The other four patients had insignificant (10–30%) irregularities noted in the coronary angiograms.

Results

Cross-clamp times (and coronary perfusion times) were longer in these patients (128 ± 27 min) than in other AVR patients (116 ± 37 min) with stentless bioprostheses.

Table 25.1 Clinical characteristics of six patients with postoperative coronary stenosis following implant of a stentless porcine aortic valve

Gender	4M:2F
Age (years)	61–78 (mean 70.3)
Valve lesion	AS (4)
	AI (2)
Valve sizes	25 mm (5)
	27 mm (1)
Concomitant CABG	2 patients
Cardioplegia	Continuous antegrade (5)
	Continuous retrograde (1)

AI, aortic insufficiency; AS, aortic stenosis; CABG, coronary artery bypass graft.

One of the six patients (H.M.) died of acute myocardial infarction 4 months after surgery. Postmortem examination revealed gross cardiomegaly (600 mg) and marked left ventricular hypertrophy, with bilateral ostial stenosis (RCA 90%, LMCA 50%) from apparently old atherosclerotic plaques, without encroachment by nearby pannus from the adjacent stentless valve edges (Figure 25.1). The remainder of the patient's coronary arteries were grossly free of plaque. The pathologist carefully documented the lesions as atherosclerotic and not reactive hyperplasia.[4]

Another patient (S.O.), with severe double vessel disease preoperatively who received saphenous vein grafts to the LAD and RCA, had recurrent angina postoperatively. Coronary angiography demonstrated a new distal 80% LCX lesion; the patient's symptoms are well controlled on the usual medical therapy. Of the remaining four patients, one (H.B.) had received a saphenous vein graft to the RCA for double vessel disease (80% prox RCA, 50% prox LCX) and presented with new mid-distal 99% left main stenosis; the patient later received an LAD graft. In only one instance (M.S.) was there a new ostial lesion (99% ostial RCA). There were four instances (M.S., M.D., J.K. H.B.) of mid-distal left main stenosis (with adjacent LAD and LCX in one). Three of these four patients underwent reoperation and one had angioplasty to provide revascularization and all survived. The stentless porcine bioprosthetic implant was not examined at reoperation in any patient. The coronary stenoses in these six patients are listed in Table 25.2 and are illustrated in selective angiographic frames seen on repeat angiography in Figure 25.2.

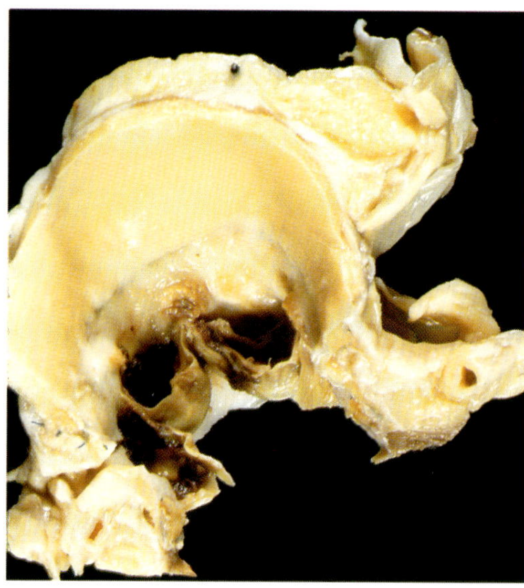

Figure 25.1 Gross pathology of patient H.M. who died 4 months postoperatively of acute myocardial infarction. The valve leaflets were pliable and there was no encroachment of the coronary orifices by pannus. The proximal coronary stumps did reveal apparently old, unrecognized atherosclerotic lesions.

Table 25.2 New coronary stenoses documented in patients after SPV implant

M.S.	50% distal LMS 80% prox. CX 99% ostial RCA	Reop. for SVG to RCA, LAD
M.D.	60% distal LMS 95% prox. LAD	Angioplasty
H.M.	50% ostial LMS 90% ostial RCA	Died of acute myocardial infarction
J.K.	90% distal LMS	Reop. for LIMA–LAD SVG to Int.
H.B.	99% mid LMS	Prior SVG to RCA Reop. SVG to LAD
S.O.	80% distal LCX	Prior SVG to LAD, RCA

Comment

Ostial injury from compression necrosis due to older, non-compliant, balloon cannulae has been recognized as a cause of postoperative coronary stenosis.[1] This is now uncommon due to the design and materials of cannulae in present use. However, high coronary perfusion pressure and flow can conceivably damage the intima or disrupt a plaque with resultant intimal hyperplasia and stenosis (a process similar to restenosis after angioplasty). We postulate that cannula and/or perfusion injury are the cause of recurrent angina in those patients with mid-distal left main coronary stenosis, especially with involvement of the bifurcation vessels (four patients).

Nonetheless, there *are* numerous opportunities to injure the proximal coronary vessels during a subcoronary stentless valve implant: extensive dissection around the base of the aorta and around the proximal vessels, a very low transverse aortotomy, a high upper valve margin encroaching on the ostium, the suturing of the upper valve margin about the coronary orifice, partial obstruction of an orifice by malposition of a commissural post, direct suture injury of the coronary ostium, or significant, exhuberant pannus and tissue creep from the valve edge. One or more of these factors may account for the new coronary stenoses in the one patient who had continuous retrograde cardioplegia (but who returned with 60% distal left main and 95% proximal LAD stenosis). It is more likely that accelerated or progressive coronary atherosclerosis is responsible. This may also account for the unrecognized stenoses in the one patient who died suddenly of acute myocardial infarction and the distal LCX lesion in the patient with prior double bypass.

The new aortic and coronary flow patterns after AVR may be implicated in rapid progression of atherosclerosis. Local tissue injury from even a well-seated valve may precipitate local platelet and fibrin deposition causing turbulent flow near the coronary orifice. In only one patient (M.S.) did the angiographic appearance of new ostial right coronary stenosis suggest tissue overgrowth from the adjacent valve or commissural post malposition. However, since the patient initially refused reoperation, successful angioplasty was performed and a stent deployed with ease, suggesting there was no obstruction from the valve or fibrous tissue overgrowth from the valve edge.

Antegrade blood cardioplegia is employed by many surgeons who also favour intubation of the coronary orifices as a visual aid during alignment and suture of the subcoronary implant. Nonetheless, it is prudent to suggest, even for those surgeons who utilize retrograde coronary sinus perfusion (in which no cannula obviously should injure the proximal coronary), that surgeons exercise great caution in

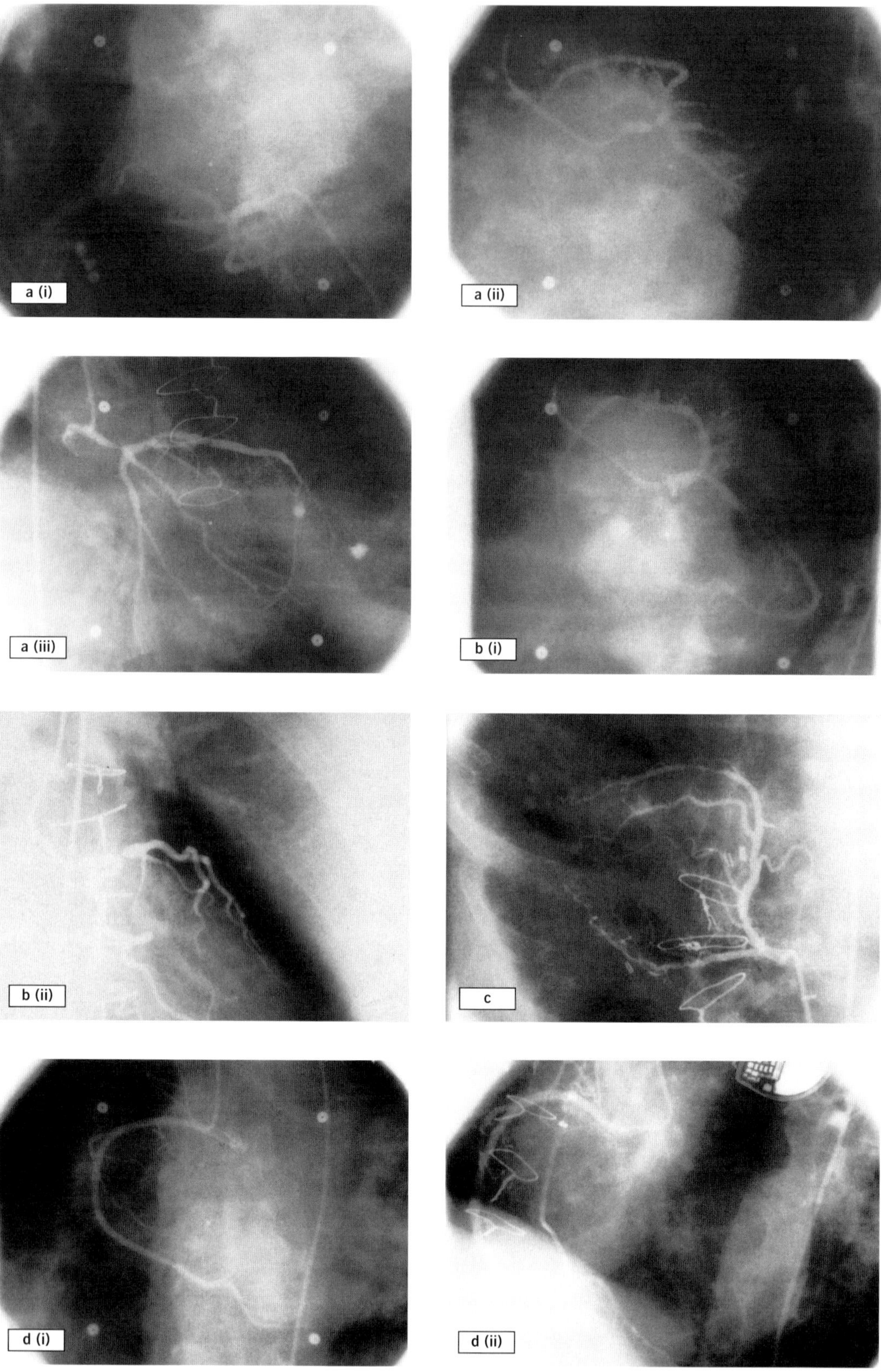

Figure 25.2 (a–g) New coronary stenoses depicted angiographically in patients after SPV implant. Patient (pt) J.K. pre-(a[i]) and post-op angios (a[ii], a[iii]) showing progression from normal left main to significant stenosis. Pt M.D. pre (b[i]) and post-AVR angio (b[ii]) showing distal LMS. Pt S.O. post-AVR angio (c) showing distal LMS. Pt M.S. pre-op normal RCA (d[i]) and post-op ostial disease (d[ii]) with catheter damping requiring sinus flush. Pre-op modest LMS (e[i]) with progression (e[ii]) post-AVR to significant LMS with involvement of bifurcation. Pt H.M. pre-op normal RCA (f[i]) and post-AVR ([f[ii]) progression to proximal RCA stenosis. Pt H.B. pre-op LCA (g[i]) with subsequent proximal to mid LMS (g[ii]) post-op.

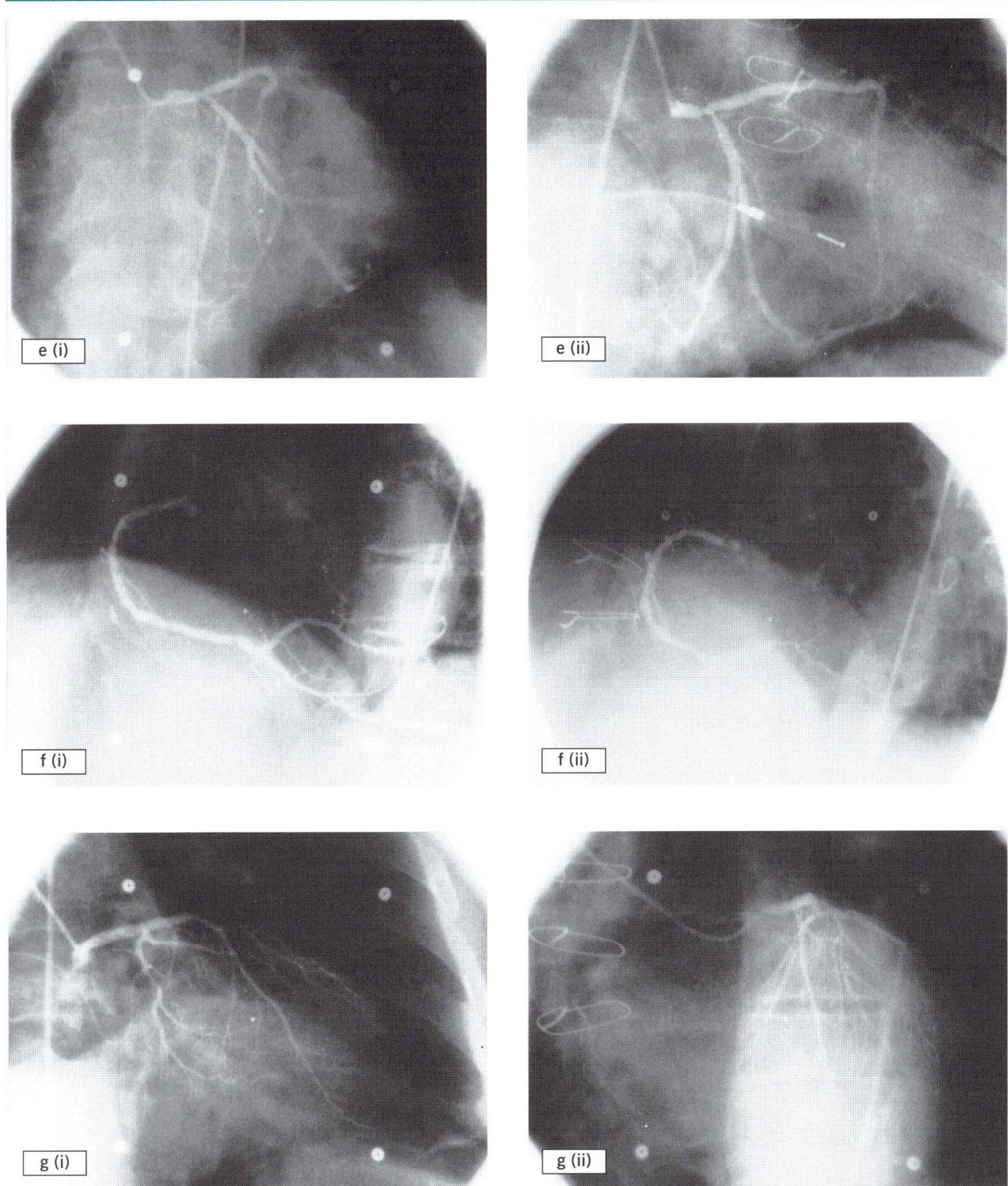

dissection about the base of the aorta, avoid dissection around the proximal coronary vessels and keep sutures and commissural posts well away from the coronary orifices. In the presence of antegrade coronary perfusion, it is probably safer to use intermittent[5] rather than continuous cardioplegic infusion to minimize any possible compression injury and to monitor carefully cardioplegia perfusion pressures and flow to diminish the possibility of intimal disruption. It is our belief that this unusual cluster of six patients with angina post-AVR primarily represents perfusion injuries and/or random progression of coronary atherosclerosis rather than complications of the stentless valve implant.

References

1. Trimble A S, Bigelow W G, Wigle E D, Silver M D 1969 Coronary ostial stenosis as a late complication of coronary perfusion in open heart surgery. J Thorac Cardiovasc Surg 57(6): 792–795

2. Menashe P, Kewal S, Fauchet M *et al* 1982 Retrograde coronary sinus perfusion: a safe alternative for ensuring cardioplegic delivery in aortic valve surgery. Ann Thorac Surg 34: 647–658
3. Menashe P, Subayi J B, Piwnica A 1990 Retrograde coronary sinus cardioplegia for aortic valve operations: a clinical report of 500 patients. Ann Thorac Surg 49: 556–564
4. Butany J 1996 Personal communication
5. Bernhard W F, Schwartz H F, Malick N P 1960 Intermittent cold coronary perfusion as an adjunct to open heart surgery. Surg Gynecol Obstet 111: 744–750

Aortic valve replacement through minithoracotomy with the stentless U.S.L. porcine valve: the ideal pathway for elderly patients?

J. A. Navia, L. Diodato, J. L. Navia and R. Pizarro

During the last year, experimental and clinical interest in minimally invasive coronary artery bypass grafting procedures has grown. These procedures have been extended to valvular patients with minimally invasive open operations with limited thoracotomies.

The benefits of a minimal access approach with less surgical trauma have been adopted by an increasing number of surgical specialties.

What really constitutes a 'minimally invasive approach' has yet to be established.[1] We see a great advantage in combining two benefits in elderly patients:

1. Less surgical trauma: by using a right anterior mediastinotomy approach (Figure 26.1) via an 8–10 cm vertical parasternal incision, with excision of a small segment of the third and fourth costal cartilages, or by a second approach, with transverse sternal transection at the level of the third rib interspace, with dissection and mobilization of both internal thoracic arteries without dividing them.
2. The use of the stentless Unique Suture Line (U.S.L.) porcine aortic valve (BioSud S.A., Buenos Aires, Argentina).[2] Due to its ease of implant, it can be done through a minimal incision. It gives the benefits of a bioprosthesis, avoiding anticoagulation treatment to elderly patients, and good haemodynamic performance of a stentless valve in the small aortic annulus.

Indications considered for valve replacement by minimally invasive techniques are given in Table 26.1.

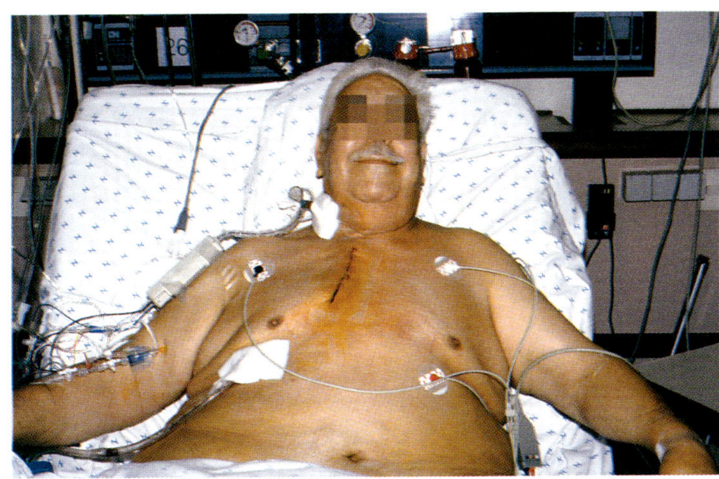

Figure 26.1 Right vertical parasternal incision (8–10 cm) at the level of the 3rd and 4th intercostal spaces.

Table 26.1 Indications for valve replacement: minimally invasive technique
All adult age
Preference in elderly patients above 70 years old
Obesity
Emphysema
COPD
Diabetes
Cachectic patients
Osteoporosis
Previous chest irradiation
Reoperation after:
MVR with severe enlargement of right cavities
Reconstruction of sternal wound (mediastinitis sequelae)

COPD, chronic obstructive pulmonary disease; MVR, mitral valve replacement.

Surgical procedure

The operation is applicable to most patients with aortic valve disease, especially those elderly patients suffering from aortic calcific stenosis. The use of the stentless U.S.L. valve is contraindicated when the aortic annulus or the ascending aorta is dilated, i.e. in aortic annuloectasia, Marfan's syndrome.

To reduce the trauma of valve surgery, a 8–10 cm right parasternal incision is made and the third and fourth costal cartilages are partially resected. The pericardium is partially opened and secured against the incision edges. A wide exposure of the ascending aorta, superior vena cava and right atrial appendage is obtained (Figure 26.2).

Cardiopulmonary bypass is commenced with an ascending aortic arterial cannula and a two-stage venous cannula placed in the right atrium, unless mitral or tricuspid procedure is required; in these cases dual caval cannulation is employed. Another cannulation site is suggested if the ascending aorta is short in length, or if severe calcific aortic wall or distal peripheral vascular diseases are present (Table 26.2).

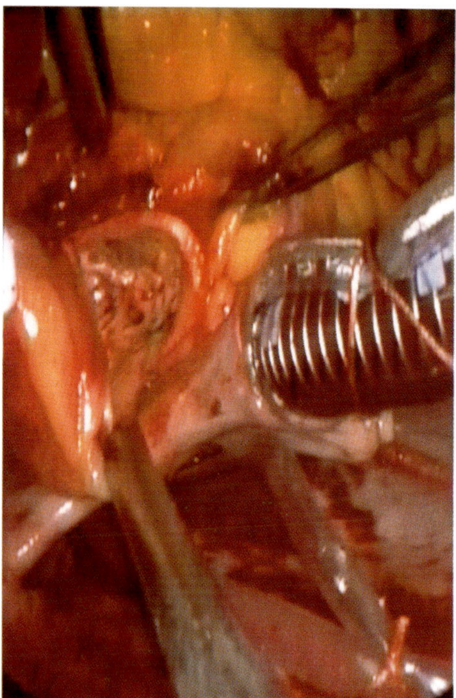

Figure 26.2 A wide exposure of the ascending aorta, superior vena cavae and right atrial appendage through parasternal incision.

A left ventricular vent is used to maintain a bloodless operative field, with a cannula introduced through the right superior pulmonary vein. Antegrade normothermic blood cardioplegic infusion is used for myocardial protection, delivered into the aortic root for pure aortic stenosis or into the coronary ostia in the presence of aortic regurgitation. Either one is combined with retrograde infusion through the coronary sinus with a cardioplegia cannula inserted by a blind manoeuvre or assisted by intraoesophageal echo.

Before the aorta is cross-clamped, arterial flow is momentarily decreased, allowing a perfect clamp placement.

A transverse aortotomy 5 mm above the sinotubular junction and at least 5 mm above the origin of the right coronary artery is

Table 26.2 Cannulation methods
Ascending aorta + right atrial two-stage cannula
Femoro-femoral bypass
Axillary artery + right atrium or femoral vein

performed. The aortic valve is excised, a meticulous decalcification of the annulus is carried out, and the implantation of the exactly fitting size of the stentless U.S.L. valve is performed, in the subcoronary position.

The 'scalloped' design of the valve and the wavy shape of the tiny suture ring allow for a single suture line, interrupted or continuous according to the patient native ring size. The surgical technique is similar to the one used for a regular stented valve implantation. The single suture line at the tiny Dacron ring and fixation of the post with interrupted single horizontal mattress suture with Teflon pledgets across the aortic wall make the surgical technique simpler. The aortic incision is closed in the regular fashion (Figures 26.3, 26.4).

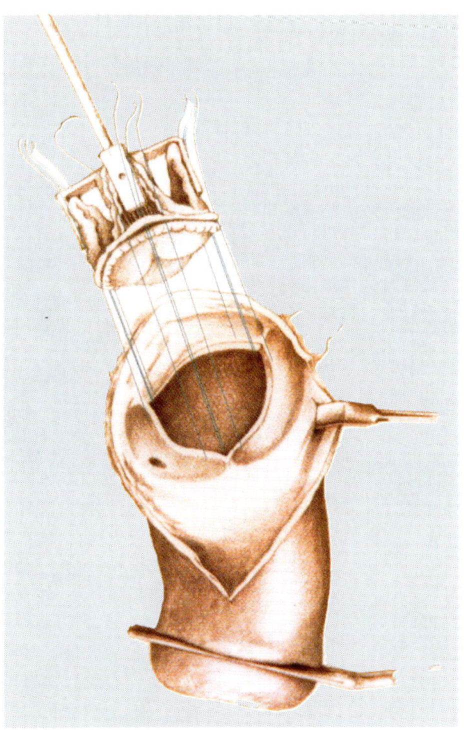
Figure 26.3 Valve fixation with interrupted single stitches.

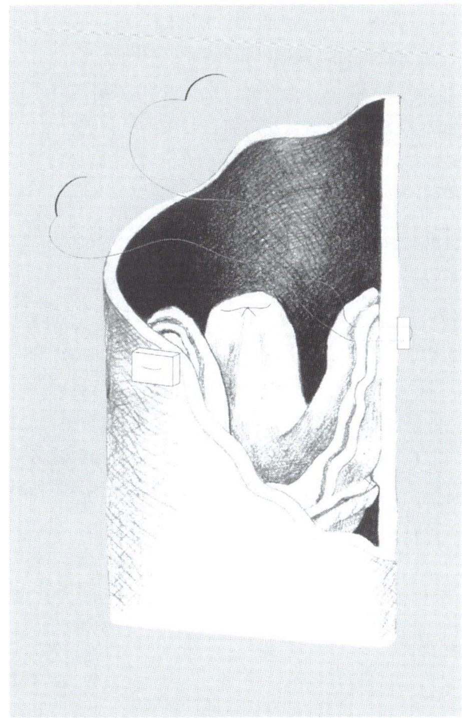
Figure 26.4 Post fixation with single horizontal mattress stitches across the aortic wall, tied over Teflon pledgets in each strut.

Results

From August 1996 to November 1997, both minimally invasive approaches were used in 50 patients. Three underwent tricuspid valve replacement for infective endocarditis, 15 received mitral valve replacement (MVR) (including four reoperations) and 32 underwent aortic valve replacement (AVR). Twenty of these 32 patients were elderly, mean age 74.7 (range 68–86) years old, 12 men and eight women. All patients underwent AVR for senile calcific aortic stenosis.

All elderly patients could receive a stentless U.S.L. porcine valve because of the easy insertion through the minimally invasive thoracotomy. The valve sizes implanted were 19, 20, 21, 22 and 23 mm in diameter, due to the small calcific annulus (Table 26.3).

There were two hospital deaths (10%) in the overall elderly group, one due to peptic ulcer perforation, the other to pulmonary infection. The amount of postoperative bleeding was 442 ml/24 h (average). The mean length of stay (LOS) was 5.8 ± 1.5 days.

Table 26.3 Minimally invasive thoracotomy for AVR in elderly patients with the stentless U.S.L. valve

		Surgical procedure (n = 20)	
Preoperative diagnosis	**No. patients**	**Valve size implanted (mm)**	**Hospital mortality**
	2	19	
	4	20	
Senile calcific aortic stenosis	9	21	10%
	2	22	
	3	23	

Ischaemic time (average) 78′ ± 12′. Bleeding postop. 442 ml/24 hr (average). Length of stay between 4th and 5th postop. days.

All patients followed the general protocol of the stentless U.S.L. porcine valve and underwent clinical and colour Doppler echocardiography follow-up. No periprosthetic leak or aortic regurgitation was found and all patients are postoperatively in NYHA class I in the short period of follow-up.

Discussion

The results reported here in a small group of elderly patients with minimally invasive thoracotomy confirm the results of larger series.[3,4]

No conversion to median sternotomy was required in this patient group. Elderly patients were out of bed very soon after operation, mobilization without problems was realized, and absence of chest pain and excellent stability were observed.

We think that one of the major advantages of the parasternal approach is chest stability; this surgical technique avoids the distortion and sometimes disruption of the sternum, the costoclavicular articulation (Figure 26.5) or joint as sometimes seen in the regular median sternotomy. The minimally invasive parasternal approach allows for a complete movement of the arms, without any problems in COPD or acute respiratory disease during chest physiotherapy, especially with reference to elderly patients.

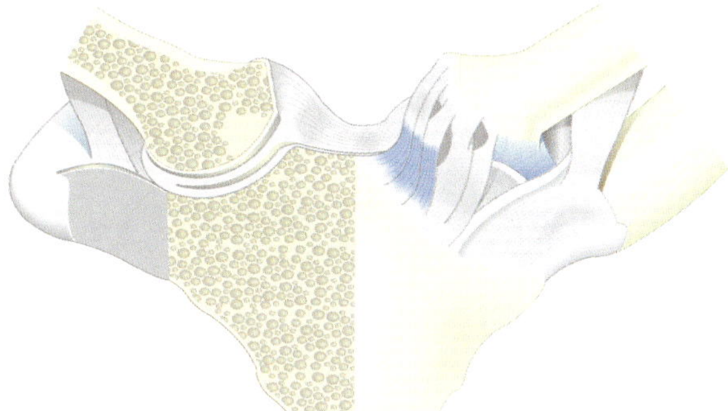

Figure 26.5 Sternum costoclavicular junction.

Conclusion

The authors believe that with increased surgical experience, the minimally invasive thoracic approach for AVR using the stentless U.S.L. valve will have a major impact on the management of elderly patients, with less morbidity and mortality, lower cost, and greater postoperative comfort for the patients.

References

1. Reitz A 1997 Less invasive cardiac surgery. Delivered at the 33rd Postgraduate program of The Society of Thoracic Surgeons (Abstracts), February 21, San Diego, CA, USA
2. Navia J 1989 Valvular surgery – presentation of the stentless porcine valve design. Symposium of the Cleveland Clinic Foundation during the XIII Inter-American Congress of Cardiology, Rio de Janeiro, Brazil, July 23–28
3. Cosgrove D M, Sabik J F 1996 Minimally invasive approach for aortic valve operations. Ann Thoracic Surg 62: 596–597
4. Cosgrove D M, Sabik J F, Navia J 1997 Minimally invasive valve surgery. (Abstract 63) 33rd Annual meeting of The Society of Thoracic Surgeons. February 3–5, San Diego, CA, USA

CHAPTER 27

The pericardial stentless bioprosthesis: preliminary results of a modified procedure for implantation

Y. De Bruyne and M. Joris

The first aortic homograft valves were implanted in subcoronary position by Ross in 1962[1] and by Barratt-Boyes in 1964.[2] The results were good but the lack of availability of these homografts and the appearance of the more easily implanted glutaraldehyde-preserved stented porcine valves made many surgeons use these bioprostheses. In the presence of a stent, whatever its geometry may be, a transvalvular gradient is unavoidable, more stress is exercised on the leaflets of the prosthesis and durability is diminished.

For several years, we have seen a renewed interest in the use of stentless valves as the absence of the stent should improve haemodynamic function and prolong life expectancy of the valvular substitute. Several surgeons started clinical trials using different types of these stentless valves which were made of different tissues and prepared in different ways.[3–10] All these stentless valves have been showing enhanced haemodynamic performance, but the technique of implantation is more demanding and time consuming than the technique currently in use for stented bioprostheses. Results at short and medium term are influenced by this implantation technique.[11,12] We report our experience with one of these stentless valves and describe the way we modified its implantation technique.

Materials and methods

Valve description

By choice we use the stentless pericardial aortic valve manufactured by Sorin Biomedica (Figure 27.1).

The valve is made of two separate sheets of glutaraldehyde-treated bovine pericardium. It is fixed by a low-pressure, progressive glutaraldehyde fixation process, allowing the maintenance of the integrity of the collagen fibres of the tissue. The first sheet is shaped into three leaflets without contact with any solid surface. The suture to the second sheet is positioned in accordance with an optimized geometric design to minimize the stress on the tissue at the level of the commissures.

Patient population and operative data

From September 1993 to December 1996, 37 pericardial stentless bioprostheses were implanted in 37 patients. Table 27.1 shows the preoperative clinical data of these patients. Table 27.2 shows the operative data. We divided the patients into three groups according to the operative technique used:

Table 27.1 Preoperative clinical data of the patient population

37 patients		
Male/female: 26/11		
Age (years): 68±6 (53–83)		
Aortic valve lesions		
Stenosis	16	(43%)
Regurgitation	10	(27%)
Mixed	11	(30%)
Endocarditis	5	(13.5%)

Table 27.2 Operative data of the patient population

Size of implanted valves (mm):	
21	1
23	7
25	12
27	17
Associated procedures:	
CABG	13
Mitral repair	1

CABG, coronary artery bypass graft.

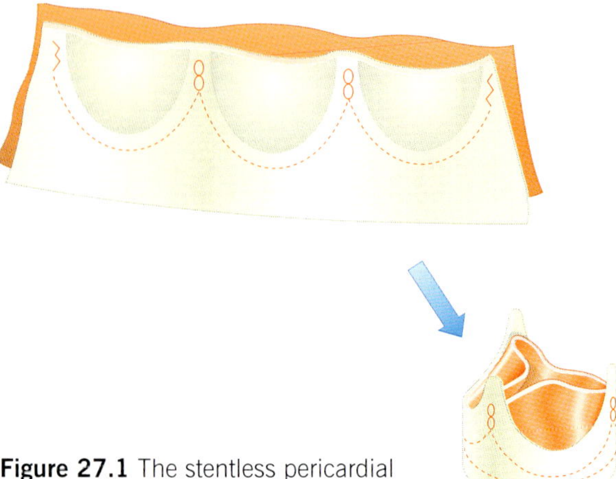

Figure 27.1 The stentless pericardial aortic valve (Sorin Biomedica).

1. Group A: classical (8/37). This group corresponds to the first eight patients operated upon by a classical subcoronary technique with this prosthesis.
2. Group B: banding (19/37). An adequate periaortic Dacron banding was added to the classical implantation.
3. Group C: vascular prosthesis (10/37). In this group not only the valve was replaced but also a part of the ascending aorta.

Operative strategy

In the first group of eight patients (group A) two patients developed an aortic regurgitation: one moderate and one severe. The latter needed reoperation 8.5 months after his first operation. At that moment we thought that our operative technique had to be reconsidered.

We have been looking for answers to two important questions concerning the implantation of the stentless aortic valve:

1. How to avoid regurgitation?
2. How to diminish the transvalvular gradient?

Aortic regurgitation after implantation of a stentless prosthesis can be influenced by two factors: the diameter of the sinotubular junction and the alignment of the commissures. If the diameter of the sinotubular junction increases, the cylindrical configuration of the prosthesis is altered and regurgitation occurs (Figure 27.2). When the commissures are distorted, the cusps of the valve move at different levels and this induces regurgitation (Figure 27.3). Both mechanisms can be avoided by a periaortic banding around the aorta at the level of the sinotubular junction or by replacing a part of the ascending aorta by a vascular prosthesis, the proximal suture of which supports the valvular commissures. The banding is used when the aorta is not dilated. When the ascending aorta is dilated, part of it is replaced by a vascular prosthesis (Figure 27.4).

Two important observations drew our attention to the transvalvular gradient. First, we focused on the reduction of the valvular obstruction. Not only did we perform a thorough decalcification of the aortic wall, but we also scalloped the prosthesis as much as possible, more particularly in its inferior part, to avoid folding of its tissue during implantation. However, one should be aware that maximal scalloping of the prosthesis increases the risk of a non-cylindrical implantation which makes the control

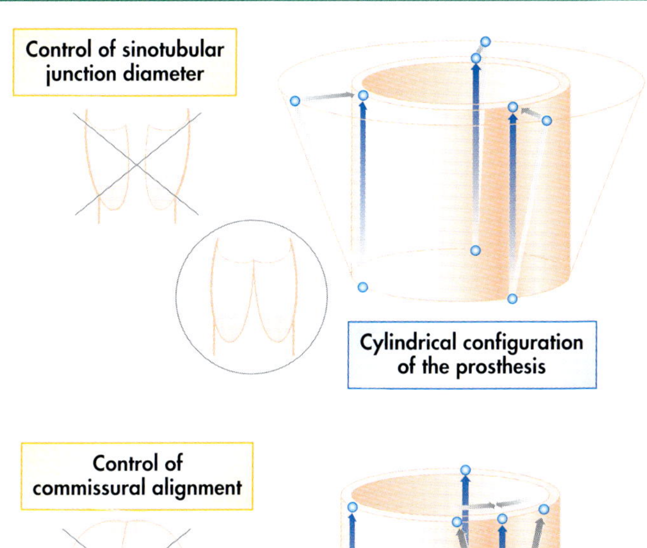

Figure 27.2 Influence of the sinotubular junction diameter on aortic regurgitation.

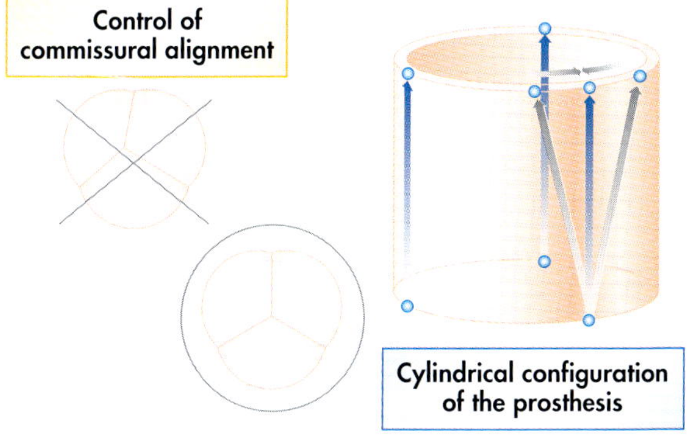

Figure 27.3 Commissural distortion causes aortic regurgitation.

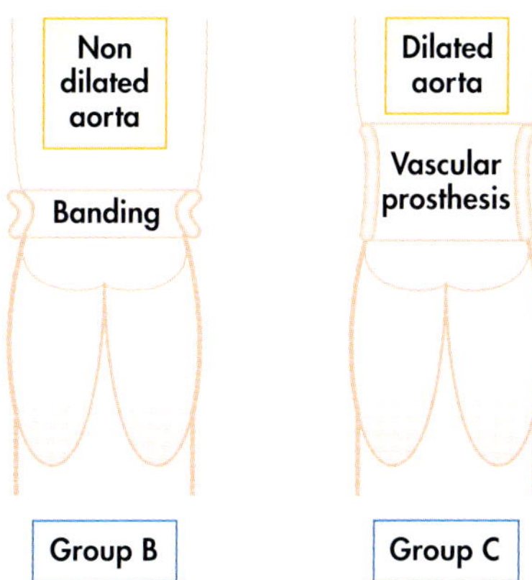

Figure 27.4 The aortic diameter determines the choice of operative technique.

of the diameter of the sinotubular junction even more useful (Figure 27.5). Secondly, we believe in the possibility of the persistence of a perivalvular space between the prosthesis and the aortic wall. To avoid this we injected GRF glue in this space (Figure 27.6). The key points which prompted us to modify our technique are summarized in Figure 27.7.

Banding technique

In a group of 19 patients we added to the aortic valve replacement an appropriate periaortic banding.

After incision of the aorta by an S-shaped aortotomy ending at the middle of the non-coronary sinus, the diseased valve is excised and

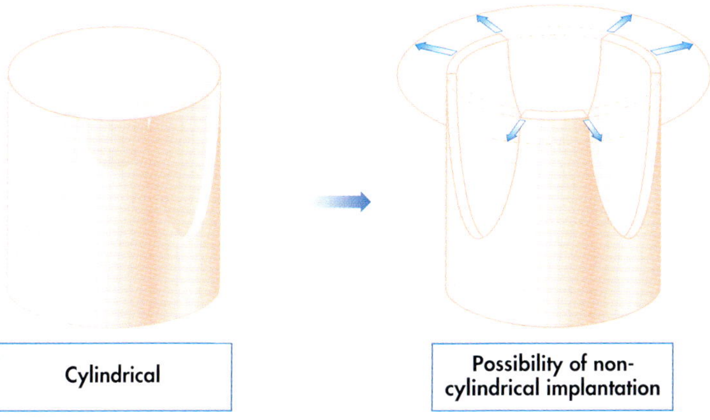

Figure 27.5 Risk of maximal scalloping of the prosthesis.

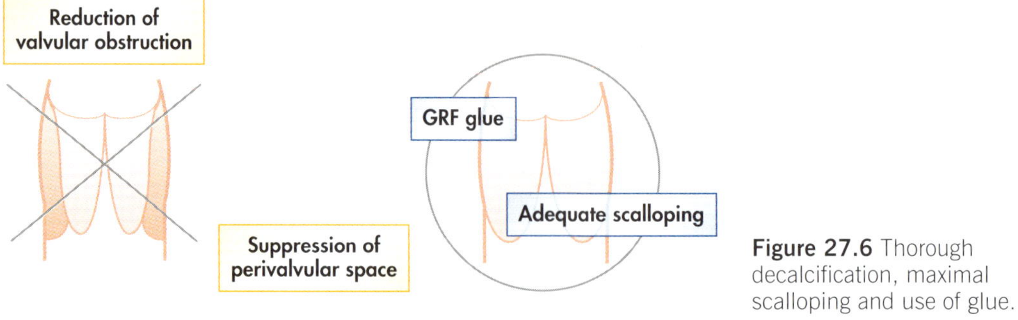

Figure 27.6 Thorough decalcification, maximal scalloping and use of glue.

the aortic wall is extensively freed of calcifications. Three stay sutures are applied just above the three commissures. The size of the prosthesis is chosen according to the diameter of the aortic annulus. The inferior part of the prosthesis is adequately trimmed to obtain a horizontal edge. The proximal or inflow suture line at the level of the aortic annulus consists of three running sutures of 4/0 polypropylene, each of them starting at the midpoint of the bottom of the Valsalva sinuses. The pericardial valve can be easily invaginated in the left ventricle using the technique of Barratt-Boyes which facilitates this suture. After repositioning the pericardial valve into the aorta, the outer wall of the stentless prosthesis is scalloped, leaving a small rim to allow a proper distal suture line. This suture line consists of three running sutures, with 5/0 polypropylene, each of them starting from the midpoint of each sinus and directed towards the top of the commissures. At this level the needle is passed across the aortic wall to anchor the periaortic Dacron strip previously prepared and positioned. Its length is defined by the formula: $C = 3.5 \times$ (prosthesis ϕ) (taking into consideration the perimeter of the prosthesis and the thickness of the aortic wall) and its width is approximately 1 cm. Every third is marked before suturing the Dacron strip.

GRF glue is then injected in the perivalvular space between the host aortic wall and the pericardial prosthesis. By means of the balloon of a urinary catheter, the prosthesis is applied to the aortic wall. Only at this moment are the three knots of the distal suture tied outside the aortic wall.

The aortotomy is closed by a 4/0 polypropylene running suture and the loose ends of the periaortic banding are fastened by separate stitches.

Vascular prosthesis

When the ascending aorta is found dilated (diameter > 40 mm at the sinotubular junction) we perform a partial replacement of the aorta (10 patients). We start with a transection at the sinotubular junction. After excising the pathological part of the ascending aorta, the aortic valve is replaced in the same way as described above

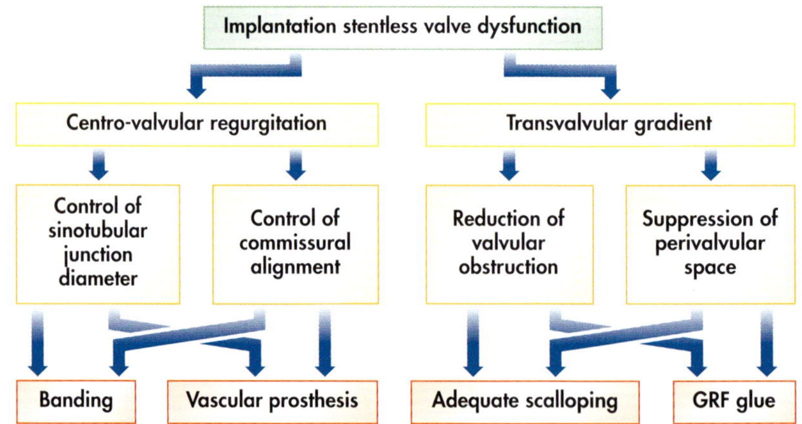

Figure 27.7 The theoretical considerations leading to the four main technical modifications.

without the presence of the Dacron banding. Sometimes a plicature of the aortic wall is required to accommodate the sizes. The size of the prosthetic valve never exceeds ϕ 27 mm (in our series of 10 patients, one patient received a 25 mm valve and nine a 27 mm one).

A vascular prosthesis with a diameter usually 1 mm more than that of the prosthesis is then sutured just above it, by means of two running suture lines with 4/0 polypropylene. The proximal suture line supports the valvular commissures and in this way an adequate geometry of valve and aorta can be preserved (Figure 27.8).

The cross-clamping times of the different procedures are listed in Table 27.3.

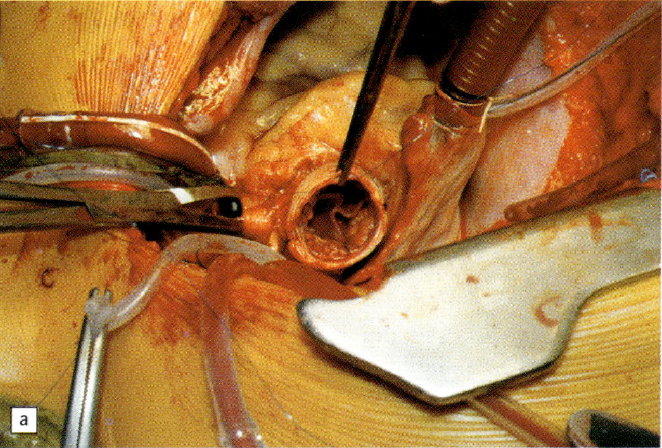

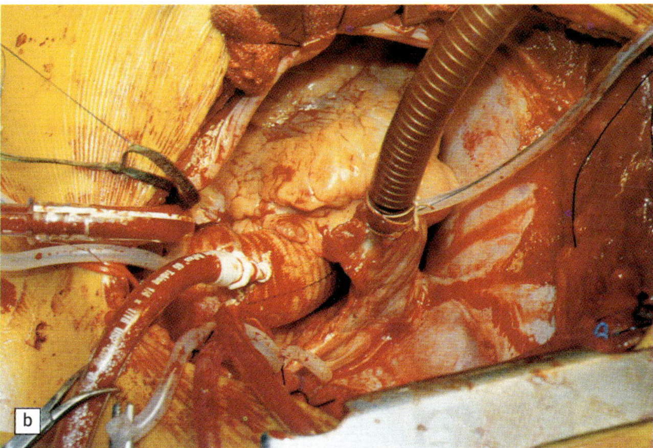

Figure 27.8 (a) Operative view of the position of a stentless prosthetic valve inside the vascular prosthesis. (b) Final result after aortic valve replacement associated with a partial replacement of the ascending aorta.

Results

Survival

Survival details are shown in Table 27.4.

In group A one patient died, in the early postoperative period, of pulmonary problems. Another patient died of cardiogenic shock 2 months after his operation. At autopsy, the morphology of his aortic prosthesis was perfectly normal. The survival in group A after a mean follow-up time of 22 months is 75%.

Among the 19 patients of group B, one died in the immediate postoperative period. He was a patient operated upon as an emergency for endocarditis. He never recovered from his sepsis and died in multiple organ failure. Another patient died 7 months after his operation from a pulmonary problem. The survival in group B after a mean follow-up time of 12 months is 89%.

In group C one of the ten patients died in the early postoperative period of a pulmonary problem. There were no late deaths and survival after a mean follow-up time of 12 months is 90%.

There were no valve-related deaths. Most of the patients in this study were elderly and often in poor general condition.

Haemodynamic assessment

Almost all patients (33/37) had a transoesophageal echocardiography in the early postoperative hours under general anaesthesia. Transthoracic colour-flow Doppler echocardiography was performed 3–6 months and 1 year after the operation by different cardiologists. The results are listed in Table 27.5.

The best results were obtained in group C, in which none of the patients has yet developed more than trivial regurgitation. In group B with the banding technique, three patients presented trivial regurgitation in the immediate postoperative period and

Table 27.3 Cross-clamping times of the different procedures

	Simple valve replacement	Replacement associated with other procedures
Group A	95±20	107±14
Group B	93±18	119±17
Group C	98±15	140

Table 27.4 Survival in the different groups

	Group A	Group B	Group C
Number of patients	8	19	10
Early mortality	1 pulmonary 13%	1 sepsis 5%	1 pulmonary 10%
Late mortality	1 cardiogenic 13%	1 pulmonary 5%	0 0%
Valve-related mortality	0	0	0
Survival	75%	89%	90%
Mean follow-up	22 months	12 months	12 months

Table 27.5 Regurgitation at postoperative echocardiography

	Group A				Group B			Group C	
	Known	None or trivial	Moderate	Severe	Known	None or trivial	Moderate	Known	None or trivial
Postop	7/8	100%	0%	0%	17/19	100%	0%	9/10	100%
3–6 months	4/6	50%	25%	25%	14/18	100%	0%	6/9	100%
> 1 year	3/5	100%	0%	0%	6/17	83%	17%	3/9	100%

one of them progressed towards a moderate regurgitation after 1 year. The results were less good in group A, before modification of the technique, and here one patient developed a moderate regurgitation and a second one needed reoperation for severe regurgitation.

For the whole patient population, only one patient presented a significant transvalvular gradient. This patient, who had been operated upon by the banding technique, developed a maximal transvalvular gradient of 32 mmHg.

Conclusions

The pericardial stentless bioprosthesis can be used in any pathological condition requiring an aortic valve replacement and with very satisfying haemodynamic results.[13]

When the ascending aorta is not dilated, an appropriate periaortic banding seemed useful to secure an adequate geometrical valve implantation. In the presence of a dilated ascending aorta, the combined replacement of the aortic valve and a part of the ascending aorta seems to be a good alternative for a root replacement. We are aware that this is a small series with a short-term follow-up. Long-term follow-up is needed to evaluate the durability of the valve and the beneficial effect of the modified procedure.

References

1. Ross D N 1962 Homograft replacement of the aortic valve. Lancet 2: 487–488
2. Barratt-Boyes B G 1964 Homograft aortic valve replacement in aortic valve incompetence and stenosis. Thorax 19: 131–150
3. David T E, Pollick C, Bos J 1990 Aortic valve replacement with stentless porcine aortic bioprosthesis. J Thorac Cardiovasc Surg 99: 113–118
4. David T E, Feindel C M, Bos J, Sun Z, Scully H E, Rakowski H 1994 Aortic valve replacement with a stentless porcine aortic valve. A six year experience. J Thorac Cardiovasc Surg 108: 1030–1036
5. Wong K, Shad S, Waterworth P D, Khaghani A, Pepper J R, Yacoub M H 1995 Early experience with the Toronto stentless porcine valve. Ann Thorac Surg 60: S402–S405
6. Westaby S, Amarasena N, Long V *et al* 1995 Time-related hemodynamic changes after aortic replacement with the Freestyle stentless xenograft. Ann Thorac Surg 60: 1633–1639
7. Pillai R, Spriggings D, Amarasena N, O'Regan D J, Parry A J, Westaby S 1993 Stentless aortic bioprosthesis? The way forward: early experience with the Edwards valve. Ann Thorac Surg 56: 88–91
8. O'Brien M F 1995 Composite stentless xenograft for aortic valve replacement: clinical evaluation of function. Ann Thorac Surg 60: S406–S409
9. Hvass U, Chatel D, Assayag P *et al* 1995 Ann Thorac Surg 60: 5414–5417
10. Del Rizzo D F, Goldman B S, Christakis G T, David T E 1996 Hemodynamic benefits of the Toronto stentless valve. J Thorac Cardiovasc Surg 112: 1431–1446
11. Kon N D, Westaby S, Amarasena N, Pillai R, Cordell A R 1995 Comparison of implantation techniques using Freestyle stentless porcine aortic valve. Ann Thorac Surg 59: 857–862
12. O'Brien M F 1995 The Cryolife–O'Brien composite aortic stentless xenograft: surgical technique of implantation. Ann Thorac Surg 60: S410–S413
13. Casabona R, De Paulis R, Zattera G F *et al* 1992 Stentless porcine and pericardial valve in aortic position. Ann Thorac Surg 54: 681–685

VII Design and Construction

CHAPTER 28

Future developments in stentless bioprosthetic heart valves

W. Mirsch

Stentless aortic valves show excellent short- and mid-term results. After receiving a Toronto SPV valve, patients experience near-normal gradients and more rapid regression of left ventricular mass hypertrophy than seen with stented valves.[1–12] These benefits may lead to improved patient survival. The focus is now on long-term outcomes. The success of the current generation of stentless aortic valves signals the beginning of a new era of prosthetic heart valves. These new valve designs will closely mimic the structure and function of the tissues they replace.

Prosthetic heart valve performance can be broken down into four main categories: haemodynamics, durability, implantability and complications (such as thromboembolic events, endocarditis, etc.). While current generations of heart valves provide good clinical outcomes, significant improvements can be made. The author believes this will be achieved through the development of new prosthetic heart valves with anatomical design, and physiological and biological function.

Unique stentless designs for specific implant requirements, such as subcoronary aortic, full root replacement, and mitral valves, will meet patient needs and reduce bypass and cross-clamp times. New processing techniques reduce calcification and improve biocompatibility. Modifications to synthetic components can reduce the potential for prosthetic valve endocarditis, and advances in biotechnology offer the potential for a 'living' valve replacement. It is the role of researchers, engineers and clinicians to improve patients' lives with continued technological advancement.

Haemodynamic performance

The early promise of stentless aortic valves was improved haemodynamic performance over stented valves. The assumption was that implanting a larger valve and using the native aorta to support the valve would decrease gradients. Clinical results show a marked improvement in haemodynamic performance. Figure 28.1 presents data collected 2 years postoperatively on 282 patients enrolled in a clinical investigation of the Toronto SPV valve. Mean systolic gradients, stratified by size, are shown versus cardiac outputs. The graph demonstrates that more than 90% of all patients receiving a Toronto SPV valve have a mean gradient of less than 10 mmHg, regardless of size or cardiac output.

The graph in Figure 28.2 shows the mean gradient versus cardiac output for patients who received the 27 mm valves, the most common size. Plotting one valve size allows comparison of valve performance across the range of cardiac outputs. The data show that gradients appear unrelated to cardiac output.

Figure 28.3 demonstrates this trend for all the smallest valve sizes. Again, these valves have low gradients, with no apparent relationship to cardiac outputs. The author believes the Toronto SPV valve's superior haemodynamic performance results from anatomical design and physiological performance.

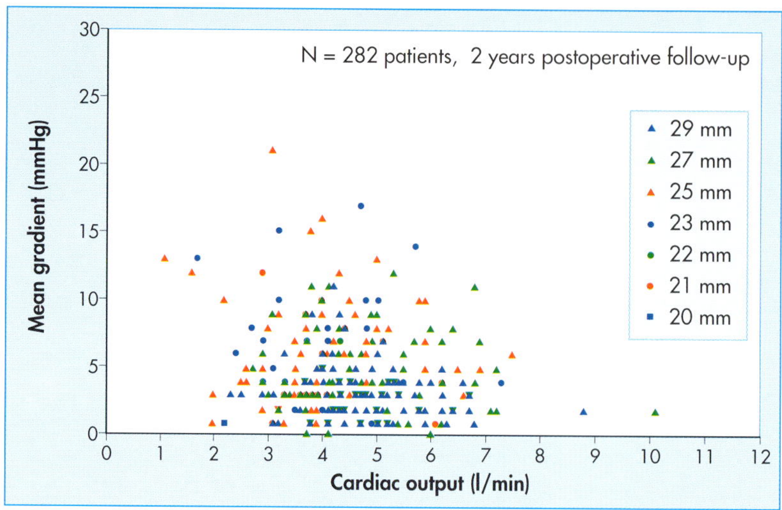

Figure 28.1 Mean gradients versus the cardiac outputs for all patients enrolled in the clinical trial at 2 years after receiving the Toronto SPV valve.

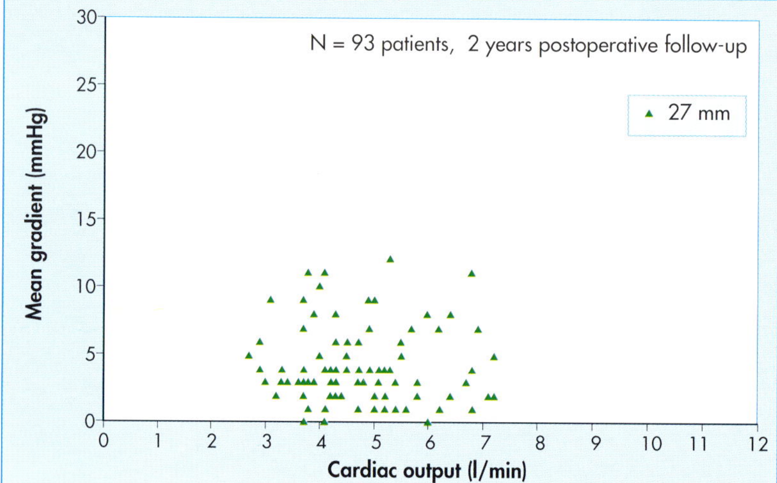

Figure 28.2 Mean gradients versus the cardiac outputs for patients receiving size 27 mm valves enrolled in the clinical trial at 2 years after receiving the Toronto SPV valve.

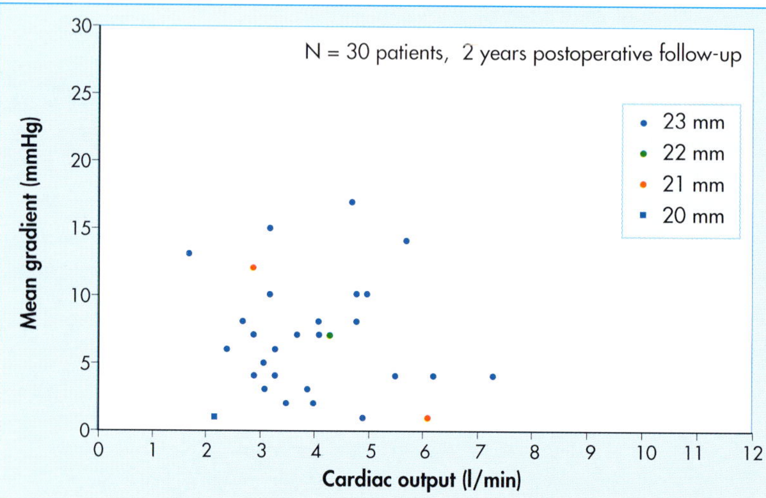

Figure 28.3 Mean gradients versus the cardiac outputs for patients receiving size 23 mm and smaller valves enrolled in the clinical trial at 2 years after receiving the Toronto SPV valve.

The Toronto SPV valve also has a very low incidence of insufficiency. Figure 28.4 is a graph showing the regurgitation observed in patients 2 years after receiving a Toronto SPV valve. Nearly 95% of all patients have trivial or no regurgitation. These excellent results can be attributed to the sinotubular junction sizing technique, developed by Dr. Tirone David, which ensures proper coaptation of stentless valve leaflets.

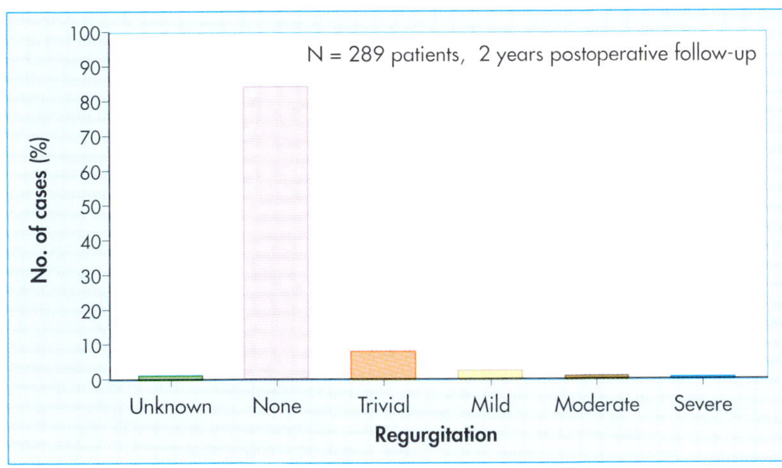

Figure 28.4 Incidence of aortic insufficiency for all patients enrolled in the clinical trial at 2 years after receiving the Toronto SPV valve.

Antimineralization technology

The next challenge for stentless valves is the demonstration of long-term durability. While animal studies and *in vitro* accelerated wear testing indicate that the reduction in aortic stentless valves' stress levels may lead to improvements in longevity, additional anticalcification measures are needed. To that end, St Jude Medical, Inc. and Dr. Robert Levy, at the University of Michigan, collaborated on the BiLinx technology, the first antimineralization treatment developed specifically for a stentless valve. This treatment, under development for several years, relies on secondary processing of glutaraldehyde cross-linked tissue.[13–18]

Optimum stentless valve function requires flexible prosthetic tissue. Therefore, an antimineralization treatment for stentless valves must address calcification of both aortic wall and leaflet tissue to ensure maximum performance and longevity. Figure 28.5 contains representative histology from a rat subdermal implant study of the BiLinx technology. The control samples for the aortic wall and leaflet tissues are heavily mineralized, as demonstrated by the material staining black in these von Kossa-stained sections. By contrast, the treated tissues, aortic wall and leaflet are devoid of mineralization.

Figure 28.6 is a plot of calcium levels in explants from this study at the two implant durations, 21 and 63 days. The control leaflet and aortic wall tissues yielded

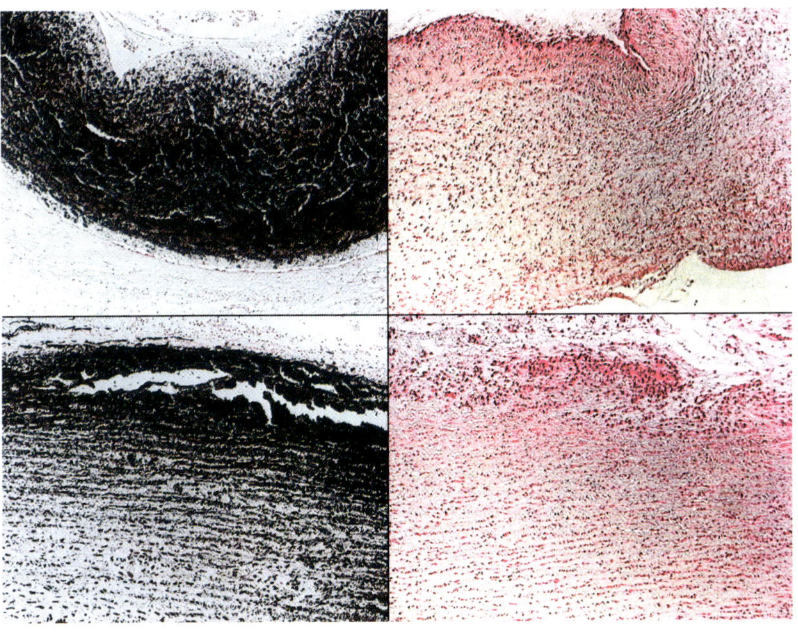

Figure 28.5 Representative histology from rat subdermal implant study of BiLinx technology. Control samples (left column) stain heavily for mineralization, whereas treated samples (right column) are devoid of mineral deposits. Treatment is effective on both leaflet (top row) and aortic wall tissues (bottom row). (von Kossa stain, × 100.)

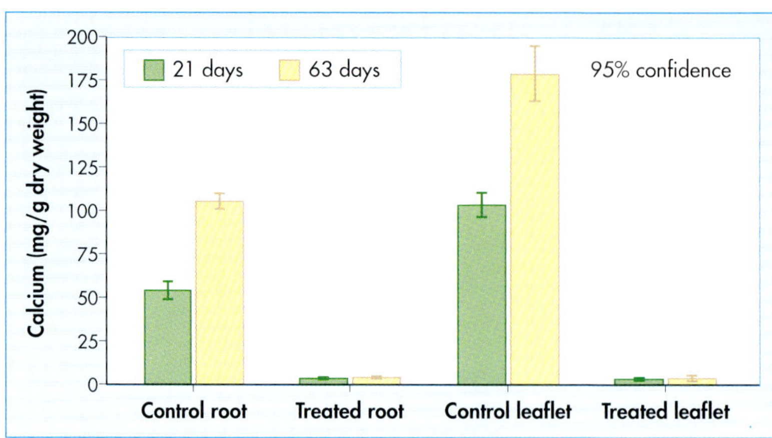

Figure 28.6 Graph of elemental analysis from rat subdermal implant study of BiLinx technology. Control samples had significant calcium deposition at 21 days and increased by the 63-day time point. The treated samples had baseline levels of calcium, which remained stable for the duration of the study. Treatment is effective on both leaflet and aortic wall tissues.

significant calcium levels. The treated tissues, by contrast, had baseline calcium levels at both explant points. The BiLinx technology has demonstrated efficacy in the rat subdermal model and is currently under evaluation in large animals with valve implants.

With an antimineralization process effective for both leaflet and aortic wall tissues, St Jude Medical, Inc. is developing a full root version stentless aortic valve for those patients with significant aortic disease, for whom a subcoronary implant would be contraindicated. Figure 28.7 shows a prototype of this device, which has a polyester inflow covering and ligated porcine coronary arteries.

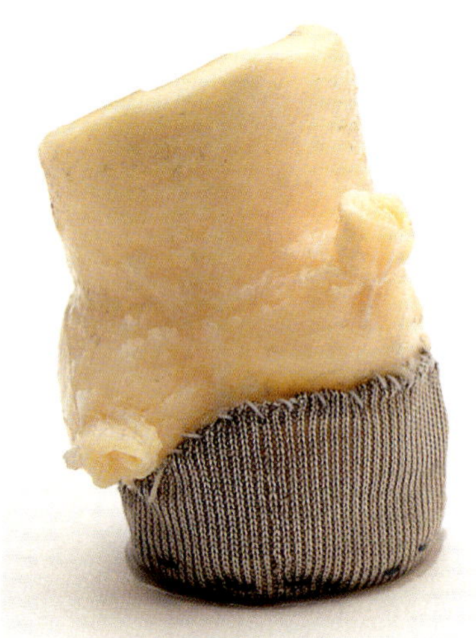

Figure 28.7 Prototype full aortic root replacement with BiLinx technology under development at St Jude Medical Valve Division.

Stentless mitral valves

The next step in stentless valve utilization will be with stentless mitral valves. Currently, stented bioprosthetic valves fare poorly in the mitral position. These valves are based on aortic valve anatomy and do not utilize the stress dissipation mechanisms of native mitral valves. As with stentless aortic valves, experience with allograft mitral valves is helping to define clinical methodology.[19] Stentless mitral valves must be based on healthy native mitral valve anatomy.

Figure 28.8 shows a diagram of the native mitral valve. The mitral valve is a complex structure, using the chordae tendineae to maintain an annular–papillary connection, which is used for proper ventricular function and stress dissipation.[20] The annulus of the mitral valve is D-shaped and the leaflets are asymmetric, with the anterior leaflet being significantly larger than the posterior leaflet. Figures 28.9 shows two stentless mitral valves currently under evaluation in clinical research.

The SJM Biocor bioprosthetic heart valve was developed by Dr. Mario Vrandecic, at the Biocor Institute, in Belo Horizonte, Brazil. It is comprised of a porcine mitral valve with bovine pericardium used to facilitate suturing at the annulus and papillary muscles. This design retains all of the anatomy of the porcine valve, including the porcine chords. The valve is implanted with the chordal attachment on the top of the patient's papillary muscles. This valve has limited clinical experience in centres in Brazil and around the world.[21]

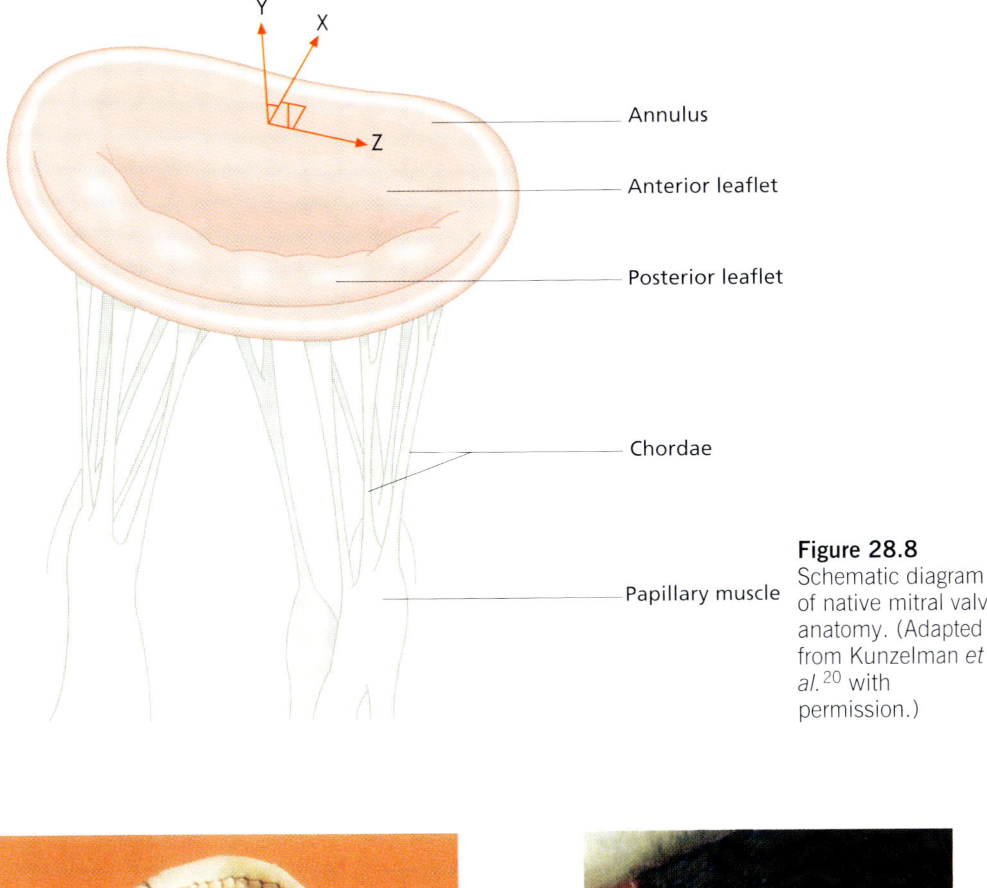

Figure 28.8 Schematic diagram of native mitral valve anatomy. (Adapted from Kunzelman *et al.*[20] with permission.)

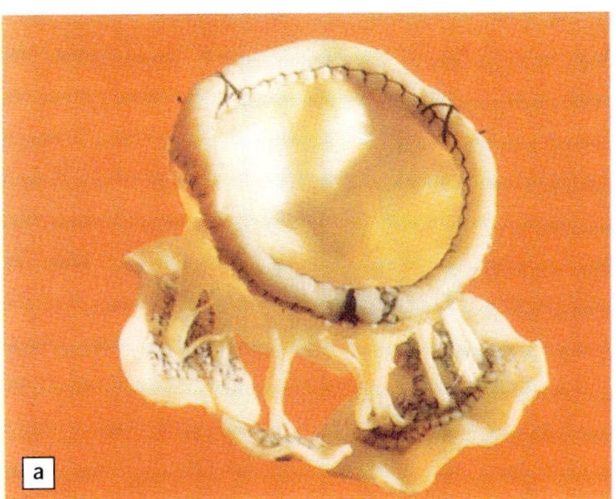

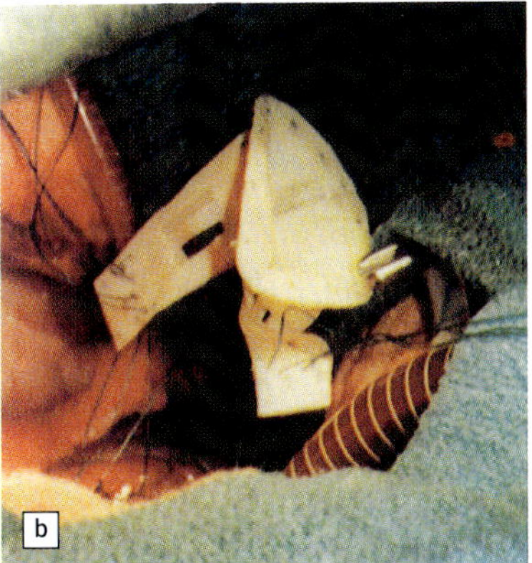

Figure 28.9 Stentless mitral valve bioprostheses with human clinical experience: (a) SJM Biocor™ bioprosthetic heart valve. (Photograph courtesy of St Jude Medical, Inc. All rights reserved.); (b) Quadricusp stentless mitral valve.

The Quadricusp stentless mitral valve was developed by Dr. Robert Frater, of Glycar, Inc. Its design uses bovine pericardium, which is cut and fabricated to emulate native mitral valves. It has a D-shaped annulus and the chordae tendineae are an integral part of the leaflets. This valve has four leaflets, instead of the two in native mitral valves. The posterior leaflet is formed with three leaflets of pericardium, creating a complex, three-dimensional structure with the inherently two-dimensional material. Papillary attachment is on the side of the papillary muscles to allow for variable annular–papillary distances. The Quadricusp stentless mitral valve is also treated with an antimineralization process, using propylene glycol, that neutralizes the cytotoxicity associated with glutaraldehyde tanned materials. This valve is just beginning clinical evaluation and has only been implanted in a few patients at this time.

Antimicrobial technology

Prosthetic valve endocarditis is a catastrophic occurrence patients may face. In developed countries, 2–4% of patients receiving prosthetic valves develop endocarditis. In the developing world, the incidence is much higher. Under the best of circumstances, 20–50% of those patients die.[22,23] Typically, the infection involves the synthetic fabric of the prostheses.

Stentless valves are beginning to be used in many cases in which allografts were previously indicated. Frequently, these valves are implanted in patients with active endocarditis. As with allografts, stentless valves can be useful for covering defects that can be generated by aggressive debriding of infected tissue. The implantation of stentless bioprostheses into patients with active endocarditis makes the treatment of synthetic components to reduce infection potential critical.

A new technology, named Silzone coating, uses ion-beam-assisted deposition of elemental silver onto the polyester fabric used in valve construction to reduce the potential for prosthetic valve infection (Figure 28.10). Silzone coating was developed by Spire Corporation (Bedford, MA, USA) and can be used on stentless valves, stented valves, annuloplasty rings, and the sewing cuffs of mechanical heart valves. The use of Silzone coating on sutures and pledgets is also being explored.

Silzone coating uses the surface properties of metallic silver to inhibit microbial growth. *In vitro* studies have demonstrated Silzone coating's ability to kill a variety of microbes known to be involved in endocarditis, including: *Staphylococcus epidermidis, Staphylococcus aureus, Streptococcus pyogenes, Candida albicans* and *Klebsiella pneumoniae*. Figure 28.11 shows an agar plate, cultured with *Staphylococcus epidermidis*, that has a St Jude Medical mechanical heart valve with a sewing cuff with Silzone coating placed on it. The bacteria on the agar were killed in the area of the Silzone coating.

Short-term animal implant studies, using mechanical valves, compared the healing characteristics of Silzone coating on polyester fabric with untreated control fabric. Composite cuffs were fabricated that were half Silzone coating on polyester fabric and half control polyester fabric. The valves were implanted in the mitral position in weanling sheep for 30 days. Figure 28.12 shows a photograph of a sectioned heart block containing one of these valves. The entire cuff is well healed and covered with pannus tissue.

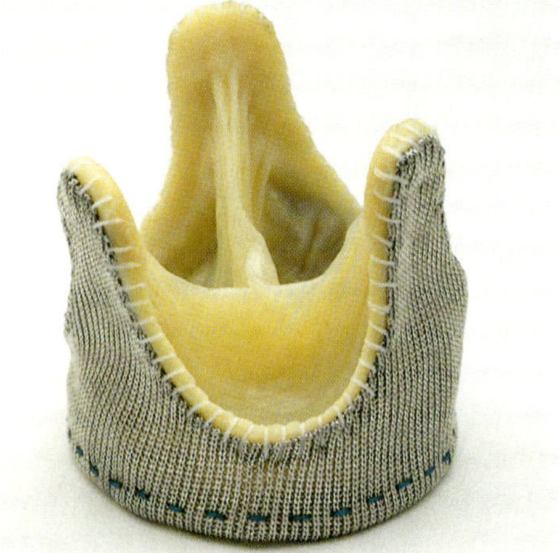

Figure 28.10 Toronto SPV® valve with Silzone coating on polyester fabric. (Photograph courtesy of St Jude Medical, Inc. All rights reserved. Toronto SPV is a registered trademark of St Jude Medical, Inc.)

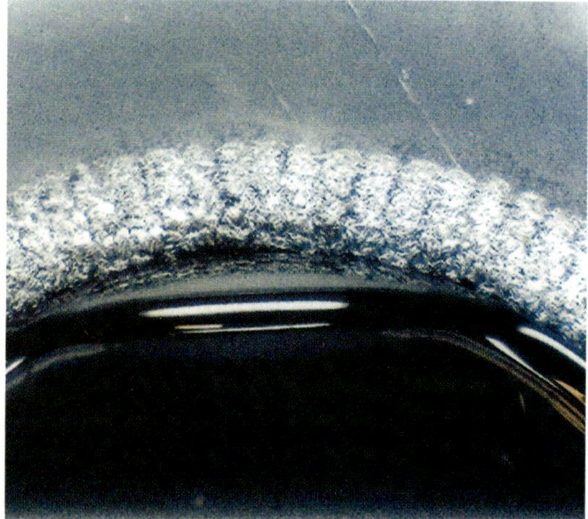

Figure 28.11 *in vitro* study of Silzone coating's efficacy for killing *Staphylococcus epidermidis* on contact.

Figure 28.13 contains 10 × histology sections that have been stained with H&E. Both types of fabric are well healed with fibroblast infiltration and collagen formation. These *in vivo* studies indicate that Silzone coating on polyester sewing cuffs elicits a host response similar to the current polyester material used in mechanical valve sewing cuffs. Additional studies are ongoing to provide preclinical evaluation of stentless and stented bioprosthetic heart valves made with Silzone coating on their synthetic fabric. This technology will soon be available to inhibit microbial colonization and infection of prostheses during the critical phase before the fabric is well healed.

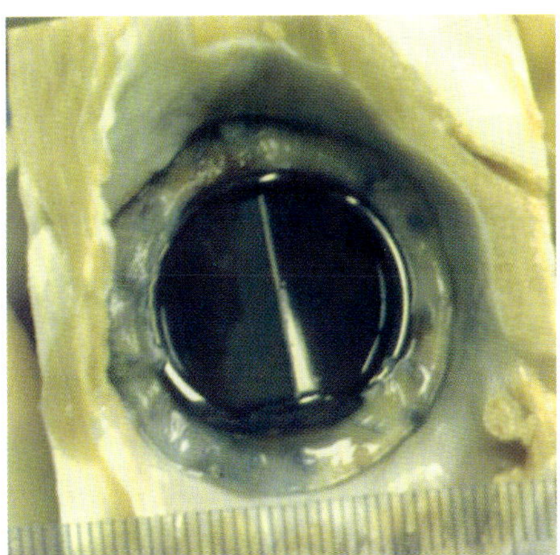

Figure 28.12 Photograph of explanted St Jude Medical mechanical heart valve with composite sewing cuff using untreated polyester fabric on one half and Silzone coating on the other half. Entire cuff is well healed after 30 days in mitral position of juvenile sheep.

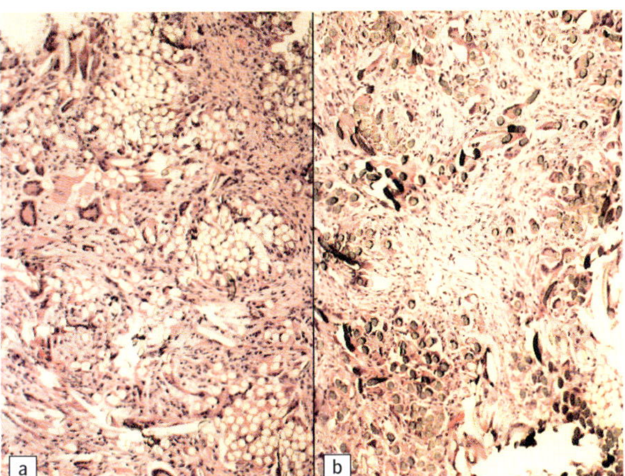

Figure 28.13 Representative histology slides from 30-day sheep mitral implants of composite sewing cuffs using (a) untreated and (b) Silzone coating on polyester fabric. Both samples are well healed with fibroblast infiltration, collagen formation and minimal foreign body response. (H&E stained, × 125.)

Improved biocompatibility

Bioprostheses do not typically have surface coverage by host endothelium. This is a result of residual toxicity, associated with residual glutaraldehyde leaching from the tissue and unreacted aldehyde groups on the tissue surface. Some of the new processes that were developed to mitigate the mineralization potential of the cross-linked tissue also improved the biocompatibility.

Figure 28.14 shows three images obtained from an *in vitro* endothelial cell adhesion assay. For these studies, live endothelial cells were fluorescently labelled and then exposed to sample bioprosthetic tissues for 1 hour. The control tissue has fewer attached endothelial cells, and those cells maintained spherical shapes. The BiLinx technology and propylene glycol-treated tissues, by contrast, had more cells attached and those cells spread to create a nearly confluent monolayer. Since endothelial cells are extremely sensitive to the cytotoxic effects of glutaraldehyde, the treated tissues demonstrate improved biocompatibility.

Figure 28.15 shows histological sections of tissues with the same treatments after *in vitro* culturing for a longer time. The control tissue has no endothelium, while the BiLinx and propylene glycol-treated tissues have endothelial cells attached and spread on their surfaces. The tendency for these treated tissues spontaneously to generate a living endothelium *in vivo* is being evaluated in large animal studies.

Tissue engineering

If a living cell component can be generated on bioprosthetic tissue, these products can be considered first-generation tissue-engineered heart valves. The endothelial cell

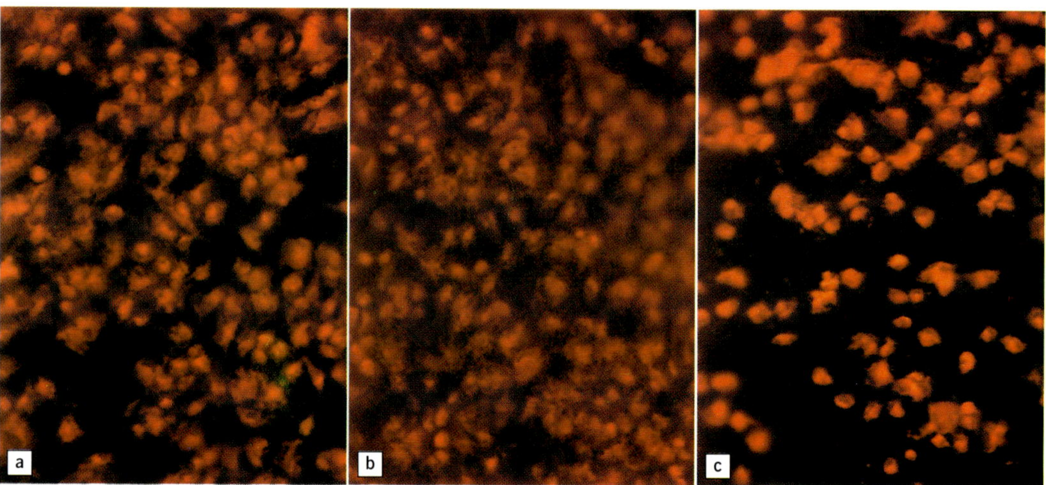

Figure 28.14 Images of fluorescently stained endothelial cells adherent to bioprosthetic surfaces. Samples treated with BiLinx technology (a) and propylene glycol (b) show excellent biocompatibility; endothelial cells on control sample (c) are fewer in number and spherical in shape. (× 160.)

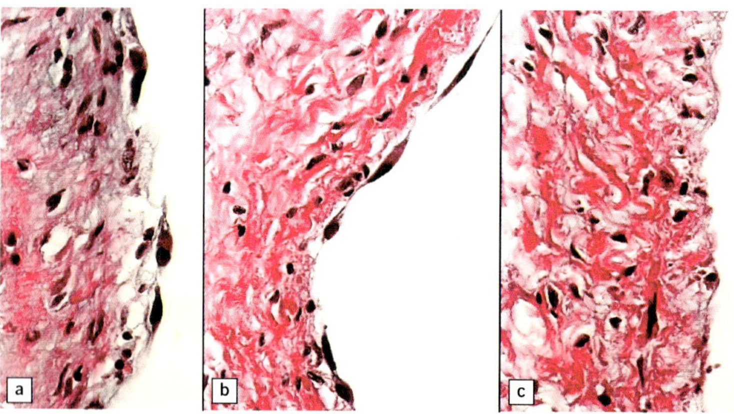

Figure 28.15 Histological sections of tissue cultured *in vitro* with endothelial cells. Samples treated with BiLinx technology (a) and propylene glycol (b) have endothelial cells attached and spread on surface; control sample (c) is devoid of attached endothelial cells. (H&E stain, × 400.)

component may improve valve performance by decreasing thrombogenicity and the potential for microbial colonization of the bioprosthetic device. The term 'tissue engineering' has been used to describe a broad range of activities. It can be simply interpreted as the incorporation of living cells into the structure of prosthetic devices. The living cells' biological function enhances performance of the implant over non-cellularized implants.

Bioprosthetic heart valves with living cells throughout their matrix could repair damage to matrix proteins and extend durability. Ultimately, valves that grow with paediatric recipients would eliminate redo procedures to replace outgrown prostheses. Tissue engineering has the potential of delivering some or all of these promises.

There are many possible permutations for tissue-engineered heart valves. The matrix could be derived from xenograft tissue, such as porcine aortic valves, or a synthetic, resorbable matrix such as polylactic acid could be used. The use of xenograft tissue requires removal of cells existing in the matrix to minimize immune responses to the implant and provide room for cellular incorporation.

Early feasibility work with porcine valves successfully replaced the porcine cells with human fibroblast cells. Figure 28.16 shows histology samples from a study conducted in collaboration between St Jude Medical, Inc. and Advanced Tissue Sciences, Inc., of La Jolla, CA, USA. In this study, porcine aortic valves were decellularized with a proprietary process and then recolonized *in vitro* using a human dermal fibroblast cell line.

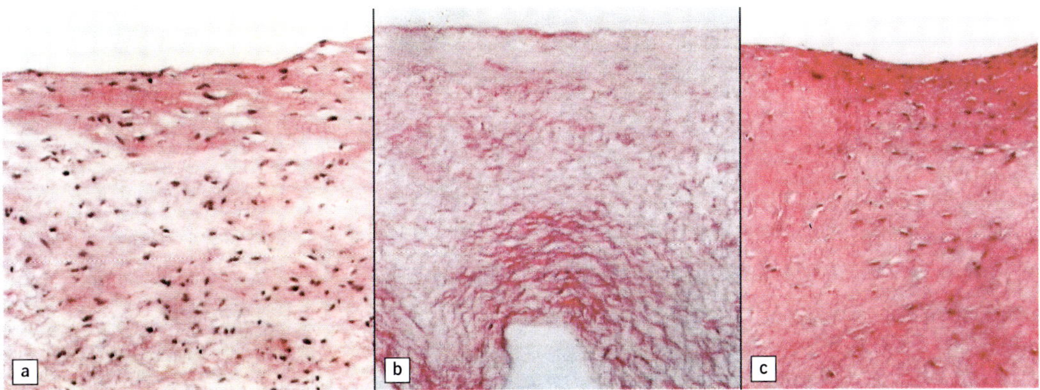

Figure 28.16 Histological sections from *in vitro* tissue engineering feasibility study. Porcine leaflets (a) were decellularized using proprietary process (b), and then recellularized using human dermal fibroblast cells (c). (H&E stain, × 40.)

Other researchers have used biodegradable matrices to construct valve leaflets *in vitro* and then implanted them in the pulmonary valve position in sheep. Explanted samples revealed new collagen formation and increased mechanical strength.[24]

There are also several strategies for cellular colonization. *In vitro* culture systems could establish growth with cells from a 'universal' cell line or autologous cells obtained from the patient prior to surgery. Conversely, the device could be provided as an acellular implant, which would colonize *in situ* with host cells from the surrounding tissues. Clearly, extensive research remains to resolve the technical issues of establishing the correct cell population and function in the matrix. However, biotechnological progress continues and future generations of heart valves will benefit from the increased understanding.

This is an evolutionary time for heart valve prostheses. The clinical success of stentless valves and the advantages offered to patients affirm that anatomical design and physiological function result in a superior valve replacement. Future generations of devices will be difficult to distinguish from healthy native structures. New technologies may increase the durability and reduce the potential for infection of glutaraldehyde-fixed bioprosthetic heart valves. Continued advances in biotechnology offer improvements over allografts, and may ultimately provide a tissue-engineered device to grow with patients after paediatric reconstructions.

References

1. Del Rizzo D F, Goldman B S, Christakis G T, David T E 1996 Hemodynamic benefits of the Toronto stentless valve. J Thorac Cardiovasc Surg 112: 1431–1446
2. Jin X Y, Zhang Z M, Gibson D G, Yacoub M H, Pepper J R 1996 Effects of valve substitute on changes in left ventricular function and hypertrophy after aortic valve replacement. Ann Thorac Surg 62: 683–690
3. Mohr F W, Walther T, Barylei M *et al* 1995 The Toronto SPV bioprosthesis: one year results in 100 patients. Ann Thorac Surg 60: 171–175
4. Wong K, Shad S, Waterworth P D, Khaghani A, Pepper J R, Yacoub M H 1995 Early experience with the Toronto stentless porcine valve. Ann Thorac Surg 60: S402–S405
5. Jin X Y, Gibson D G, Yacoub M H, Pepper J R 1995 Perioperative assessment of aortic homograft, Toronto stentless valve, and stented valve in the aortic position. Ann Thorac Surg 60: S395–S401
6. Del Rizzo D F, Goldman B S, David T E *et al* 1995 Aortic valve replacement with a stentless porcine bioprosthesis: multicenter trial. Can J Cardiol 11: 597–603
7. David T E, Feindel C M, Bos J, Sun Z, Scully H E, Rakowski H 1994 Aortic valve replacement with a stentless porcine aortic valve. A six year experience. J Thorac Cardiovasc Surg 108: 1030–1036
8. Walther T, Falk V, Autsbach R *et al* 1994 Hemodynamic assessment of the Toronto SPV bioprosthesis by echocardiograhy. J Heart Valve Dis 3: 657–665
9. Goldman B S, David T E, Del Rizzo D F, Sever J, Bos J 1994 Stentless porcine bioprosthesis for aortic valve replacement. J Cardiovasc Surg 35: S105–S110

10. Del Rizzo D F, Goldman B S, Joyner C P, Sever J, Fremes S E, Christakis G T 1994 Initial clinical experience with the Toronto stentless porcine valve. J Card Surg 9: 379–385
11. David T E, Bos J, Rakowski H 1992 Aortic valve replacement with the Toronto SPV bioprosthesis. J Heart Valve Dis 1: 244–248
12. David T E, Pollick C, Bos J 1990 Aortic valve replacement with stentless porcine aortic bioprosthesis. J Thorac Cardiovasc Surg 99(1): 113–118
13. Vyavahare N, Hirsch D, Lerner E *et al* 1997 Prevention of bioprosthetic heart valve calcification by ethanol preincubation. Circulation 95: 479–488
14. Levy R J, Schoen F J, Flowers W B, Staelin S T 1991 Initiation of mineralization in bioprosthetic heart valves: studies of alkaline phosphatase activity and its inhibition by $AlCl_3$, or $FeCl_3$ preincubations. J Biomed Mater Res 25: 905–935
15. Webb C L, Schoen F J, Flowers W E, Alfrey A C, Horton C, Levy R J 1991 Inhibition of mineralization of glutaraldehyde-pretreated bovine pericardium by $AlCl_3$. Am J Pathol 138: 971–981
16. Webb C L, Nguyen N M, Schoen F J, Levy R J 1992 Calcification of allograft aortic wall in a rat subdermal model. Am J Pathol 141: 487–496
17. Webb C L, Flowers W E, Horton C, Schoen F J, Levy R J 1990 Long-term efficacy of Al^{3+} for prevention of bioprosthetic heart valve calcification. ASAIO Trans 36: M408–M410
18. Webb C L, Flowers W E, Boyd J, Rosenthal E L, Schoen F J, Levy R J 1990 Al^{+++} binding studies and metallic cation effects on bioprosthetic heart valve calcification in the rat subdermal model. ASAIO Trans 36: 56–59
19. Acar C, Tolan M, Berrebi A *et al* 1996 Homograft replacement of the mitral valve. J Thorac Cardiovasc Surg 111: 367–380
20. Kunzelman K S, Cochran R P, Chuong C, Ring W S, Verrier E D, Eberhart R D 1993 Finite element analysis of the mitral valve. J Heart Valve Dis 2: 326–340
21. Vrandecic M P, Gontijo B F, Fantini F A *et al* 1995 Heterologous mitral valve transplant: the first 50 patients clinical analysis. Eur J Cardiothorac Surg 9: 69–74
22. Cowgill L D, Addonizio V P, Hopeman A R, Harken A H 1987 A practical approach to prosthetic valve endocarditis. Ann Thorac Surg 43: 450–457
23. Lytle B W, Priest B P, Taylor P C *et al* 1996 Surgical treatment of prosthetic valve endocarditis. J Thorac Cardiovasc Surg 111: 198–210
24. Shinoka T, Ma P X, Shum-Tim D *et al* 1996 Tissue engineered heart valves. Circulation 94(Suppl II): II164–II168

CHAPTER 29

Acellular porcine pulmonary and aortic heart valve bioprostheses

D. N. Ross, J. Hamby, S. Goldstein and K. Black

Stentless heart valve designs, which omit sewing rings and struts, should provide optimal bioprosthetic graft haemodynamic function, more like that of heart valve homografts. Presently, two stentless porcine bioprostheses are being developed at CryoLife Inc. to take advantage of the lower expected transvalvular gradients and larger orifice size predicted for stentless valves. The design of the CryoLife–O'Brien 300 glutaraldehyde-fixed heart valve (Figure 29.1) incorporates the novel approach of forming a composite valve from three geometrically and size-matched non-coronary leaflets and wall derived from three separate porcine aortic valves to provide symmetrical leaflet opening. The second of these stentless bioprostheses is the Ross pulmonary heart valve, a glutaraldehyde-fixed porcine pulmonary root (Figure 29.2). The native porcine pulmonary valve does not have a singular muscle bar on its leaflets, and with its thinner and more pliable leaflets, it should share with the CryoLife–O'Brien 300 valve the potential to maximize functional valve orifice area. In fact, excellent haemodynamic function has been demonstrated for aortic valve replacements utilizing fixed pulmonary roots.[1]

Although the absence of stent and sewing ring should have an obvious impact on the flow characteristics of these valves, an additional expected benefit should be in calcification reduction. The lack of a stent should have a direct impact on decreased valve durability due to stress concentration-related leaflet mineralization.[2,3] What remains to be addressed is the issue of reducing the anticipated calcification of glutaraldehyde-fixed leaflets. Although alterations in fixation chemistry may have an impact on valve calcification, the role of heart valve cells and soluble proteins as participants in the mineralization process has been demonstrated by a number of studies. Detergents such as sodium dodecyl sulphate[4,5] should remove phosphoproteins, and phospholipids are partially successful in reducing glutaraldehyde-fixed tissue calcification. Similarly, aluminium salts inhibit fixed tissue calcification, apparently by binding to phosphorus-containing cellular remnants.[6–8] Finally, extraction of pericardium with chloroform/methanol prior to glutaraldehyde fixation resulted in less calcification as compared to unextracted fixed tissue.[9]

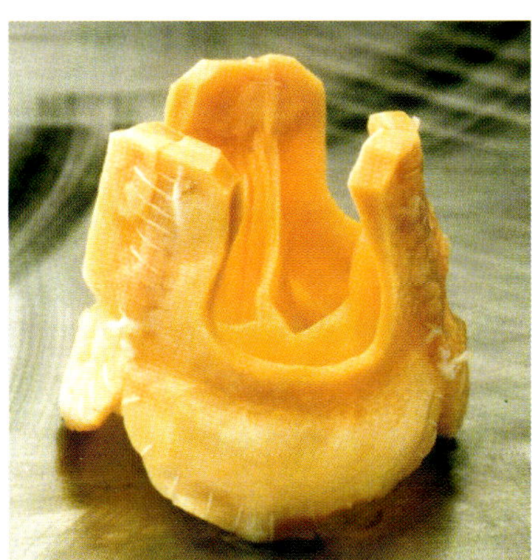

Figure 29.1 The completed CryoLife–O'Brien Model 300 stentless valve.

This study evaluates the concept of decellularization of tissues prior to fixation as a means of limiting calcification of bioprosthetic heart valves. *In vivo* modelling of calcification in subdermal implants in rats,[10] as well as in orthotopic implants of glutaraldehyde-fixed porcine valves in sheep,[11] reflects the progression of the pathological calcification of

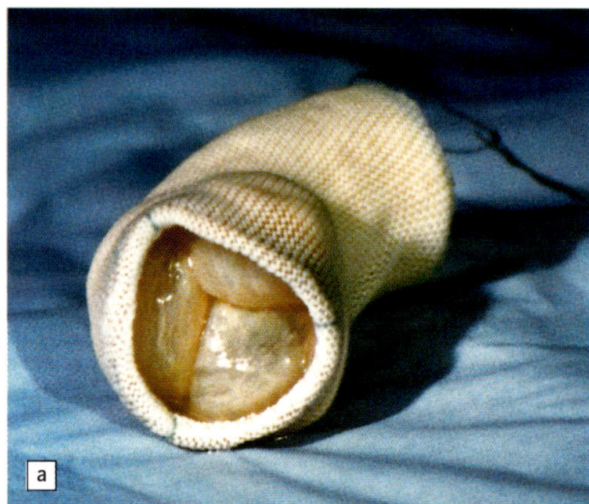

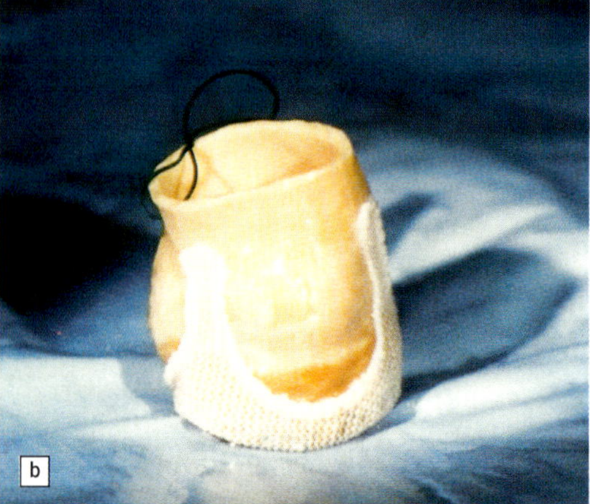

Figure 29.2 The Ross pulmonary heart valve bioprosthesis as a full root design (a) and as a mini-root design with minimal Dacron skirt (b).

the leaflets which are known to occur clinically,[12,13] namely, the earliest calcium deposits can be localized to the membranous components of the interstitial cells which include likely calcium binding sites in phosphoproteins and phospholipids.[14,15] It is these repositories of organic phosphorus which may provide the phosphorus necessary to nucleate calcium phosphate deposits. In this regard, it should be noted that the calcium content of porcine pulmonary leaflets and vascular conduit is lower than in paired aortic valve tissues and the cellularity of the pulmonary valve is less than that of the aortic counterpart.[16]

We have developed a decellularization procedure which can be applied to heart valves and other connective tissue structures. When applied to porcine aortic or pulmonary heart valves, both the leaflet and vascular conduit components can be rendered histologically acellular. The effect of this decellularization process on tissue biomechanics and the influence of decellularization on glutaraldehyde-induced tissue calcification have been studied. We find that decellularization markedly influences the extent of calcification in leaflet tissue from both types of heart valves while preserving biomechanical properties suitable for the clinical utilization of the decellularized grafts.

Materials and methods

Porcine heart valves

Porcine hearts were shipped at 4°C in sterile PBS and the aortic and pulmonary valves dissected within 24 h of slaughter. These tissues were treated with antibiotics for 48 h at 37°C to effect a reduction in bioburden. The disinfected tissues were either cryopreserves [10% (v/v) DMSO and 10% (v/v) fetal bovine serum, –1°C/min] or were decellularized by a procedure involving treatment with hypotonic medium followed by digestion with a mixture of nucleases. After decellularization, the valves were either cryopreserved as above or chemically fixed in 0.35% (w/v) glutaraldehyde at 2 mmHg in phosphate buffered saline (pH 7.4). The fixed tissues were not cryopreserved, but were stored in 0.35% glutaraldehyde solution.

Prior to any examination (calcification, biomechanics, histology), the cryopreserved tissues were thawed rapidly to prevent ice recrystallization. Cryopreservation medium was eluted from the thawed valves with 500 ml of lactated Ringer's solution containing 5% dextrose. The glutaraldehyde-fixed tissues were washed three times each with 200 ml of normal saline.

In vivo static calcification

Calcification of treated tissues was assessed *in vivo* by subdermal implantation in rats. Weanling male Sprague–Dawley rats were obtained from Charles Rivers Laboratories; animals averaged 136 ± 18 g in weight at implantation. The heart valves were dissected to provide aortic and pulmonary leaflets and vascular conduit sections, each 0.5 cm^2. With the rats anaesthetized, 2 cm diameter pouches were formed in the dorsal subcubitis, four per animal, and sections of tissues inserted. Tissue samples were recovered at 1 month post-implantation for determination of calcium content.

Method for calcium determination in tissue samples

Tissues were washed in sterile calcium- and magnesium-free phosphate buffered saline, three times, 10 ml each. The pieces were dried overnight in a centrifugal evaporator (Savant Speed-Vac). After recording dry weight, the tissues were digested in 10 ml of 25% (v/v) HNO_3 for at least 24 h at 70°C. An aliquot of the digest solution was diluted in 0.2 M HCl containing 1% (w/v) lanthanum nitrate. Finally, calcium content was measured using a Perkin-Elmer 300 atomic absorption spectrometer linear between 0.2 and 20 μg Ca^{2+}/ml.

Biomechanics testing

Aortic and pulmonary leaflets were die cut in the circumferential dimension to provide 'dog-bone'-shaped specimens, 0.5 cm wide at midsubstance. The thickness of each sample was derived from the average of three measurements taken with a low-mass pin attached to a conductance circuit and digital caliper. Leaflets were mounted at a standard gauge length of 1 cm. All testing was carried out with the tissue in Hank's balanced salt solution maintained at 37 ± 2°C. Each specimen was preconditioned to a load of 150 g until successive load-elongation curves were superimposable (approximately 20 cycles). The following measurements were then taken:

1. low-load elongation to derive stress–strain relationships while imposing up to 150 g load on the tissue at an extension rate of 10 mm/min, a rate that reflects previously reported studies of leaflet biomechanics;[17,18]
2. examination of viscoelastic properties of the specimens in a stress–relaxation study (tissue elongated to a load of 150 g and following residual loads for up to 1000 s). We determined both the percentage of initial load remaining at these time points as well as the rate of stress–relaxation (i.e. the slope of the % stress remaining versus time), and
3. ultimate uniaxial tensile testing to tissue failure. At least eight specimens of each tissue were examined.

Histochemistry

Samples of fresh and explanted tissues were immersed in 10% sucrose solution for 4–18 h at 4°C. After brief fixation in 10% formalin, the pieces were placed in moulds and frozen in OCT using a liquid nitrogen bath. Cryosections, 6–10 μm thick, were cut using an IEC (Needham Heights, MA, USA) cryostat. Sections were then either stained with haematoxylin and eosin or stained specifically for calcium according to the method of von Kossa. Sections were viewed and photographed using a Nikon Optiphot microscope.

Statistics

Statistical differences in the group means of biomechanical parameters were assessed by independent *t*-tests. A *p*-value of 0.05 was chosen as the level of significant differences. Calcium data were analysed according to ANOVA testing carried out with the statistical program for the IBM-PC, SPSS-PC.

Results

Biomechanics: low-load testing, extensibility and low modulus

The biomechanical properties of strips of aortic and pulmonary porcine heart valve leaflets were compared between fresh-cryopreserved and decellularized-cryopreserved tissues. Fresh aortic and pulmonary leaflets were found to have significant differences in extensibility; pulmonary leaflets had extension 2.3-fold greater than aortic leaflets ($p < 0.01$). However, the elastic moduli of these tissues were not different pre-decellularization (10.6 ± 1.1 vs 9.15 ± 0.64, $p = 0.255$ (Figure 29.3). With decellularization, the extensibility of the two leaflet types became indistinguishable (30.4 ± 2.5 vs 30.2 ± 3.3, $p = 0.981$). The elastic modulus of the aortic leaflets was unchanged by decellularization ($p > 0.5$, as compared to the fresh tissue). By contrast, pulmonary leaflet tissues were markedly stiffened by decellularization, with the elastic modulus rising by 660% ($p < 0.05$). As a result, the elastic modulus of decellularized pulmonary tissue was 550% greater than that of the decellularized aortic leaflet.

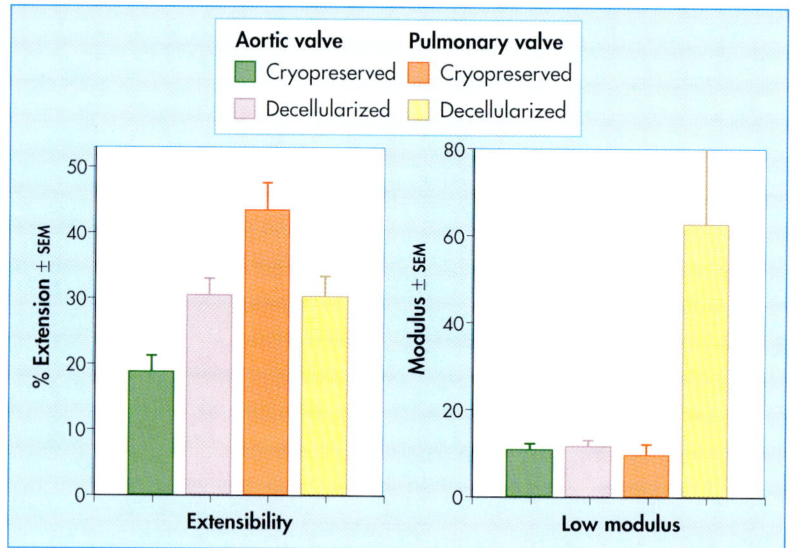

Figure 29.3 Low-load biomechanics testing of porcine heart valve leaflets. Aortic and pulmonary porcine heart valves were either cryopreserved or decellularized according to techniques described in the text. Following decellularization, tissues were cryopreserved. After thawing the valves, the leaflets were excised, cut in the circumferential dimension, preconditioned to a 150 g load, and examined for load–elongation relationships. The derived values for extensibility (left panel) and elastic modulus (right panel) are given.

Stress–relaxation testing

The initial (10 s) and the final (1000 s) rates of stress–relaxation for fresh aortic and pulmonary leaflets were comparable and not statistically different ($p = 0.103$ and $p = 0.115$, respectively) (Figure 29.4). For decellularized tissues, only the initial rate of stress–relaxation of aortic leaflets was obtained; this was no different from the fresh tissue value. The increased stiffening of the pulmonary leaflets with decellularization, which was observed with low-load testing, was reflected by a higher final level of stress remaining (increase from 64.1 ± 2.18% to 81.5 ± 2.5%). The relaxation slope for the pulmonary leaflets was reciprocally changed by decellularization, decreasing from 9.8 ± 0.8 in the fresh tissue to 4.7 ± 1.5 in the treated tissue.

Ultimate tensile testing: failure load, maximum stress and elastic modulus (Figure 29.5)

In fresh tissues, the aortic leaflets failed at twice the load at which the pulmonary valve tissue failed ($p < 0.001$). However, there was no statistical difference of maximum

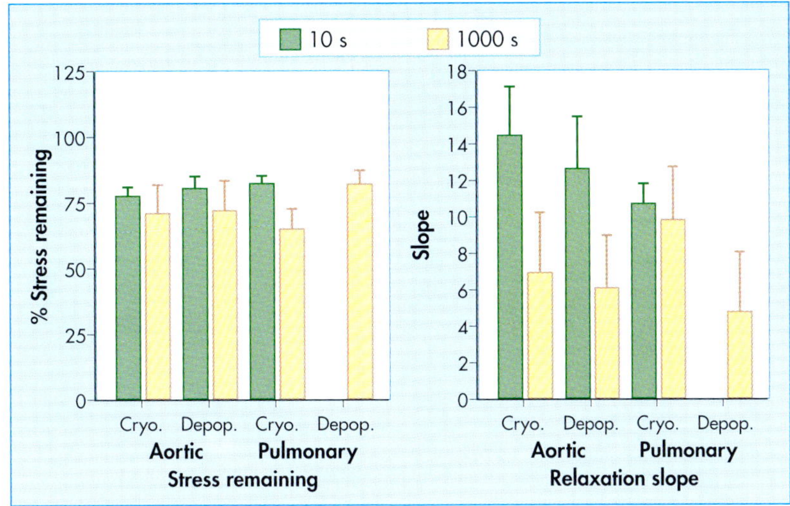

Figure 29.4 Stress–relaxation biomechanics testing of porcine heart valve leaflets. Following low-load testing, circumferential strips of aortic and pulmonary porcine heart valve leaflets were loaded to 150 g and maintained at constant extension. The decay in apparent load was followed and the percentage stress remaining and relaxation slope were calculated at 10 s and 1000 s after initial loading.

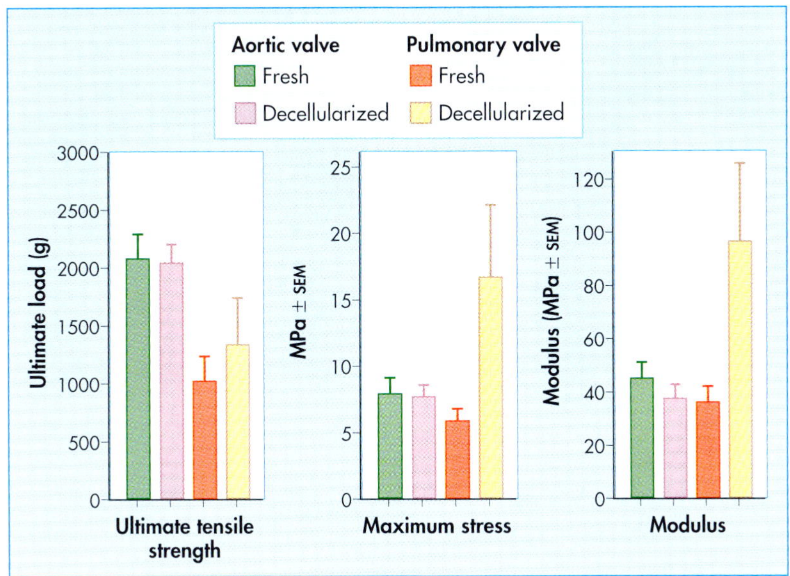

Figure 29.5 Ultimate tensile strength testing of porcine heart valve leaflets. Following stress-elongation testing, circumferential strips of aortic and pulmonary porcine heart valve leaflets were loaded to failure. The measured load (left panel), calculated stress at failure (middle panel), and tissue modulus at failure (right panel) are shown.

stress at failure of the aortic and pulmonary leaflets (8.0 ± 1.2 MPa vs 6.0 ± 0.9 MPa, p = 0.202). The moduli of the fresh leaflets were also not statistically different (p = 0.333).

Decellularized aortic leaflets failed at the same load and maximum stress as did the fresh tissue. The failure load of pulmonary leaflets rose slightly but not significantly, but there was almost a tripling of the stress at failure.

The stiffening of pulmonary leaflets observed with low-load testing was again reflected when the tissue was loaded to failure. The modulus of pulmonary leaflets taken to failure increased 2.6-fold after decellularization; by contrast, the elastic modulus of the decellularized aortic leaflets declines slightly (45.5 ± 6.2 MPa vs 38.3 ± 5.2 MPa).

Tissue calcification

The extent of calcification of porcine heart valve tissues at 1 month of implantation is presented in Figure 29.6. As is typical in the weanling rat subdermal implant model, glutaraldehyde-fixed leaflet calcification exceeded that of vascular wall at 1 month, regardless of the valve of origin. [In studies not shown, fixed vascular conduits calcified more slowly than the leaflets from the same valve type and the final calcium content was significantly lower ($p < 0.05$ for both aortic and pulmonary valves) over a 4-month period.]

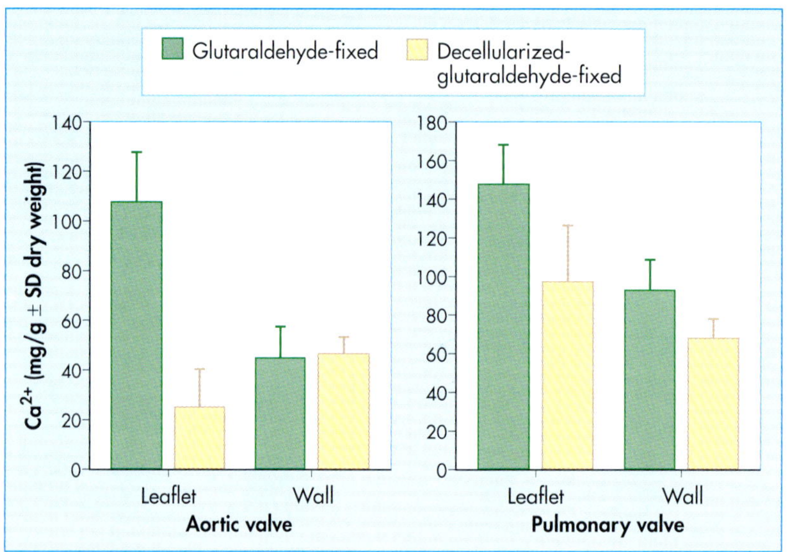

Figure 29.6 *In vivo* static calcification of porcine aortic and pulmonary heart valve tissues. Decellularized, decellularized/glutaraldehyde-fixed, or glutaraldehyde-fixed leaflets and conduits were implanted four per rat for 1 month. The tissues were explanted and processed for calcium determinations as described in the text.

The impact of depopulation prior to heart valve fixation with glutaraldehyde was seen as a decreased calcification of aortic leaflets, pulmonary leaflets or pulmonary artery (wall) (all $p < 0.05$). The effect was most pronounced for the aortic leaflet where calcium levels in decellularized tissues were less than 20% of those fixed without prior decellularization. (In studies not shown, a plateauing of tissue calcium content was seen in all the decellularized tissues by 2 months after implantation; fixed cellular tissue calcium continued to increase past this time.)

Histological examinations

Totally acellular areas of aortic and pulmonary leaflets can be shown in the 1-month explants of the decellularized tissues. Likewise, these areas of tissue matrix are free of calcium deposits (Figure 29.7). Measured tissue calcium in this group was 25 ± 14 mg/g and calcific deposits were found only in localized areas. When examined further using von Kossa's stain, specific calcium-free areas were evident. Within these areas, the calcium deposits did not appear in association with any specific structures (Figure 29.8). By contrast, the early calcification of non-decellularized glutaraldehyde-fixed tissues was always associated with cell nuclei (Figure 29.9).

Discussion

No single theory satisfactorily explains the calcification of glutaraldehyde cross-linked xenogeneic heart valve leaflets. While continued immunogenicity of the foreign tissue has been proposed,[19] calcification of glutaraldehyde-fixed tissue still occurs in T-cell-

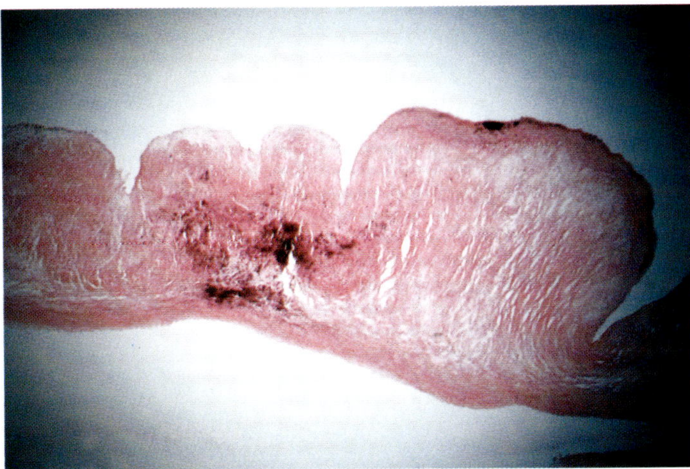

Figure 29.7 Decellularized, glutaraldehyde-fixed porcine aortic leaflet explanted after 1 month's implantation in a rat.

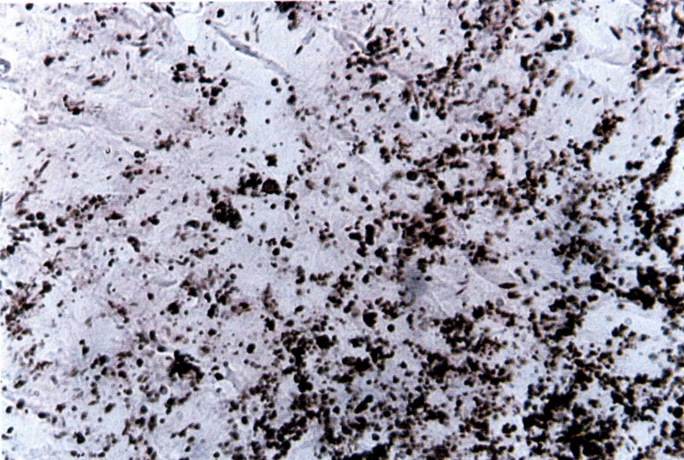

Figure 29.8 Calcified area of decellularized, glutaraldehyde-fixed leaflet.

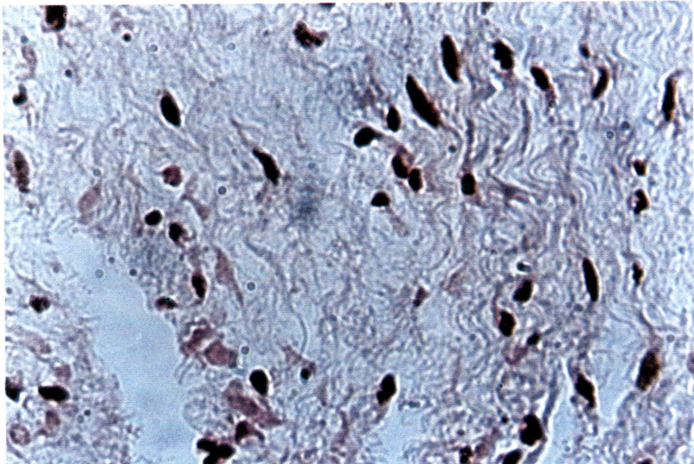

Figure 29.9 Calcified area of non-decellularized, glutaraldehyde-fixed leaflet.

deficient (athymic) mice.[20] Collagen itself is a calcium-binding molecule. Normally, the binding sites are cryptic, being covered by associated glycosaminoglycans. Once the tissues are recovered and processed, these binding sites may be available to bind calcium and allow crystal growth along the protein fibres. This might result in generalized leaflet calcification; however, calcific deposits usually grow from point sources,[21] and crystal growth along collagen fibres has been observed only infrequently.[14] However, an interplay of cyclic loading and tissue damage with the uncovering of these latent sites provides the basis for initiation of calcium deposition in regions of the leaflets subjected to stress concentration.[9] Finally, residual aldehydes in fixed tissues may have long-term cytotoxic effects; the resulting de-endothelialized surface may no longer be a barrier to calcium and protein flux into the leaflet.[22,23]

The studies described here lend support for an additional cause of calcification. We have found that treatment of either aortic or pulmonary leaflets to cause 'decellularization' limits the rate of calcium uptake by glutaraldehyde-fixed tissue. This process is assessed here by loss of staining with traditional histochemical dyes. In other studies we have examined decellularized tissues further by immunohistochemical probes for specific cell membrane and intracellular proteins and have shown a decrease in staining for these cellular elements. Therefore, the decrease in calcium uptake coincides with a reduction in the complement of cellular proteins to which calcium could bind and supports the concept that they could contribute to the calcium-binding activity in the fixed tissue. The fact that these calcium-binding sites (presumably phosphorus-containing moieties) would be affixed to the tissue by glutaraldehyde treatment should tend to enhance their long-term interaction with calcium in surrounding media.

Decellularization of tissue before glutaraldehyde fixation is as effective as post-glutaraldehyde treatments with aldehyde-reactive substances such as glutamine[24,25] or protamine sulphate[26] or presumptive phosphorus-reactive substances such as aluminium or iron salts[15] in limiting calcification in this subdermal implant model. Despite cross-linking, there are reports[19,27] that glutaraldehyde-fixed tissues remain capable of stimulating the recipient's immune system as indicated by both cellular and antibody responses. We have shown that decellularization attenuates both these responses[28] and would expect that this additional effect could result in a more durable implant.

This study also demonstrates the biomechanical properties of decellularized leaflets. The major difference between aortic and pulmonary tissues at both low and high loads is the high elastic modulus of the pulmonary leaflets. Similar to the findings of Lesson-Dietrich *et al.*,[29] cryopreserved aortic leaflets were marginally stiffer than pulmonary leaflets (45 MPa vs 38 MPa). Most notable is the 2.7-fold increase in elastic modulus that the pulmonary leaflet exhibits once decellularized. However, as is pointed out by Lesson-Dietrich *et al.*, other materials, such as bovine pericardium, which is itself a useful substrate for aortic valve bioprostheses, have elevated elastic modulus.

The stress of the decellularized aortic or pulmonary tissues at failure is not statistically different from that of the cryopreserved controls. In addition, they both exhibit failure stress comparable to glutaraldehyde-fixed porcine aortic leaflets (9.14 ± 2.4 MPa, data not shown). It would be anticipated that the ultimate failure loads of decellularized leaflets would increase to glutaraldehyde-fixed tissue levels (2710 ± 850 g) following fixation.

Conclusion

The authors have demonstrated that decellularization of either aortic or pulmonary heart valve leaflets provides an alternative to other methods which might limit bioprosthetic valve calcification. An anticipated added benefit to this approach is further reduction in tissue immunogenicity, which should add to the effect of glutaraldehyde cross-linking itself.

References

1. Gerosa G, Ross D N, Brucke P E *et al* 1994 Aortic valve replacement with pulmonary homografts. Early experience. J Thorac Cardiovasc Surg 107: 424–437
2. Bemacca G M, Fisher A C, Wilkinson R, Mackay T G, Wheatley D J 1992 Calcification and stress distribution in bovine pericardial heart valves. J Biomed Mater Res 26: 959–966
3. Bemacca G M, Mackay T G, Wheatley D J 1992 In vitro calcification of bioprosthetic heart valves: report of a novel method and review of the biochemical factors involved. J Heart Valve Dis 1: 115–130
4. Schoen F J, Levy R J, Hilbert S L, Bianco R W 1992 Antimineralization treatments for bioprosthetic heart valves: assessment of efficacy and safety. J Thorac Cardiovasc Surg 104: 1285–1288
5. Valente M, Minarini M, Maizza A F, Bortolotti U, Thiene G 1992 Heart valve bioprosthesis durability: a challenge to the new generation of porcine valves. Eur J Cardiothorac Surg 6(Suppl II): S82–S90
6. Hirsch D, Schoen F J, Levy R J 1993 Effects of metallic ions and diphosphonates on inhibition of pericardial bioprosthetic tissue calcification and associate alkaline phosphatase activity. Biomaterials 14: 371–377
7. Murphy G M, Norris P G, Young A R, Corbett M F, Hawk J L M 1993 Low-dose ultraviolet-B irradiation depletes human epidermal Langerhans cells. Br J Dermatol 129: 674–677

8. Pathak Y V, Boyd J, Levy R J, Schoen F J 1990 Prevention of calcification of glutaraldehyde pretreated bovine pericardium through controlled release polymeric implants: studies of Fe^{3+}, Al^{3+}, protamine sulphate and levamisole. Biomaterials 11: 718–723
9. Jorge-Herrero E, Fernández P, Escudero C *et al* 1996 Influence of stress on calcification of delipidated bovine pericardial tissue employed in construction of cardiac valves. J Biomed Mater Res 30: 411–415
10. Girardot M-N, Torrianni M, Dillehay D, Girardot J-M 1995 Role of glutaraldehyde in calcification of porcine heart valves: comparing cusp and wall. J Biomed Mater Res 29: 793–801
11. Schoen F J , Hirsch D, Bianco R W, Levy R J 1994 Onset and progression of calcification in porcine aortic bioprosthetic valves implanted as orthotopic mitral valve replacements in juvenile sheep. J Thorac Cardiovasc Surg 108: 880–887
12. Ferrans V J, Boyce S W, Billingham M E, Jones M, Ishihara T, Roberts W C 1980 Calcific deposits in porcine bioprostheses: structure and pathogenesis. Am J Cardiol 46: 721–734
13. Ferrans V J, Spray T L, Billingham M E, Roberts W C 1978 Structural changes in glutaraldehyde-treated porcine heterografts used as substitute cardiac valves. Am J Cardiol 41: 1150–1184
14. Fishbein M C, Levy R J, Ferrans V J *et al* 1982 Calcification of cardiac valve bioprostheses. Biochemical, histologic, and ultrastructural observations in a subcutaneous implantation model system. J Thorac Cardiovasc Surg 83: 602–609
15. Levy R J, Schoen F J, Flowers W B, Staelin S T 1991 Initiation of mineralization in bioprosthetic heart valves: studies of alkaline phosphatase activity and its inhibition by $AlCl_3$ or $FeCl_3$ preincubations. J Biomed Mater Res 25: 905–935
16. Gerosa G, David H, Valente M *et al* 1995 Wear-tested pulmonary porcine valve: mechanical properties and ultrastructural findings. In Piwnica A, Westaby S (eds) Stentless bioprostheses. Isis Medical Media Ltd, Oxford, pp 81–92
17. Lee J M, Boughner D R, Courtman D W 1984 The glutaraldehyde-stabilized porcine aortic valve xenograft. II. Effect of fixation with or without pressure on the tensile viscoelastic properties of the leaflet material. J Biomed Mater Res 18: 79–98
18. Lee J M, Courtman D W, Boughner D R 1984 The glutaraldehyde-stabilized porcine aortic valve xenograft. Tensile viscoelastic properties of the fresh leaflet material. J Biomed Mater Res 18: 61–77
19. Bajpai P 1985 Immunological aspects of treated natural tissue prostheses. In Williams D F (ed) Biocompatibility of tissue analogs, Vol. 1. CRC Press, Inc., Boca Raton, FL, pp 5–25
20. Levy R J, Schoen F J, Howard S L 1983 Mechanism of calcification of porcine bioprosthetic aortic valve cusps: role of T-lymphocytes. Am J Cardiol 52: 629–631
21. Scott J E, Haigh M 1985 Proteoglycan-type I collagen fibril interactions in bone and noncalcifying connective tissues. Biosci Rep 5: 71–81
22. Gabbay S, Kadam P, Factor S, Cheung T K 1988 Do heart valve bioprostheses degenerate for metabolic or mechanical reasons? J Thorac Cardiovasc Surg 95: 208–215
23. Schoen F J, Levy R J 1992 heart valve bioprostheses: antimineralization. Eur J Cardiothorac Surg 6(Supp III): S91–S94
24. Eybl E, Grimm M, Grabenwoger M, Bock P, Muller M M, Wolner E 1992 Endothelial cell lining of bioprosthetic heart valve materials. J Thorac Cardiovasc Surg 104: 763–769
25. Moritz A, Grimm M, Eybl E *et al* 1990 Improved biocompatibility by postfixation treatment of aldehyde fixed bovine pericardium. ASAIO Trans 36: M300–M303
26. Golomb G, Ezra V 1991 Prevention of bioprosthetic heart valve tissue calcification by charge modification: effects of protamine binding by formaldehyde. J Biomed Mater Res 25: 85–98
27. Salgaller M L, Bajpai P K 1985 Immunogenicity of glutaraldehyde-treated bovine pericardial tissue xenografts in rabbits. J Biomed Mater Res 19: 1–12
28. Goldstein S, Brockbank K 1993 Effects of cell removal upon heart valve leaflet mechanics and immune responses in a xenogeneic model. Second International Congress on Xenotransplantation (Abstracts), p 29
29. Lesson-Dietrich J M, Boughner D R, Vesely I 1995 Porcine pulmonary and aortic valves: a comparison of their tensile viscoelastic properties at physiologic strain rates. J Heart Valve Dis 4: 88–94

CHAPTER 30

Anticalcification treatments for stentless bioprostheses

T. Walther, V. Falk, B. Günther, A. Diegeler, T. Rauch, J. A. M. van Son and F. W. Mohr

At present, no ideal artificial heart valve is available.[1–3] In the aortic position, bioprostheses are the valve of choice in patients older than 70 years. They are advantageous in terms of haemodynamics, thrombogenicity, risk of bleeding and need for anticoagulation.[4–6] However, limited durability is the greatest problem of bioprostheses.[7–9] Valve failure is mainly due to structural degeneration from tissue and cell calcification, caused by multiple factors.[10–13]

Bioprostheses are xenografts from porcine valves or from bovine pericardium. To avoid any immunological reaction and to achieve an optimally stable material, the xenograft tissue has to be denaturated by cross-linking before implantation.[9,13] Glutaraldehyde is the standard fixative, with no other process in view.[9,14] Nevertheless, it became apparent that glutaraldehyde itself is in part responsible for calcification of the xenograft tissue and that the residual cells are the main target for calcification.[15–17]

Current research to improve valve performance and durability has developed in two directions: change of the valve design from conventional to stentless bioprostheses, and the development of additional anticalcificant treatments.[12,18] The stentless design leads to a more flexible device that is much closer than the conventional stented bioprostheses to the native aortic valve. The stentless aortic bioprostheses consist of valve leaflets and aortic root tissue.

All new anticalcificant treatments aim to wash residual glutaraldehyde out of the device. Thereafter, either additional surfactants are applied[15,19–21] or methods to block calcification at the cellular level or to extract the cells are used.[13,19] Clinically, stentless bioprostheses are gaining increasing acceptance and are implanted with good results.[6,22–24] Several stentless aortic bioprostheses from different companies are now available.

In this experimental study, samples from different stentless aortic bioprostheses treated with No-React (Biocor), Aminooleic acid (AOA) (Medtronic Freestyle) and BiLinx (St Jude Medical Toronto II) were compared to a standard glutaraldehyde fixation process (Toronto SPV valve) used as a control group. Whereas with No-react and AOA different surface binding substances are used after tissue processing, the BiLinx method aims at inhibiting calcification at the cellular level. At present, details of the different treatments are not fully disclosed.

The aim of the study was to evaluate independently the effectiveness of the different new anticalcification treatments upon aortic valve leaflets and upon the aortic root.

Methods

Animal model

Subcutaneous implantation of tissue samples in weanling rats is an established animal model to test calcification. Eight to 12 weeks of implantation are equivalent to many years of implantation in humans.[12,25] In this experimental model it is extremely important to use 21-day young rats only. In older animals the calcium metabolism would be different and therefore would not resemble years of clinical implantation.

In this study all animals received human care in compliance with the *Principles of Laboratory Animal Care* (NIH publication 85–23, revised 1985). Consent was obtained from the German governmental offices according to the *Tierschutzgesetz* after outlining the study protocol in detail.

Experimental set-up

Thirty weanling 21-day-old male Sprague–Dawley rats were used at the animal research facility of the University of Leipzig. Under sterile conditions, the stentless bioprosthetic valves were rinsed according to the usual intraoperative rinsing process with sterile saline three times for 5 min each. Then the prostheses were cut into aortic root samples of 1 × 1 cm; valve leaflets were cut into two pieces each.

All operations were performed under general anaesthesia using ketamine 100 mg/kg i.m. and xylazine 5 mg/kg i.m.

Each animal was then shaved at the dorsal thorax, positioned horizontally on the table, scrubbed and sterilely draped. Four horizontal incisions of 1 cm each were performed and four separate subcutaneous pouches prepared.

Afterwards the samples were carefully positioned in the pouches to avoid any folding. The skin was then stitched using 3/0 Prolene.

Each animal had four different implants, one from each valve. Thus, 15 animals received aortic valve leaflet and the other 15 aortic root tissue. The implants were separate throughout the whole study, with no interactions or lateral movements seen at explantation.

Explantation was performed at 3 weeks in one-third of the animals (n = 10) to detect any early calcification and at 12 weeks in the remaining 20 animals. These 12 weeks of subcutaneous implantation are sufficient to achieve maximum calcification resembling about 10 years of implantation in humans.

New anticalcification treatments

Most of the new treatments available aim at some additional process besides glutaraldehyde fixation of the xenograft tissue. The application of surfactants is one approach whereas other methods try to avoid calcification at the cellular level or even to excise the cells completely. Unfortunately, at present not all methods are fully disclosed.

The BiLinx method will be available soon with the Toronto SPV II (St Jude Medical) stentless bioprosthesis. It is said to affect both leaflets and aortic root and therefore to inhibit calcification completely. Tissue processing using glutaraldehyde is performed first. The additional method aims at inactivating calcium binding sites and at interfering with the enzymatic process forming hydroxyapatite crystals. Clinically it is not yet available.

The No-React treatment is used for the Biocor (Belo Horizonte, Brazil) stentless bioprosthesis.[21] After aldehyde cross-linkage, a detoxification process of solutions made from natural endogenous substances is used and, finally, a surfactant is applied. The whole method is not fully disclosed.

The Amino-oleic acid (AOA) method is used for the Freestyle (Medtronic) stentless bioprosthesis.[15,19,20] Glutaraldehyde is used for tissue fixation and afterwards the AOA surface treatment is applied.

The control group in this study consisted of the Toronto SPV valve that has a standard glutaraldehyde low-pressure fixation.

Post-implantation analyses

The calcium analyses were performed using an inductively coupled plasma spectrophotometer (ICP) at a laboratory (W. Mirsch, St Jude Medical, St Paul, MN, USA). Samples were transported in 0.5% HEPES buffered glutaraldehyde solution to ICP analysis. The examiner was blinded for the type of prosthesis. No information regarding preliminary results was available before the end of the study.

Histological examination of the explanted probes was performed at our hospital using hematoxylin and eosin and van Kossa staining on 2 μm and 4 μm slices. The sample for the histological examination was taken from the lateral aspect of each implant. Results are given as mean ± standard deviation. Statistical analysis was performed using the SPSS statistical package (SPSS Inc., Chicago, IL, USA); the Student's *t*-test was applied.

Results

Surgery

There were neither infections nor any animal deaths during the whole study. All probes could be easily located at explantation. Randomization and transportation did not lead to any drop-outs.

Histology did not reveal inflammmatory responses with any of the implants. At the surface some oedema was recognized. Furthermore, macrophages were seen, revealing some diffuse foreign body reactions at most implants.

Calcium analysis

Calcium analysis is shown for aortic valve leaflet and aortic root tissue independently. The results are shown in Tables 30.1 and 30.2 for 3- and 12-week explants. Calcium is given in mg/g dry weight.

In summary, there was a relevant reduction of aortic valve leaflet calcification with all three methods examined in comparison with the control group. The effectiveness could be demonstrated after 3 as well as after 12 weeks of implantation. At the aortic root implants, lower levels of calcification were found with the BiLinx treatment. Both

Table 30.1 Calcium analysis (ICP) from 3-week explantation

3-week explantation	Aortic valve leaflet	Aortic root
BiLinx	1.8 ± 0.4	3.2 ± 0.4
No-React	0.2 ± 0.1	24.9 ± 5.9
AOA	0.4 ± 0.1	32.0 ± 2.8
Control	100.1 ± 35.5	63.4 ± 5.2

Data are given for five samples each; the calcium level is shown in mg/g dry weight.

Table 30.2 Calcium analysis (ICP) from 12-week explantation

12-week explantation	Aortic valve leaflet	Aortic root
BiLinx	1.4 ± 0.4	2.5 ± 0.4
No-React	0.4 ± 0.1	138.8 ± 30
AOA	0.4 ± 0.2	115.5 ± 11.8
Control	228.5 ± 29	129.3 ± 16.2

Data are given for 10 samples each; the calcium level is shown in mg/g dry weight.

methods in which surfactants are applied to the xenograft tissue showed no relevant differences of calcification levels in comparison with the control group. Statistical analysis of the results is shown in Table 30.3.

Table 30.3 Statistical analysis of the levels of calcification at 3- and 12-week explantation

Aortic valve leaflet	
3-week	No-React < AOA < BiLinx << Control
12-week	No-React = AOA < BiLinx << Control
Aortic root	
3-week	BiLinx << No-React < AOA < Control
12-week	BiLinx << AOA < Control = No-React

< shows statistically significant differences ($p<0.05$) whereas << shows highly significant differences ($p<0.01$).

Discussion

The beneficial impact of additional anticalcification treatments to achieve a better longevity for stentless bioprostheses is well accepted. Given that calcification is the most important clinical problem with the implantation of bioprostheses, it is obvious that new treatments are required. Less or even no calcification would lead to a significant clinical improvement for the patients in term of a better valve performance and longer durability. Preclinical testing of different implants can be easily performed using a subcutaneous animal model. The comparision of different implants yields some valuable results for further clinical application of stentless bioprostheses. This is the first study comparing different anticalcification treatments independently.

Animal model

The animal model used in this study was very useful to achieve standardized results. With the separate implantation of samples from all four valves into each individual rat, very reliable data could be obtained, excluding any additional external impact upon the level of calcification. The amount of calcification seen in the control group in this study underlines that this model is absolutely correct and that it is justified to draw some conclusions on *in vivo* calcification.

Nevertheless, when evaluating the results it has to be mentioned that subcutaneous implantation in rats is only an experimental model and the first step for comparison of different anticalcification treatments. There are no haemodynamic conditions in this model, therefore the next step for testing would be implantation in sheep. Nevertheless, this model is relatively simple and allows excellent comparison of different implants. Therefore, subcutaneous implantation in rats holds a standard position in the initial testing of different anticalcification techniques that have been developed.

Stentless bioprostheses

The haemodynamic and functional advantages of stentless aortic bioprostheses using the aortic sinuses as a physiological stent are well known. Stentless aortic bioprostheses have a complex interaction of valve leaflets and aortic root. Effective anticalcification treatment of both valve leaflet and aortic wall tissue is important to prevent failure of this functional unit. Whereas in this study the level of calcification could be exactly determined, no conclusion on the importance of that functional unit to prevent further calcification can be drawn. The more flexible design with a preserved uncalcified aortic root may have an additional benefit when implanted in patients.

New anticalcificant treatments

In this study all new anticalcification treatments, no matter whether applying surfactants or inhibiting calcification at the cellular level, were shown significantly to reduce calcification of the aortic valve leaflets. Looking at the level of calcification, the two treatments applying surfactants were shown to be somewhat more effective. Nevertheless, there is no clinically relevant difference in calcification considering the small difference of 1 mg/g dry weight only. Therefore, all three methods examined in this study are effective for aortic valve leaflets.

Aortic root tissue is histologically different from the valve leaflets. Therefore, it could be anticipated that any anticalcification treatment for the aortic root must have a different mechanism. In this study the three methods tested were differently effective in their anticalcification property on the aortic root. Only the BiLinx treatment proved to be effective with low levels of calcification of the aortic root. There were no clinically relevant differences in the level of calcification of the two methods applying surfactants when compared to the control group. Thus both methods applying surfactants can not effectively inhibit calcification of the aortic root. To improve these methods, a more intense tanning or a change of the preparation may be required.

Clinical conclusions

Even though not all anticalcification methods are fully disclosed, it is extremely important to compare them to find the best stentless valve clinically available. The results of this independent comparative study justify the clinical use of effective anticalcificant treatments in future patients.

In addition to the new anticalcification treatments, the impact of the stentless design on long-term valve performance should be further evaluated. Because aortic valve leaflet and aortic root are a functional unit in stentless aortic bioprostheses, a complex anticalcificant treatment is required. The BiLinx method, if clinically available, would be the best method to address the whole stentless aortic valve at this time. New anticalcification treatments are promising to provide better structural integrity and thus to achieve longer valve durability.

References

1. Collins J J 1991 The evolution of artificial heart valves. Editorial. N Engl J Med 324: 624–626
2. Wernly J A, Crawford M H 1991 Choosing a prosthetic heart valve. Cardiol Clin 9: 329–338
3. Davila J C 1989 Where is the ideal heart valve substitute? What has frustrated its realization? Ann Thorac Surg 48: S20–S23
4. Cohn L H, Allred E N, DiSesa V J, Sawtelle K, Shemin R J, Collins J J 1984 Early and late risk of aortic valve replacement. J Thorac Cardiovasc Surg 88: 695–705
5. Jamieson W R 1993 Modern cardiac valve devices – bioprostheses and mechanical prostheses: state of the art. J Card Surg 8: 89–98
6. Walther T, Falk V, Autschbach R *et al* 1994 Hemodynamic assessment of the stentless Toronto SPV™ bioprosthesis by echocardiography. J Heart Valve Dis 3: 657–665
7. Treasure T 1995 Which prosthetic valve should we choose? Curr Opin Cardiol 10: 144–149
8. Magilligan D J 1988 The future of bioprosthetic valves. ASAIO Transactions 34: 1031–1032
9. Burman S O 1989 Heterologous heart valves: past, present and future. Ann Thorac Surg 48: S75–S76
10. Turina J, Hess O M, Turina M, Krayenbuehl H P 1993 Cardiac bioprostheses in the 1990s. Circulation 88: 775–781
11. Schoen F J 1988 The future of bioprosthetic valves. A pathologist's perspective. ASAIO Trans 34: 1040–1042
12. Schoen F J, Levy R J 1994: Pathology of substitute heart valves: new concepts and developments. J Card Surg 9(Suppl): 222–227
13. Courtman D W, Pereira C A, Kashef V, McComb D, Lee J M, Wilson G J 1994 Development of a pericardial acellular matrix biomaterial: biochemical and mechanical effects of cell extraction. J Biomed Mater Res 28: 655–666

14. Levy R J 1994 Editorial: Glutaraldehyde and the calcification mechanism of bioprosthetic heart valves. J Heart Valve Dis 3: 101–104
15. Chen W, Schoen F J, Levy R J 1994 Mechanism of efficacy of 2-amino oleic acid for inhibition of calcification of glutaraldehyde-pretreated porcine bioprosthetic heart valves. Circulation 90: 323–329
16. Gong G, Ling Z, Seifter E, Factor S M, Frater R W M 1991 Aldehyde tanning: the villain in bioprosthetic calcification. Eur J Cardiothorac Surg 5: 288–293
17. Golomb G, Schoen F J, Smith M S, Linden J, Dixon M, Levy R J 1987 The role of glutaraldehyde-induced cross-links in calcification of bovine pericardium used in cardiac valve bioprostheses. Am J Pathol 127: 122–130
18. David T E, Ropchan G C, Butany J W 1988 Aortic valve replacement with stentless porcine bioprostheses. J Card Surg 3: 501–505
19. Chen W, Kim J D, Schoen F J, Levy R J 1994 Effect of 2-amino oleic acid exposure conditions on the inhibition of calcification of glutaraldehyde cross-linked porcine aortic valves. J Biomed Mater Res 28: 1485–1495
20. Gott J P, Pan-Chih, Dorsey L M A *et al* 1992 Calcification of porcine valves: A successful new method of antimineralization. Ann Thorac Surg 53: 207–216
21. Abolhoda A, Yu S, Oyarzun R, McCormick J R, Bogden J D, Gabbay S 1996 Calcification of bovine pericardium: glutaraldehyde versus No-React biomodification. Ann Thorac Surg 62: 169–174
22. David T, Feindel C M, Bros J, Sun Z, Scully H E, Rakowski H 1994 Aortic valve replacement with a stentless porcine aortic valve. A six year experience. J Thorac Cardiovasc Surg 108: 1030–1036
23. Westaby S, Amarasena N, Ormerod O, Amarasena C, Pillai R 1995 Aortic valve replacement with the Freestyle stentless xenograft. Ann Thorac Surg 60: S422–S427
24. Mohr F W, Walther T, Baryalei M *et al* 1995 The Toronto SPV bioprosthesis: one-year results in 100 patients. Ann Thorac Surg 60: 171–175
25. Schoen F J, Levy R J, Hilbert S L, Bianco R W 1992 Antimineralization treatments for bioprosthetic heart valves. Assessment of efficacy and safety. J Thorac Cardiovasc Surg 104: 1285–1288

CHAPTER 31

Anticoagulation for stentless aortic bioprostheses

S. Westaby

The aims of anticoagulation in heart valve surgery are to prevent thrombus formation on the prosthesis and thromboembolism (from any source) whilst minimizing the risk of bleeding. Prosthesis-specific anticoagulation tailors the dosage level by taking into account the type of valve together with patient-related risk factors. All mechanical valves require lifelong anticoagulation, but at differing levels according to the valve mechanism.[1] For bioprostheses, progressive improvements in technology are aimed at eliminating anticoagulation altogether without risk of thromboembolism.[2] Avoidance of anticoagulation conveys the enormous benefit of eliminating any risk of anticoagulant-induced bleeding.

There are three fundamental questions surrounding anticoagulant policy after aortic valve replacement:

1. Is anticoagulation necessary and for how long?
2. When should anticoagulation be started?
3. What is the optimal level of anticoagulation for a particular individual with a particular prosthesis?

These questions are answered against the background of the pathophysiology of thromboembolism after aortic valve replacement.

Pathophysiology of thromboembolism

The long-term risk of thromboembolism is defined, first in terms of patient-related and secondly in terms of prosthesis-related factors.[1,3] Temporary short-term issues, such as perioperative alteration in blood coagulability and time for resolution of surgical injury, are also relevant. For bioprostheses, patient-related factors are predominant in determining the need for long-term anticoagulant treatment. The principal patient-related risk factors for thromboembolism are atrial fibrillation, an enlarged left atrium, low cardiac output, and old age.[4] Those who have suffered a previous embolus are at increased risk and thromboembolism is more likely with pregnancy, the taking of oral contraceptives, cigarette smoking, hypertension, diabetes, hyperlipidaemia and with increased fibrinogen levels or abnormalities of coagulation.[5]

Whilst less critical than for mechanical valves, anticoagulation must also be considered for bioprostheses. The normal anatomy and flow characteristics of pulmonary autografts and homografts in the aortic position convey a much lower risk of thromboembolism than stented xenografts or pericardial valves (hybrids of tissue and synthetic materials). The obstructive nature of the valve stent generates turbulent flow, whilst the sewing ring is covered by thrombus which matures to vascular fibrous tissue. The sewing ring eventually develops an endothelial covering with some antithrombotic effect.[6] Xenograft cusps are chemically fixed with glutaraldehyde and have little thrombotic potential in the high-flow, high-pressure aortic position. By contrast, the risk of valve thrombosis is five times higher and the risk of thromboembolism approximately twice as great in the mitral position.[7] The risk of thromboembolism doubles with multiple valve replacement.

Fresh, cryopreserved or antibiotic-sterilized homografts may still be covered with some viable thromboresistant endothelium, at least for a short time after implantation. Nevertheless, the early risk of thromboembolism may not be absent even after pulmonary autograft or homograft implantation, since the collective risk depends on Virchow's triad:

1. changes in surfaces in contact with the blood (i.e. injured native tissue and the prosthesis);
2. changes in blood flow (turbulence or stagnation caused by the prosthesis);
3. changes in coagulability (after cardiopulmonary bypass and surgical injury).

Any valve operation has the potential for thromboembolism through surgical injury to the aorta and aortic annulus. Suture lines predispose to microthrombosis early after valve replacement until the damaged tissues are endothelialized. Cardiopulmonary bypass adversely affects the dynamic balance between coagulation, fibrinolysis and endothelial cell function by depressing the levels of the natural anticoagulant antithrombin III.[8] General alterations in coagulability associated with surgical injury are further complicated by foreign surface interaction, hypothermia, heparin and protamine interaction, or the use of aprotinin.[9]

Is anticoagulation required after bioprosthetic aortic valve replacement?

Over the last three decades, numerous publications have reported the risks of thromboembolic and anticoagulation-related complications after aortic valve replacement. Differences in valve prostheses, patient populations, anticoagulation regimens, indices of anticoagulation status, definitions of complications, methods of follow-up and statistical analysis, and a dearth of randomized clinical trials allow few definitive conclusions to be drawn. Recommendations concerning the need for and level of anticoagulation have largely come from observational studies.[10,11]

There is general consensus that all patients with a mechanical prosthesis require lifelong anticoagulation at a level determined by the type of valve and patient-related factors. The need for anticoagulation with pulmonary autografts or aortic and pulmonary homografts is less well defined, but in general, anticoagulation seems unnecessary at any stage for patients in sinus rhythm (despite Virchow's triad). The physiological function of pulmonary autografts and homografts, together with the absence of stents and sewing rings, result in a very low incidence of thromboembolism in the absence of patient-specific problems.[12,13] A very small risk of thromboembolism is outweighed by the risk of anticoagulant-related bleeding for this group. Nevertheless, with time, a degenerating calcified homograft becomes more prone to thromboembolism, and the need for anticoagulants should be considered as the haemodynamic performance decreases, particularly in the presence of atrial fibrillation or dilated cardiac chambers.

For patients with stented bioprosthetic valves in sinus rhythm, there is a general consensus that anticoagulants should be given for 3 months after surgery, then discontinued in a stepwise manner.[7,14] The recommended level of anticoagulation during this period is an international normalized ratio (INR) of 2.0–3.0. In a randomized comparison of low (INR 2.0–2.5) and moderate (INR 2.5–4.0) anticoagulation for 3 months after bioprosthetic replacement, Turpie reported no difference in the incidence of thromboembolism but a significantly reduced incidence of bleeding with the lower INR.[15] In most cardiac surgical centres, the standard practice is to commence anticoagulation on the morning after operation when the chest drains are removed, though this provides inadequate anticoagulation for several days.[16] The incidence of embolism is higher in the first 30 days after aortic valve replacement than in the longer term because of Virchow's triad. Consequently, some groups recommend the use of antiplatelet agents or intravenous heparin given on the first or second postoperative day, until adequate levels of anticoagulation are achieved.[17] Currently, there is no evidence from randomized trials that these policies are more efficacious than the standard practice. Early heparinization also conveys the risk of bleeding or cardiac tamponade within the first 48 h of surgery.

The stentless aortic bioprostheses

Realization that the superlative haemodynamics of the aortic homograft and pulmonary autograft need not be reserved for the young has prompted detailed re-evaluation of the stentless porcine xenograft first used in the 1960s. Given that stent mounting leads to suboptimal valve geometry, obstructive turbulent flow and the presence of synthetic surfaces in blood contact, stentless valves should lessen the risks of thromboembolism. For a specified external diameter, effective orifice areas are larger and the pressure drop lower than for stented valves.[18] The native aortic wall and aortic sinuses also provide non-turbulent flow virtually equivalent to the aortic homograft. In addition, the complete relief of increased ejection resistance for aortic stenosis patients has a significant early beneficial impact on left ventricular function which is not seen with stented bioprostheses.[19] Stentless valves provide a significant increase in left ventricular stroke volume and left ventricular stroke work index compared to stented bioprostheses. These changes are based on underlying improvements in left ventricular systolic and diastolic function, with particular advantage for patients with a small (<23 mm) aortic root.

David has case-matched Toronto SPV valve patients with those receiving the Hancock II valve.[20] When the duration of follow-up exceeds 5 years, the actuarial survival of patients with the stentless valve is 93% versus 86% for the stented valve. Proportional hazard analysis shows valve-related complications to be three times less in the stentless valve patients, which suggests that improved haemodynamic function translates directly into better event-free survival. Survival curves for elderly patients with stentless bioprostheses are now similar to those of younger patients after homograft implantation.

Both the Toronto SPV valve and the Freestyle valve have a thin layer of cloth covering at the inflow, but this has very little interface with blood flow. In addition, no suture knots need be exposed within the aortic lumen. The combination of better haemodynamic profile with no stent or foreign material in the blood path suggests that anticoagulation with warfarin is unnecessary. Patient-related risk therefore predominates with these valves and clinical experience is required to increase confidence. For the Toronto SPV valve, data on thromboembolic events from six centres were presented at the Food and Drugs Agency Advisory Panel Meeting (September 1997). The patient population comprised 577 adults, 67% of whom were males, with a mean age of 65.6 years. Total follow-up was 1081 patient-years, with a mean follow-up of 1.9 years. All thromboembolic or bleeding events were classified according to Edmunds *et al.*[21] There were 11 thromboembolic events with an early (<3 months) rate of 0.9% and a late thromboembolic rate of 0.5% per patient-year (linearized rate). Only 12% of patients were discharged on anticoagulation, predominantly at one centre that routinely used warfarin for 3 months. This was associated with four serious anticoagulant-related bleeding events, two of which were intracerebral haemorrhage resulting in death.

Table 31.1 Thromboembolic rates for stentless aortic valves: the Toronto SPV valve (1081 patient years) and the Freestyle (864 patient years). Presented to the Food and Drug Administration (USA) Advisory Panel Meeting, September 16, 1997 by St Jude Medical, Inc. and Medtronic Inc.

	Toronto SPV valve	**Freestyle**
Early TE* rate	0.9%	1.7%
Late TE rate	0.5% per patient year	0.7% per patient year
Anticoagulation at discharge	12.0%	32.0%

* Permanent neurological event. Transient ischaemic attacks excluded.

At the same meeting, similar data were presented for the Freestyle valve (Table 31.1). Again, thromboembolic events were infrequent, with a similar incidence of major anticoagulant-related haemorrhage for those who received warfarin. In the author's series of 200 consecutive Freestyle valves in patients over 65 years, warfarin was initially prescribed for 3 months, as for stented bioprostheses. However, two early patients suffered stroke through intracerebral haemorrhage and there were no convincing thromboembolic events. The early anticoagulation policy was therefore discontinued in favour of aspirin 75 mg daily for the first 3 months. Since that time, only patients in atrial fibrillation have received anticoagulation, and there have been no documented thromboembolic events or bleeding. The balance of evidence would therefore suggest the following strategy for stentless aortic xenograft patients:

1. Patients with atrial fibrillation or other significant risk factors for thrombosis should receive full anticoagulation with warfarin at an INR of 2.5–3.0. In those with residual mitral pathology or a mitral valve prosthesis, the INR should be 3.0–3.5.
2. For those with isolated aortic valve replacement in sinus rhythm with no patient-related risk factors, there should be no formal anticoagulation. We prescribe aspirin 75 mg daily for 3 months pending endothelialization of surgical sites. We omit this in patients intolerant to aspirin.
3. Currently, the authors do not use heparin in the perioperative period, because of a small risk of haemopericardium.

It is important that these recommendations be reviewed with time and in the light of further clinical experience. When xenograft cusps stiffen and calcify, providing obstructive flow, anticoagulants may then be indicated.

References

1. Butchart E G, Lewis P A, Bethel J A, Breckenridge I M 1991 Adjusting anticoagulation to prosthesis thrombogenicity and patient risk factors. Circulation 84(Suppl III): III61–III69
2. McGoon D C 1984 The risk of thromboembolism following valvular operations; how much does one know? J Thorac Cardiovasc Surg 88: 782–786
3. Horstkotte D, Schulte H, Bircks W, Strauer B 1993 Unexpected findings concerning thromboembolic complications with anticoagulation after complete 10 year follow-up of patients with St Jude Medical prostheses. J Heart Valve Dis 2: 291–301
4. Gohlke-Barwold C, Acar J, Oakley C *et al* 1995 Guidelines for prevention of thromboembolic events in valvular heart disease. Eur Heart J 16: 1320–1330
5. Cannegieter S C, Rosendaal F R, Wintzen A R *et al* 1995 Optimal oral anticoagulant therapy in patients with mechanical heart valves. N Engl J Med 333: 11–17
6. Berger K, Sauvage L F, Woods S J, Wesolowski S A 1967 Sewing ring healing of cardiac valve prostheses. Surgery 61: 102–117
7. Stein P D, Frantrowitz A 1989 Antithrombotic therapy in mechanical and biological prosthetic heart valves, and saphenous vein bypass grafts. Chest 95(Suppl): 107S–111S
8. Schipper H G, Roos J, van der Meulen F, ten Cate J W 1981 Antithrombin III deficiency in surgical intensive care patients. Thromb Res 21: 73–80

9. Kesteven P J 1990 Haemostatic changes during cardiopulmonary bypass. Perfusion 5(Suppl): 9–19
10. Hirsh J, Fuster V 1994 Guide to anticoagulant therapy. Part 2. Oral anticoagulants. AHA Medical/Scientific Statement Special Report. Circulation 89: 1469–1480
11. Hirsh J, Dalen J E, Deykin D, Poller L 1992 Oral anticoagulants; mechanisms of action, clinical effectiveness, and optimal therapeutic range. Chest 102(Suppl): 312S–326S
12. Ross D, Jackson M, Davies J 1991 Pulmonary autograft aortic valve replacement: long term results. J Card Surg 6(Suppl): 529–533
13. O'Brien M F, Stafford E G, Gardner M A *et al* 1995 Allograft aortic valve replacement; long-term follow-up. Ann Thorac Surg 60: S65–S70
14. BCSH Haemostasis and Thrombosis Task Force 1990 Guidelines on oral anticoagulation: second edition. J Clin Pathol 43: 177–183
15. Turpie A G, Gunstensen J, Hirsh J *et al* 1988 Randomised comparison of two intensities of oral anticoagulant therapy after tissue valve replacement. Lancet 1: 1242–1245
16. Taggart D P, Westaby S 1997 Anticoagulation after aortic valve replacement – the Oxford approach. In: Piwnica A, Westaby S (eds) Surgery for acquired aortic valve disease. ISIS Medical Media, Oxford, pp 298–303
17. Turpie A G, Gert M, Laupacis A *et al* 1993 A comparison of aspirin with placebo in patients treated with warfarin after heart valve replacement. N Engl J Med 329: 524–529
18. Westaby S, Huysmans H A, David T E 1998 Stentless aortic bioprostheses: compelling data from the Second International Symposium. Ann Thorac Surg 65: 235–240
19. Jin X Y, Westaby S, Gibson D *et al* 1997 Left ventricular remodelling and improvement in Freestyle valve haemodynamics. Eur J Cardiothorac Surg 12: 63–69
20. David T E, Feindel C M, Bos J, Sun Z, Scully H E, Rakowski H 1994 Aortic valve replacement with a stentless porcine aortic valve. A six year experience. J Thorac Cardiovasc Surg 108: 1030–1036
21. Edmunds L H Jr, Clark R E, Cohn L H, Grunkemeier G L, Miller D C, Weisel R D 1996 Guidelines for reporting morbidity and mortality after cardiac valvular operations. The American Association for Thoracic Surgeons Ad Hoc Liaison Committee for Standardizing Definitions of Prosthetic Heart Valve Morbidity. Ann Thorac Surg 62: 932–935

INDEX

M

N

O

P